retro spectro scope

Insights into Medical Discovery

Julius H. Comroe, Jr.

Von Gehr Press   Menlo Park, California

To my wife Jeanette

First published in 1977 by the Von Gehr Press,
P.O. Box 7654, Menlo Park, CA 94025
ISBN 0-9601470-1-2
Library of Congress catalog card number: 77-088230
Printed in USA

These essays originally appeared in the
American Review of Respiratory Disease
Copyright 1975, 1976, 1977
by the American Lung Association

Cover design by Aida Cordano

Preface

For more than 40 years, I've been a medical educator and researcher — for 16 of these years, Director of the University of California's rather large Cardiovascular Research Institute in San Francisco. Naturally, I've had some thoughts — even a few convictions — on how to create a favorable environment in which carefully selected scientists can do their best research. But I was sure that I didn't know *for sure!*

Suddenly I found that a lot of very important people — Presidents of the United States (guided by their budget analysts), Congressmen, Nobel Laureates, heads of foundations — knew *for sure* how to get the most for the medical research dollar and how to plan and generate medical breakthroughs. Since I *didn't* know (because I hadn't done any honest-to-goodness research on research — research on the process of discovery — and I couldn't find reports of objective studies done by others), I thought it was time to learn something for sure. I decided that, for a start, I would determine how recent life-saving advances in some branches of medicine and surgery had actually come about. I've now spent most of the last five years trying to find out; I've put in this volume some of what I've learned.

Don't panic. There's not a statistic or a table of data in this little book; these have been, or will be, presented elsewhere. And I've used only one instrument, one with a long name (the *Retrospectroscope*), a device that enables one to look backwards in many directions, from the level of brightness of today to the murkiness or darkness of decades or centuries ago when "breakthroughs" were rewarded by burning at the stake instead of by the Nobel Prize. I've used this instrument to find the seeds and roots of modern miracles (none of which appears to have occurred by spontaneous generation), and to learn why and how we've moved from ignorance to life-saving knowledge. I suppose it might be called "Santayana's Scope," for it was he who said: "Those who cannot remember the past are condemned to repeat it."

As you will see, everywhere that I have turned the Retrospectroscope, it has shown that scientists depend on the work of other scientists who depended on the work of still others. Turned in some directions, especially outside of medical laboratories, it has revealed that crucial discoveries, essential to later *medical* miracles, were often made by those not directly concerned with diagnosing or curing or preventing disease, and that the work of many of these was judged to be impractical, impossible, irrelevant or absurd at the time of discovery. Thus, answering the esoteric question "What makes the sky blue?" has become as important to medical advance as answering an engineering question "Why can't a vacuum pump raise a column of water to more than 34 feet high?", or the frivolous question "Are all four hoofs of a trotter ever off the ground at the same time?", or the tantalizing question "Why do human pathogenic bacteria disappear when human sewage is tilled into the soil?"

No matter where I've turned it, the Retrospectroscope has not disclosed a simple or royal road to success in medical discovery. Those involved had many motives, many goals and used many approaches. Some have moved in a straight line — directly to their goal. But the Retrospectroscope has found others who, in their later years, told "like it really was" the story of their earlier discoveries; we learn from them that scientists are human, take wrong turns, travel tortuous paths and sometimes arrive because of someone else's speculation or unrelated observation, or by chance (*plus* sagacity). We also learn that occasionally a discovery is premature for all except the one who made it and it gets lost for years; that some scientists have had an important discovery staring them in the face and have not grasped its meaning; that some commissions, Geheimrats, scientists and clinicians, by their authoritarian (and incorrect) pronouncements, have unknowingly retarded scientific advance for decades, until some brash scientist challenged authority and put the show back on the track in the right direction. We learn that many important discoveries have been made by youngsters — medical or even college students. We also learn that some scientists are resistant to new discoveries, even those who, when much younger, suffered the discouragement or anguish of having their own unorthodox (but correct) ideas scoffed at.

I started looking in the Retrospectroscope to get more insight into "how to get the most for the medical research dollar." There are vast areas still to be examined; there's not a word in this book about cancer, or mental health, or even recombinant DNA. Nevertheless, what I have seen and set down may give you more insight into the complex world of discovery and discoverers. Perhaps you'll even get a Retrospectroscope of your own and use it; as an instrument to aid in shaping future research policy, I think you'll agree that it is more helpful than a crystal ball.

JULIUS H. COMROE, JR.

Contents

What Makes the Sky Blue?

Charles E. Wilson, a former president of General Motors, President Eisenhower's Secretary of Defense from 1953 to 1957, and a determined opponent of basic research, will long be remembered by scientists for his classic phrase, "I don't care what makes the grass green." Wilson might just as well have said, "I don't care what makes the sky blue." John Tyndall, the British physicist, *did* care what made the sky blue and this look into the Retrospectroscope shows how blue sky, of all things, paid off for biomedical research.

Born in 1820, Tyndall became professor of natural philosophy in the Royal Institution in 1853; in 1867, when Michael Faraday died, Tyndall succeeded him as Superintendent of the Institution. Tyndall made notable scientific contributions to the fields of diamagnetism, light, sound, and radiant heat. In addition, he was a gifted lecturer and writer and probably did more than any person of his time to make the great scientific discoveries of the nineteenth century intelligible and even fascinating to the general public. This special talent brought him an invitation to lecture in America in 1872-73; his book, *Six Lectures on Light,* that grew out of these went through 5 editions by 1895 and earned for Tyndall £6,000-7,000 (quite a sum in those days), all of which he used as a fund to encourage original research in the United States.

But back to blue sky. The idea that the color of the sky is due to the action of finely divided matter that creates a turbid atmosphere, through which we on earth look toward the darkness of space, dates back to Leonardo da Vinci. Newton, Goethe, Clausius, Stokes, and others also studied this phenomenon. But the cause of the blue color of the sky was, in the 1860s, still one of the enigmas of meteorology. Tyndall in 1869 conducted experiments with a glass tube about 36 inches long and 3 inches in diameter into which he introduced vapors. When he illuminated them with a strong condensed beam from an electric lamp, they "decomposed" and he now had a tube filled with fine particles. Sometimes these were

so fine that their "diameters constitute but a very small fraction of the length of a wave of violet light." When he plunged the room into darkness and focused his powerful beam of light on the tube, a sky-blue cloud now filled the tube.

With this dramatic, easily repeatable evidence in hand, he could now extrapolate from the glass tube in his laboratory to the blue sky and say:

> Suppose our atmosphere surrounded by an envelope impervious to light, but with an aperture on the sunward side through which a parallel beam of solar light could enter and traverse the atmosphere. Surrounded on all sides by air not directly illuminated, the track of such a beam through the air would resemble that of the parallel beam of the electric lamp through an incipient cloud. The sunbeam would be *blue*, and it would discharge laterally light in precisely the same condition as that discharged by the incipient cloud. In fact the azure revealed by such a beam would be to all intents and purposes that which I have called a "blue cloud." (1).

As one would expect of the Superintendent of the Royal Institution, Tyndall performed controls using particle-free air and made the fascinating observation that air containing only pure gases *and no particles* acted like a vacuum, in that in a dark room it remained pitch black when "illuminated" by a powerful electric beam. It immediately became obvious to Tyndall that we perceive light only when light waves strike particles in their path (as when the beam from a powerful projector becomes visible in a dark theatre only because it hits myriads of dancing particles of dust).

Tyndall soon put his discovery to work. Louis Pasteur in 1862 (2) had announced a revolutionary new concept. Pasteur insisted that there was no such thing as spontaneous generation; germs (no matter how small) came from other germs. His experimental proof convinced many scientists, but the new doctrine shattered beliefs that were centuries old and aroused much vigorous opposition. Some of Pasteur's opponents in-

2

sisted that bacteria did in fact generate spontaneously because bacteria appeared where the most powerful microscopes could not detect a preexisting generation. Tyndall came to Pasteur's aid with a test for optically pure, uncontaminated air—certain to be free of both inorganic dust and organic germs because it could not scatter light (3).

Numerous experiments showed optically pure air to be incapable of developing bacterial life. In properly protected vessels, previously boiled infusions of fish, flesh, and vegetable, freely exposed to air that had been proved to be optically pure by the invisible passage of a powerful electric beam, remained permanently pure and unaltered, whereas the identical liquids, exposed afterwards to ordinary dust-laden air, soon swarmed with bacteria. Tyndall wrote:

It seemed that this simple method of examination could not fail to be of use to workers in the field. They had hitherto proceeded less by sight than by insight, being in general unable to see the physical character of the medium in which their experiments were conducted. . . . The optical deportment of the floating matter of the air proves it to be composed, in part, of particles of this excessively minute character [that passed sensibly unimpeded through forty layers of the best filtering paper]. The concentrated [light] beam reveals them collectively, long after the microscope has ceased to distinguish them individually. They are,

moreover, organic particles, which may be removed from the air by combustion. In the presence of such facts, any argument against atmospheric germs, based upon their being beyond the reach of the microscope, loses all validity.

"Why is the sky blue?" thus paid off handsomely for the new science of bacteriology.

"Why is the sky blue?" also paid off for pulmonary medicine. Lord Lister had pointed out that air that had passed through the lungs had lost its power of causing putrefaction, and, as a strong proponent of the germ theory of disease, he attributed the purification of air to the filtering action of the lungs. Tyndall provided experimental proof by showing that air from the upper airways scattered light but air from the deepest parts of the lung did not. He darkened a room containing dusty air and focused a powerful beam of light on the end of a glass tube through which the subject breathed (figure 1). When the subject inspired the dusty room air, the inhaled particles scattered the intense beam of light as the air entered the glass tube en route to the airways and alveoli. When the subject expired, Tyndall observed at first a diminution in scattered light. But toward end-expiration, a perfectly black gap broke the white track of the light beam owing to the total absence from the end-expired air of any matter that could scatter

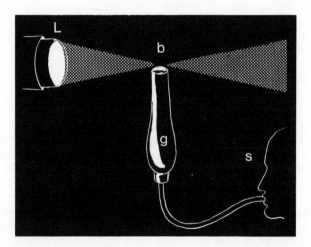

Fig. 1. A lens (L) focuses a powerful beam of light on the end (b) of a glass tube (g) through which the subject (s) breathes. The room is darkened and the air is dusty for optimal demonstration of light scattering. When mid- to end-expired gas reaches b, this region becomes perfectly black because this gas contains no light-scattering particles. Tube g is warmed to prevent condensation of water vapor. (Redrawn from Tyndall [3]).

light (the glass tube had been warmed to prevent condensation of water vapor) (3). This was the first experimental demonstration of the defense mechanisms of the airways—of the ability of the airways (by mechanisms then unknown) to remove particles from inspired air before they reached alveolar gas. I believe it was also the first "single-breath test" used to demonstrate or evaluate a function of the lung. Light-scattering methods have, since Tyndall, played an important role in quantifying particles responsible for air pollution and for estimating the clearance of various-sized particles by pulmonary defense mechanisms.

(Light scattering theory has also been put to other uses. In wartime, in the early 1940's, La Mer devised technics for determining the precise size of particles and built smoke generators that could produce uniform aerosols made of particles of any desired size; his work permitted large scale production of smoke screens with maximal obscuring power and their effective use against aerial bombing. In peacetime, light-scattering technics have been used by astronomers to learn about the density and distribution of matter in the universe, by physicists and chemists to determine the size of particles and the weight of molecules and by microbiologists to measure the size of viruses in their natural state.)

Tyndall then became interested in one particular type of the particles known to float in air—atmospheric germs:

> I wished . . . to obtain clearer and more definite insight as to the diffusion of atmospheric germs. Supposing a large tray to be filled with a suitable organic infusion and exposed to air. Into it the germs would drop and, could the resulting organisms be confined to the locality where the germs fell, we should have the floating life of the atmosphere mapped, so to speak, in the infusion.

In 1877 (3), he set up trays with 10 rows of 10 tubes in each and soon had his catch—both bacteria and molds.* One of the molds was Penicilli-

---

* In these experiments on germs that fell into clear broth, Tyndall again made use of light scattering for the early detection of bacterial growth. However, here he used the method of his close friend and colleague, Faraday, who in 1857 demonstrated that exceedingly fine particles of gold suspended in apparently clear liquid "are easily rendered evident, by gathering the rays of the sun (or a lamp) into a cone by a lens, and sending the part of the cone near the focus into the fluid; the cone becomes visible, and though the illuminated particles cannot be distinguished because of their minuteness, yet the light

um. Tyndall appears to have accomplished by experiment in 1877 what Fleming happened upon in 1929, and Tyndall was probably the first to comment on antagonism between molds and bacteria. He wrote:

> The Penicillium was exquisitely beautiful. . . . In every case where the mould was thick and coherent, the Bacteria died, or became dormant, and fell to the bottom as a sediment. The growth of mould and its effect on the Bacteria are very capricious. . . . Of two tubes placed beside each other, one will be taken possession of by Bacteria, which successfully fight the mould and keep the surface perfectly clean; while another will allow the mould a footing, the apparent destruction of the Bacteria being the consequence.

Score another for "Why is the sky blue?"!

Tyndall made still another contribution to pulmonary medicine. Quite unknowingly, he was the father of the flexible bronchoscope and other techniques (such as intravascular spectrophotometry) that require a curved path of light (5). In 1854, he constructed a small box with one glass side and a glass tube (3/4" wide and 5" long) fitted into the opposite side. He then arranged to condense electric light so that it passed first through the pane of glass, then through the air-filled box and out the glass tube at the opposite side; the light formed a white disc on a screen held against the end of the tube. The top of the box was connected to a water tank on the roof; when Tyndall turned a tap, water filled the box and spouted out the glass tube in a downward curve. Now the path of the light beam was no longer straight but followed the curve. Tyndall noted that where the water flowed out of the glass tube, "the light on reaching the limiting surface of air and water was totally reflected and seemed to be washed downward by the descending liquid, the latter being thereby caused to present a beautiful illuminated surface" (6). This was a singular demonstration, under special circumstances, that light could follow a curved path. At first the path was a curved "water tube," then a glass thread, and more recently, flexible glass fibers. Tyndall's 1854 demonstration was not put to medical use until 37 years after his death when, in 1930, Lamm advocated using glass fibers in a flexible gastroscope (7); the flex-

---

they reflect is golden in character, and seen to be abundant in proportion to the quantity of solid gold present" (4). This later formed the basis for quantitative studies of turbidity of suspensions, an important measurement in many biomedical sciences.

4

ible bronchoscope of Ikeda came into use in 1968 (8).

Out of a blue sky came (1) the final blow to the theory of spontaneous generation, (2) proof of the defense mechanisms of the airways against inhaled particles, (3) quantitative tests of air pollution and of clearance of particles from inspired air, and (4) the first observations of the antibacterial action of *Penicillium*. And the "blue-sky man" also provided the theoretic basis for the flexible bronchoscope.

Now Mr. Wilson, wouldn't you really like to know what makes the grass green?

References

1. Tyndall, J.: On the blue colour of the sky, the polarization of skylight and on the polarization of light by cloudy matter generally, Philos Mag, 1869, *37*, 384-394.
2. Pasteur, L.: Mémoire sur les corpuscules organisés qui existent dans l'atmosphère, Ann Chim Phys, 1862, *64*, 5-110.
3. Tyndall, J.: II. The optical deportment of the atmosphere in relation to the phenomena of putrefaction and infection, Philos Trans, 1877, *166*, 27-74.
4. Faraday, M.: The Bakerian Lecture. Experimental relations of gold (and other metals) to light, Philos Trans R Soc Lond, 1857, 145-181.
5. Ikeda, S.: Atlas of Flexible Bronchofiberscopy, University Park Press, Baltimore, 1971.
6. Tyndall, J.: On some phenomena connected with the motion of liquids, Philos Mag, 1854, *8*, 74-76.
7. Lamm, H.: Biegsame optische Geräte, Z Instrumentenk, 1930, *50*, 579-581.
8. Ikeda, S., Yanai, N., and Ishikawa, S.: Flexible bronchofiberscope, Keio J Med, 1968, *17*, 1-18.

A Sea of Air

One of the puzzles in the early part of the seventeenth century was that a suction pump could not raise water higher than 34 feet. Galileo in his "Dialogues Concerning Two New Sciences" has one of his characters say, "I once saw a cistern which had been provided with a pump under the mistaken impression that the water might thus be drawn with less effort or in greater quantity than by means of the ordinary bucket... This pump worked perfectly so long as the water in the cistern stood above a certain level; but below this level the pump failed to work. When I first noted this phenomenon, I thought the machine was out of order; but the workman whom I called to repair it told me the defect was not in the pump but in the water, which had fallen too low to be raised to such a height; and he added that it was not possible, either by a pump or by any other machine working on the principle of attraction, to lift water a hair's breadth above eighteen cubits" (1). (A cubit, an ancient measure of length, was the length of the forearm, or cubitus, from the tip of the middle finger to the elbow. In the Scriptures, this distance was about 22 inches; later, it became 18 inches.)

We know now that, at sea level, the atmosphere presses down with a weight equivalent to that of a column of mercury about 30 inches high. Since mercury is almost 13.6 times as heavy as water, the weight of air, if unopposed, can support a column of water 406 inches, or about 18 cubits, high. Whenever the pressure of air is decreased above a segment of water (as by sucking on a straw immersed in water), the water rises in it; if a good vacuum pump replaces inspiratory effort, and creates a near-vacuum in the tube, the water will rise to almost 34 feet, but no higher.

Galileo knew of the problem of pumping water but apparently did not concern himself with it. However, his pupil, Evangelista Torricelli, did. There were few scientific publications in 1644 and Torricelli told of his experiments in a letter to Cardinal Ricci—so one can only surmise that his famous experiment was related to the practical problem of pumping water (2). Torri-

celli obviously could not experiment with a glass tube 18 cubits high but he could with one 1/14 as high. This solution was an elegantly simple one; he made the *contents* of a short tube 14 times as heavy by substituting mercury for water. Using a glass tube 2 cubits long and closed at one end, he filled it with mercury, stoppered the upper, open end with his finger, and inverted it in a basin of mercury (figure 1). When he removed his finger, the mercury column dropped to "a height of a cubit and a quarter and an inch besides" (29.75 inches, if we assume that Torricelli's cubit was 23 inches) (2). In this one series of experiments, Torricelli made four important contributions. (1) He developed an entirely new concept—"that we live submerged at the bottom of a sea of the element air, which by unquestioned experiments is known to have weight." (2) He invented the barometer, a scientific instrument for measuring the weight of the air. (3) He produced in his tube *above* the

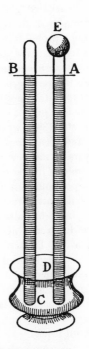

Fig. 1. Torricelli's barometer (2).

mercury column what came to be known as a Torricellian vacuum. (4) He opened the door for quantitative measurements in "pneumatics" and a renaissance in physics.

The first consequence of Torricelli's discovery provided the basis for high altitude physiology. In 1648, Pascal reasoned that, if air did indeed have weight, it must have less weight on a mountain top than at sea level; this his brother-in-law, Perier, confirmed—though with such exact data that some suspect he *calculated* the pressure rather than measured it!

The second consequence was Boyle's reasoning that if air pressing on the mercury in the dish supported the mercury in the tube, the mercury column should fall if he enclosed the dish and sucked out air above the mercury. This led to a continuing series of experiments by Boyle with ever-improved suction pumps and to the birth of experimental, quantitative physics, supported by published measurements. Boyle in 1669 constructed a U-tube with a short leg closed at the top and a long leg open at the top into which he could pour mercury. When he increased the height of the column of mercury from 29 2/16 inches to 58 13/16 inches, the volume of air trapped above the mercury in the short leg decreased from 48 units to 24 units and Boyle's law was born (3). Boyle also developed improved suction pumps to replace the Torricellian vacuum and evacuated glass chambers to learn that sound required air for its transmission. (Boyle's pumps probably were unable to lower pressures to less than 1/4 inch of mercury because he lacked modern equipment for making leak-proof seals for moving parts. It was not until an important industrial need arose for lower pressures that modern pumps were developed; the need came in the 1880s when Edison was developing the incandescent lamp [1].)

For certain advances, the new physics had to await the new chemistry in the eighteenth century—and the new physiology in the nineteenth. Dalton's law of partial pressure (1805) and his atomic theory (4), built initially on studies of gases, required the discoveries of CO_2 by Black in 1755 (5) and of O_2 by Lavoisier in 1776 (6) because these provided proof that air was composed of several elements. Poiseuille's study of cardiovascular physiology, and especially of resistance to flow through both large and very fine tubes, led him in 1828 to construct a U-tube open at both ends, fill it part way with mercury, and use it to record superimposed blood pressure;

in 1847, Ludwig added a float with a stylus to write on a rotating kymograph and created the first system to record dynamic cardiovascular events. Mountain sickness and disasters in balloons at high altitudes led Paul Bert to his classic studies in high and low pressure chambers recorded in his monograph "La Pression Barométrique" in 1878 (7).

A few years ago, engineers, wanting a more convenient term than "millimeters of mercury" (8 syllables), hit upon a one-syllable contraction of Torricelli—"torr." One torr is essentially the pressure required to support a column of mercury 1 mm high when the mercury is of standard density and subject to standard acceleration. Torr is now used by many respiratory physiologists in referring to total and partial gas pressures and serves the double purpose of simplifying speech and honoring the Italian physicist who first measured the weight of the sea of air whose bottom we inhabit.

It is true that Torricelli's experiments were built on the older science of hydrostatics and the knowledge that the pressure at the bottom of a vessel filled with water depended on the *height* of the water and not on the volume or shape of the vessel. But to paraphrase Albert Szent Gyorgi (in his definition of creative research), Torricelli looked at what everyone had looked at before, saw what everyone had seen before, but *thought* what no one else had thought before.

References

1. Harvard Case Histories in Experimental Science, vol. 1, J. B. Conant, ed., Harvard University Press, Cambridge, 1957, p. 60.
2. Torricelli, E.: On the pressure of the atmosphere, in *The Physical Treatises of Pascal*, I. H. B. Spiers and A. G. H. Spiers, tr., Columbia University Press, New York, 1937, pp. 163-166.
3. Boyle, Robert: A defence of the doctrine touching the spring and weight of the air, in *The Works of the Honourable Robert Boyle*, vol. 1, J & F Rivington and Associates, London, 1772, pp. 156-159.
4. Dalton, J.: Manchester Philosophical Society Memoires, vol. 1, 1805, pp. 244-287.
5. Black, J.: Experiments Upon Magnesia Alba, Quick Lime, and Other Alcaline Substances, William Creech, Edinburgh, 1796, 134 pages.
6. Lavoisier, A.: Essays, Physical and Chemical, ed. 2, T. Henry, tr., Frank Cass and Co., Ltd., London, 1970, pp. 407-419.
7. Bert, P.: Barometric Pressure: Researches in Experimental Physiology, M. A. Hitchcock and F. A. Hitchcock, tr., College Book Co., Columbus, Ohio, 1943, 1038 pages.

The Inside Story

Come, come, and sit you down.
You shall not budge.
You go not till I set you up a glass
Where you may see the inmost part of you.

Shakespeare
Hamlet III, iv

"No discovery of our time—or any other time—has been followed by so immediate and universal an outbreak of scientific activity" (from Silvanus Thompson's first presidential address before the Roentgen Society, November 5, 1897). What was this discovery that sped throughout the world with the speed of wireless and profoundly influenced the course of many sciences, especially Medicine?

On November 8, 1895, Wilhelm Conrad Roentgen, Professor of Physics at the University of Würzburg, passed the discharge from a large induction coil through an evacuated Crookes tube. The apparatus was in a completely darkened room and the tube was covered with black cardboard; nevertheless, at each discharge he observed that a paper screen covered with a fluorescent material became brightly illuminated. He soon found that not only black cardboard but all substances permitted the passage of "X-rays" (as he named them) but—and this is all-important—to differing degrees: a bound book of about 1,000 pages offered no hindrance, glass containing lead offered some, and lead itself, if at least 1.5 mm thick, almost blocked them. Most remarkable was his observation that "if the hand be held before the fluorescent screen, the shadow shows the bones darkly with only faint outlines of the surrounding tissues." (1)

Over the next few weeks he satisfied himself that he was not dealing with cathode or any other known type of rays and, by substituting a glass photographic plate for the fluorescent screen, he took the first roentgenogram—that of his wife's hand. He then wrote a communication to the Würzburg Physical Medical Society that the president immediately published in the December 28 Proceedings, more than three weeks before Roentgen presented his paper orally (January 23, 1896).

The response was dramatic. Roentgen, as was customary then (and now), had mailed to some of his physicist colleagues reprints of his paper and, with each, some photographic prints (his published paper contained no illustration—not even of his wife's hand, though the latter appeared miraculously in the English translation of his paper in *Science*, February 14, 1896). One colleague showed the paper and prints to a physician whose father, publisher of the Vienna *Freie Presse*, printed an article on Roentgen's discovery on January 5.*

On January 23, 1896, Roentgen gave his oral presentation to the Würzburg Society—the same day that an English translation of the December 28 report was printed in *Nature*. Albert Rudolph Kölliker, famous for his 1856 work on the electrocardiogram, presided, and in the discussion that followed the paper, it was he who proposed, with enthusiastic acclaim from the large audience, that x-rays thenceforth be called Roentgen rays (2).

Probably not even penicillin was used as rapidly and as widely as the new Roentgen rays. The

---

* In this modern age of speed, let us note humbly that in 1895-96, the total time between submission of Roentgen's paper and its world-wide acclaim by the press took no longer than 15 to 20 days (among these were the Christmas and New Year's holidays); this time includes that for review and acceptance by the editor, setting in type a 10-page article, proofreading and printing it, supplying reprints to the author, mailing reprints, delivery by a Postal Service and notice by the press!

8

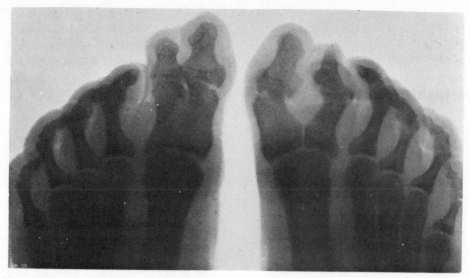

Fig. 1. A young lady, with six toes on each foot, suffered from the extra breadth of her feet. The surgeon removed the supernumerary toes "with much greater precision than if he had not had it [the skiagram] to guide him." Plate XV from Arch Clin Skiagraphy, 1896, *1*.

supply of commerically available Crookes tubes quickly ran out but almost anyone who knew a little about physics could easily assemble the equipment at little expense and go to work. Within the first year, more than 1,000 scientific papers and 50 books were published dealing entirely with Roentgen rays! A new journal, *Archives of Clinical Skiagraphy*† ("shadow writing") appeared in the spring of 1896, edited by Sydney Rowland, still a medical student (3). And a new Roentgen Society was formed in June 1897 (4).

The wide range of the uses of the new rays was amazing (5). Surgeons of course used them to examine broken bones, to study abnormal bony structures (figure 1) and to locate foreign objects. Others used them to detect, locate and characterize a wide variety of pulmonary disorders. Anatomists had a new tool to examine the human skeleton without even undressing the subject. Figure 2 shows the first radiograph of the entire skeleton taken with one exposure (produced by W. J. Morton, son of the Morton who first used ether for surgical anesthesia). The lady has removed only her corset; her hat pin, necklace, bracelet, rings, and highbutton shoes with nailed-on heels remain.

† The Archives dropped the word Clinical from its title in 1897, to emphasize its broad field of interest, and one number later it dropped Skiagraphy and became the *Archives of the Roentgen Ray.*

Within a few months, others put Roentgen rays to many uses that we often regard as more modern developments: studies of the motion and size of the human heart (6) reported first at the April 1896 meeting of the Association of American Physicians; angiographic examination of an amputated hand made after injection into its vessels of a medium opaque to x-rays (7); cine-radiography of a leg in motion (8); examination of a patient's esophagus while he swallowed nitrate of bismuth (9); and locating an aortic aneurysm (10). Walter Cannon plunged into research on Roentgen rays while still a first-year medical student at Harvard and presented his classic work on the effect of emotions on gastric motility at the May 1897 meeting of the American Physiological Society (11).

Botanists and zoologists also got into the act. Volume 1 of the *Archives of Clinical Skiagraphy* contains roentgenograms of Homarus vulgaris (lobster) and Cancer pagurus (edible crab). The 1897 *Archives of the Roentgen Ray* contained its first supplement and it was completely devoted to Marine Zoology, with 36 illustrations of the British Echinodermata (figure 3). The effect of x-rays on ascaris eggs was also studied by 1897. One reviewer could adequately describe the diversity of experimental material only by quoting Macbeth:

> Eye of newt, and toe of frog,
> Wool of bat, and tongue of dog,

Equally fascinating was the early application of the Roentgen ray to many nonbiological problems. Hedley, in his 1897 review (5), noted:

> It now also bids fair to prove useful in other "arts and crafts." It has been used, or its use suggested, in distinguishing real gems from artificial ones; to discover the fraudulent introduction of mineral substances into textile fabrics to increase their weight; to discover the contents of packages in the parcel post; to recognize explosives and contraband in baggage; to age and oxidize alcohol; to test insulation in the construction of cables; to ascertain cohesion in welding.

(I confess that I thought that filling suitcases with bombs and finding them using x-rays were unique to our present stage of civilization!) Another early use was in metallography: Heycock in 1897 (4) "placed thin slices of alloys under the rays and revealed their structure in a marvellous way"; was this the beginning of x-ray diffraction to study the structure of matter?

Harmful Effects of Roentgen Rays

For a while, most physicists and physicians thought that x-rays passed through tissues without damaging them; some individuals even used exposure to Roentgen rays to promote good health, and the feature of every charity bazaar was the x-ray booth where anyone could see the bones of his hands for sixpence (the forerunner

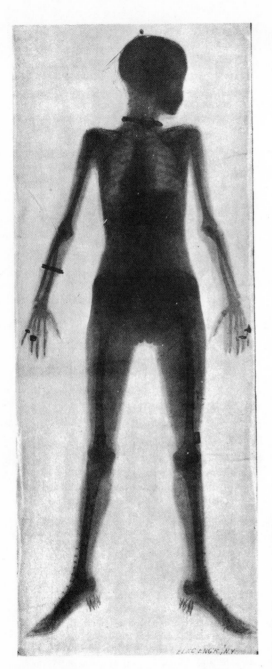

Fig. 2. First x-ray picture of the entire adult body at one exposure. The tube was 54 inches from the photographic plate. "Time, including stoppages, thirty minutes." Plate XXX b from Arch Roentgen Ray, 1897 (July), 2.

Adder's fork, and blind-worm's sting,
Lizard's leg, and howlet's wing . . .

One even noted that the light of glowworms (like Roentgen's rays) passed through aluminum and cast shadows (4).

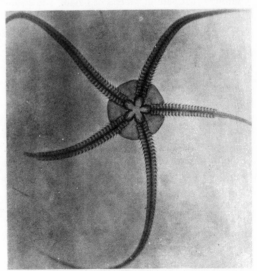

Fig. 3. X-ray photography of Ophiurus Ciliaris. From the first Supplement to Archives of the Roentgen Ray, 1897. It dealt entirely with radiography of marine biology, specifically with the British Echinodermata.

of free x-ray examination of feet by shoe store clerks!). Elihu Thomson decided to find out for himself whether the passage of x-rays harmed tissues (12):

I was interested sometime ago in regard to the effect of Röntgen rays on tissues. I had read a few times that certain people had been burned by Röntgen rays. I did not believe it. These rays went through tissue so easily that their action could not amount to anything, but it was certainly worthwhile investigating so as to know . . . I put my finger up to the clear glass window and kept the other fingers pretty well shielded by the blue glass of other parts of the tube. I exposed the finger for half an hour to the rays, a Holtz machine being the source of electricity. I put the finger up pretty close to the tube, and after half an hour I thought perhaps it was not long enough, perhaps it was not half long enough. But if there were to be any effect it would be equivalent to a few hours distance, and as I got tired I went no farther. I shut down the tube and went away. Five, six, seven, eight days passed and nothing happened, and I felt that people had been mistaken about the effect of the rays. But on the ninth day the finger began to redden; on the twelfth day there was a blister, and a very sore blister. On the thirteenth and fourteenth day after exposure, the blister had included all the skin down to the part not exposed and had gone around the finger almost to the other side. The whole of the epidermis came away and left an ulcer without any possibility of recovering its own epidermis except from the edges, and I had to go through that painful process of having a raw sore there and the epidermis growing in from the side and gradually closing up. Only three days ago was the sore actually closed, and the skin is yet very tender, and nature does not appear to have found out how to make a good skin over that finger. The skin still comes off in flakes and is very disagreeable and very tender, and there is a burning, smarting, sensation every now and then. But I am satisfied it is coming out all right. . . . This has taken six and a half weeks today.

That was written in 1896. It convinced Grubbe to devise lead shielding that same year and Price to make lead-lined gloves in 1898. But it didn't reach or convince everyone. Thomas Edison was intrigued first with "photographing" the brain. When that yielded nothing of interest, he became fascinated with the idea of fluorescent light bulbs. According to Griggs (2, p. 783), Edison began to use modified Crookes tubes as light bulbs, calling them "fluorescent lamps." The results were disastrous: ". . . I [said Edison] started in to make a number of these lamps, but I soon found that the x-ray had affected poisonously my assistant, Mr. Dally, so that his hair came out and his flesh commenced to ulcerate. I then concluded it would not do, and that it would not be a very popular kind of light, so I dropped it . . ." (Understatement of the century!)

Dally died in 1904 at the age of 39—the first fatality from x-ray "poisoning" in the United States. In April 1898, the Council of the Roentgen Society appointed the first committee to collect information on alleged injurious effects of x-rays. One of the five-man group reported in 1899, in part (13):

We may, I think, safely assert that the length of exposure necessary to produce any injury is at least three or four times that required to obtain a radiograph with the improved apparatus now at our disposal, even where the most opaque parts of the body are concerned, and then only when the patient is specially susceptible to the electrical forces which cause the injury.

It is noteworthy that the first cure of cancer by x-ray therapy was reported in 1899, three years before the first report of cancer *caused by* x-ray exposure. If the cancer-*caused* had preceded the cancer-*cured*, would the story of x-rays have stopped abruptly with the cancer-caused? (14)

Rays before Roentgen

Sylvanus Thompson wrote:

In the history of Science, nothing is more true than that the discoverer—even the greatest of discoverers—is but the descendant of his scientific forefathers, is always and essentially the product of the age in which he is born. Roentgen himself has frankly avowed the ancestry of his discoveries. He himself has stated that, being aware of the existence of unsolved problems respecting the emission of cathode rays in and by an electrically stimulated vacuum tube, he had for a long time followed with the greatest interest the researches of Hertz and of Lenard, and had determined, as soon as he should find the necessary leisure, to make some researches of his own. Behind Roentgen then, stand Lenard and Hertz; behind Hertz stand Crookes, and Varley, and Hittorf, and Sprengel and Geissler; and so back to Hauksbee, and Boyle, and Otto Guericke, into the beginnings of modern science as it emerged from the vain imaginings and occult mysteries of Mediaeval night (15).

Hedley (5) began his account with the fascinating electrical demonstrations that amused and amazed the savants of the French Court in the 1750s and the "electric egg," an ovoid glass vessel with a variable vacuum, across which leaped a spark created by an electrical machine. Then in 1838, Faraday began his systematic investigations of phenomena that occur when electric discharges pass through rarefied gases. Four years later, Abria of Boulogne, passing current from an induction coil through an "electric egg," saw the beautiful purple light that streamed from the positive to negative pole and had the extraordinary power of exciting fluorescence. In 1879, Crookes, working with much higher degrees of vacuum (one millionth of an atmosphere or less), discovered emanations from the negative pole that excited brilliant fluorescence and were deflected by a magnet; he regarded these as a stream of negatively electrified molecules or atoms flying with great velocity from the cathode. Crookes' experiments were interesting but his tube shared the oblivion of the electric egg until Hertz took it out of retirement. Hertz believed that the cathode discharge did not consist of electrified particles but was wave motion. When Hertz found that the waves passed through a thin aluminum sheet, Lenard decided to bring the cathode rays *outside* the glass tube and did it by substituting a small window of thin aluminum for a portion of the glass tube; by so doing, he made both cathode rays and true Roentgen rays available for study. Roentgen differentiated the two.

Was Roentgen's an accidental discovery? Others might have discovered them earlier, but did not. Crookes, after experimenting with his tube and developing some photographic plates, noted on his pictures marks that corresponded to his fingers; thinking the plates were defective, he returned them to the manufacturer with some strong remarks! Roentgen's research dealt with the nature of rays coming from Lenard or Crookes tubes. "Roentgen's discovery cannot in any sense be called accidental; it was the result of deliberate and directed thought. He was looking for something—he knew not precisely what. And he found it. Fortunate the discovery may well be deemed, but not fortuitous" (15).

References

1. Röntgen, W. C.: Ueber eine neue Art von Strahlen, Sitzung Physikal-Medicin Gesellschaft, Würzburg, 1895, *137*, 132-141. (English translation: Science, 1896 [Feb. 14], *3*, 227-231.)
2. Grigg, E. R. N.: The Trail of the Invisible Light from X-Strahlen to Radio(bio)logy, Charles C Thomas, Springfield, Ill., 1965.
3. Archives of Clinical Skiagraphy, vol. 1, edited by Sydney Rowland. Rebman Publishing Co., 1896.
4. Thompson, S.: Minutes of the first meeting of the Roentgen Society, June 3, 1897, Arch Roentgen Ray, 1897, *2*, 5-6.
5. Hedley, W. S.: Roentgen rays. A survey, present and retrospective, Arch Roentgen Ray, 1897, *2*, 6-12.
6. Williams, F. H.: A method for more fully determining the outline of the heart by means of the fluoroscope [sic] together with other uses of this instrument in medicine, Boston Med Surg J, 1896, *135*, 335-337.
7. Haschek, E. and Lindenthal, O. Th.: Ein Beitrag zur praktischen Verwertung der Photographie nach Röntgen, Wien Klin Wochenschr, 1896, *9*, 63-64.
8. MacIntyre, J.: X-ray records for the cinematograph, Arch Skiagraphy, 1897, *1*, 37.
9. Kummel. Ger Surg Soc, 1897 (April), Quoted by Hedley (5), p. 10.
10. Béclère, Oudin and Barthelemy: Soc Med des Hôpit, Quoted by Hedley (5).
11. Cannon, W. B.: The movements of the stomach studied by means of the Röntgen rays, Am J Physiol, 1898, *1*, 359-382.
12. Rowland, H. A., Thomson, E., Pupin, M. I., and Kennelly, A. E.: The Röntgen ray and its relation to physics: a topical discussion, Trans Amer Inst Elect Engin, 1896, *13*, 403-432 (quoted by Nelson, P. A.: Role of scientific societies in disseminating knowledge and fostering research on x-rays, Med Instrum, 1975, *9*, 260-266).
13. Payne, E.: Notes on the effects of x-rays, Arch Roentgen Ray, 1899 (Feb), *3*, 67-69.
14. Spear, F. G.: Early days of experimental radiology, Br J Radiol, 1973, *46*, 762-765.
15. Thompson, Silvanus: First Presidential Address to the Roentgen Society, Arch Roentgen Ray, 1897, *2*, 23-30.

12

Whodunit (And Why)[1]

Part I

The scientific method depends on the careful accumulation of data by objective means. However, when medical scientists testify before congressional appropriations committees, they support their case with anecdotal evidence (the "let-me-give-you-an-example" approach). In fairness to them, they've had little choice, because the scientific method has never really been used to determine the genesis of crucial scientific discoveries. Yet national biomedical science policy should be directed mainly toward creating conditions that favor discovery, and a little objectivity might help.

In the summer of 1971, Robert Dripps (then Vice President for Health Affairs at the University of Pennsylvania) and I wondered whether we could obtain objective data on how critical discoveries have come about in the past, to serve as a historical basis for predicting how equally important discoveries are likely to be made in the future.

We decided to study the ten most important clinical advances in cardiovascular-pulmonary medicine and surgery of the past 30 years and see how much first had to be learned by how many scientists working in how many fields before someone could take the final step of successful clinical application (1). In our analysis we started with more than 4,000 scientific articles, whittled them down to about 2,500, and then, with the help of consultants, reduced these to 529 key articles. A key article was defined as one that had an important effect on the direction of subsequent research and develop-

ment, which in turn proved to be important for one of the ten clinical advances. It reported new data, new ways of looking at old data, a new concept or hypothesis, a new method, a new drug, new apparatus, or a new technique that was either essential for the full development of a clinical advance or greatly accelerated it. The key article might represent basic laboratory investigation, clinical investigation, development of apparatus or essential components, synthesis of data or ideas of others, or wholly theoretic work.

Having selected these key articles, we then examined them carefully to see why their authors did the work in the first place. One question we wanted to answer was, how many of these studies were done to solve a specific clinical problem related to the prevention, diagnosis, or treatment of a specific disease, and how many were done simply to learn something completely unrelated to clinical medicine or surgery or to the genesis or course of a disease?

Our analysis showed that 217 of the 529 key articles (41 per cent) reported work that, at the time it was done, had no relation whatever to the disease that it later helped to prevent, diagnose, treat, or alleviate (2). Because this is a surprisingly large percentage—enough to have a real impact on national biomedical science policy—I think it is important to list some of the 217 for you; in other parts of this book, I refer to some in more detail.

X-rays. When, in 1895, Roentgen discovered that rays from a Crookes' tube could pass through the human hand and darken photographic plates, he was a physicist studying a basic problem dealing with the electrical nature of matter. He did not have a "mission" to look inside people and examine their lungs or hearts or coronary arteries (3a).

[1]The final report *"The Top Ten Clinical Advances in Cardiovascular-Pulmonary Medicine and Surgery between 1945 and 1975: How They Came About"* on which "Whodunit" is based is published by the U.S. Government Printing Office as Vol. 1 (158 pp.) #913-837 and Vol. 2 (433 pp.) #913-836.

13

Motion pictures. When Muybridge devised the first motion pictures in 1887, he was a photographer interested only in determining whether all four hoofs of a horse ever left the ground at the same time (3b); he had no thought of devising an apparatus that was essential to the advance of angiocardiography—x-rays weren't even discovered until December 1895. But in 1896, Macintyre combined Roentgen's and Muybridge's "pure" research and made the first ciné roentgenograms.

Lung volume. When Davy measured his own lung volume in 1800 by rebreathing hydrogen, he had no thought whatever of using it as a test to help in the diagnosis or evaluation of pulmonary disease (3c); he was simply curious.

Microvascular surgery. When two pharmacologists wanted to solve a basic problem that required complete denervation of a dog's artery *in vivo*, they went to a young research surgeon, Julius Jacobson, for advice. Jacobson knew that the only way to be sure that he had severed every nerve fiber was to remove a segment of the artery, reverse it, and sew it back in place. In trying to do this, he found that the problem was "not in the ability of the hand to sew but rather the eye to see"; to solve the problem, he applied a dissection microscope and special instruments to the task. He then went on to use the technique in clinical microvascular surgery (3d), including operations on coronary and intracranial vessels.

Pulmonary diffusing capacity. When Marie Krogh, in 1915, developed the carbon monoxide technique of measuring diffusing capacity in man, she wanted only to answer a basic physiologic question—did oxygen cross the alveolar capillary membrane only by diffusion or was oxygen secreted, at least in part, by an active process? She did answer it unequivocally (it was by diffusion alone) but she never applied her test to the clinical diagnosis of pulmonary disorders (3e).

Nitrogen meter. When John Lilly devised this instrument, it was to help the Air Force during World War II to determine when and why air leaked into oxygen masks worn by aviators (3f). Lilly reasoned that, since air contained 79 per cent N_2 and oxygen contained none, he could determine the precise moment of the leak if he had a method for continuous, almost instantaneous, measurement of the nitrogen concentration in small samples of gas drawn from the mask. With his background in physics, it took him little time to devise the nitrogen

meter. He soon saw the clinical usefulness of a nitrogen meter to determine uneven distribution of inspired gas to the lungs, but this came later, after he had solved the Air Force's problem.

Intracellular recordings of transmembrane potential differences. When, in 1936, J. Z. Young came across the giant axone of the squid, he had been studying the process of degeneration of the central stump after complete section of a nerve. In his first report on these huge axones (up to 1 mm in diameter—50 to 1,000 times thicker than mammalian nerve fibers), he mentioned that they might prove useful in studying the structure of nerve membranes and the location of inorganic ions involved in depolarization of membranes. He did not mention using the technique for measuring electrical activity in normal or diseased heart muscle fibers to obtain transcellular potential differences (3b).

Influence of calcium and potassium on cardiac contraction. When Sidney Ringer suddenly realized that calcium and potassium ions, in proper proportions, were essential for the normal rhythm and contraction of heart muscle, he was studying a basic physiologic problem in frogs (3d). He had no idea at that time that his observations would be clinically important in cardiac defibrillation, in elective cardiac arrest during open heart surgery, and in understanding the mechanism of cardiac malfunction in electrolyte disturbances in man.

Antimicrobial action of penicillin. When, in 1941, Chain re-investigated penicillin, first studied by Fleming in 1929, he considered his study to be of purely scientific interest; he had no thought of developing an antimicrobial drug for clinical use. As Chain put it in 1971, "a substance of the degree of instability which penicillin seemed to possess according to the published facts does not hold out much promise for practical application. If my working hypothesis had been correct and penicillin had been a protein, its practical use as a chemotherapeutic agent would have been out of the question because of anaphylactic phenomena which inevitably would have followed its repeated use" (3d).

Heparin, a naturally occurring anticoagulant. When McLean, a medical student working in the physiologic laboratory at Johns Hopkins Medical School, discovered heparin he was working on a basic problem (assigned to him by Professor Howell) on the biochemistry of factors favoring coagulation of blood; neither he nor Howell had an anticoagulant in mind (3d). Professor Howell continued McLean's work and, in 1916–18 (4, 5) speculated that hemophilia might be due to abnormal amounts of heparin circulating in blood, but even then he did not suggest that heparin might be used clinically.

Who was the clinician who decided that it was important to purify and concentrate heparin for clinical work? There was none. The decision to purify it came from a physiologist. Best (a co-discoverer of insulin in 1922) relates that in 1926, when he was working with Sir Henry Dale in London on problems related to histamine, he had more than his share of problems with blood that clotted in his pressure recording system. The crude heparin available then was practically useless and Best determined that on his return to Toronto he would organize a group to purify heparin (Best, C. H.: Personal communication, Nov. 23, 1972). He did, and in 1933 Charles and Scott reported that, "because of the importance of heparin in certain physiological experiments," they had tackled the problem of making heparin useful for biologic work (6). They succeeded and soon John Gibbon was using it in his physiologic experiments on the artificial heart-lung and Murray was using it clinically to manage thrombosis. But neither those who discovered heparin or purified it had a clinical problem in mind. It seems that neither physicians nor the pharmaceutical industry in the 1920s or 1930s saw a need to purify it for clinical use, just as no one earlier saw a need to purify hirudin, an anticoagulant that Abel, Rowntree, and Turner extracted from medicinal leeches (obtained from French cupping barbers) to prevent blood coagulation in their 1914 artificial kidney (7).

Cardiac catheterization. I have already mentioned (1) that when Cournand and Richards performed their first cardiac catheterizations in man, it was not to develop a new method for diagnosing or evaluating congenital or acquired heart disease. They were then pulmonary physiologists who wanted to learn more about a basic physiologic problem about how blood and air were distributed to air sacs in the lungs. To do that, they needed to know the oxygen content of mixed blood in the right atrium and the only way to get such blood was to catheterize the human heart. Soon thereafter they used their new technique to study patients with shock and congestive heart failure, as did McMichael and Sharpey-Schafer in England. And a few years later, Bing in Baltimore, Dexter in Boston, and Warren in Atlanta began to use the cardiac catheter to diagnose specific defects in patients with congenital cardiac disease.

Recently, Cournand has written about the first cardiac catheterization in animals (8), which he attributes to Claude Bernard, the famous French physiologist. Bernard wanted to settle a then-controversial matter: Was animal heat produced in the lungs by the chemical reactions involving exchange of O_2 and CO_2 (as Lavoisier maintained) or was it produced by combustion occurring in all tissues of the body (as Magnus maintained)? Bernard decided to learn whether the temperature of left ventricular blood (that had just passed through the lungs) was greater than that of right ventricular blood. In 1844, he passed a long mercury thermometer down a carotid artery of a horse into its left ventricle and one down the jugular vein into the right ventricle and settled the mat-

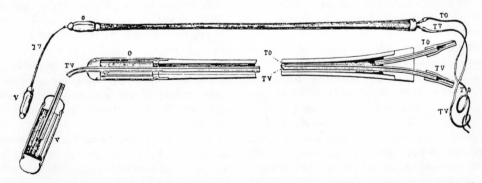

Fig. 1. Chauveau and Marey's double-lumen tube for cardiac catheterization and measurement of intracardiac pressures in dogs (1861). (*Top*) Complete instrument. (*Bottom*) Enlarged drawings of three sections of it (10).

ter in favor of Magnus (9). In 1847, Bernard passed a glass tube through the right jugular vein of a dog and measured right ventricular pressure.

Most physiologists credit Chauveau and Marey with being the first (in 1861) to use cardiac catheterization in animals to measure intracardiac pressures (10); certainly they were the first to make systematic and continuous measurements of atrial and ventricular pressures and were the first to design and use a double-lumen catheter for simultaneous recordings from two intracardiac locations (figure 1).

None of this research, from Bernard to Chauveau and Marey to Cournand and Richards, was clinically oriented; it was all done to solve basic physiologic problems.

Some additional key discoveries that were not clinically oriented were:

Flow-directed cardiac catheter. The "Swan-Ganz catheter" (11), now widely used in the management of acutely ill cardiac patients, is usually listed as a clinically oriented venture, although the investigators credit Lategola and Rahn (12) with the development and use of a quite similar catheter 17 years earlier. Lategola and Rahn were pulmonary physiologists interested in solving physiologic problems in dogs. Since the title of their 1953 paper, "A self-guiding catheter for cardiac and pulmonary arterial catheterization and occlusion" didn't mention dogs, it should have brought cardiologists to their laboratory in droves—but no one applied it clinically until 1970.

Bronchospirometer. While discussing catheters, let us not forget that Henry Head in 1889 (13) devised a double-lumen tube for separating gas entering and leaving the right lung from that ventilating the left lung (figure 2). He was a physiologist who worked on animals. His work was not oriented toward the diagnosis of clinical problems, although his apparatus was later widely used for several decades in determining differential lung function.

Direct measurement of arterial blood pressure. Although the indirect (Riva-Rocci) method of estimating arterial blood pressure in man is by far the most widely used in clinical medicine (and the apparatus for making indirect measurements is now a standard item in drugstores and mail order catalogs), direct measurement is routine in intensive care units and many operating rooms. The first direct measurement was made in 1733 by an English clergyman, Stephen Hales. He used a 9-foot-long glass tube

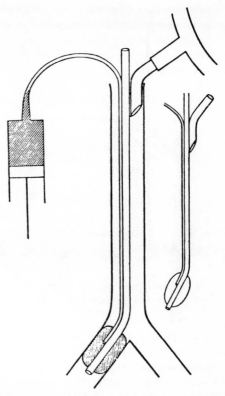

Fig. 2. Head's double-lumen tube with inflated balloon for separating gas flow into and out of the right and left lungs of a dog (1889) (13).

attached by a brass connection to a flexible windpipe of a goose and measured blood pressure in the femoral and carotid arteries of horses (14). Why did he do it? In his dedication "to the King's Most Excellent Majesty," Hales wrote:

> As the beautiful fabric of this world was chiefly framed for and adapted to the use of man, so the greater insight we get into the nature and properties of things, so much the more beneficial will they be to us, the more will our real riches thereby increase, the more also will man's original grant of dominion over the creatures be enlarged. [This must have been one of the earliest statements on cost:benefit analysis of pure research.]

In brief, Hales was curious about nature. Earlier, he had been intrigued by the fact that sap rises to the very top of even tall trees and he made measurements of sap pressure at various distances from the ground (15). I suppose a logical next step was to measure how high the sap that circulated in the tubes of animals would rise. Hypertension was not yet recognized as a disease in Hales's time, and attaching a 9-foot glass tube to a man's carotid artery was not a

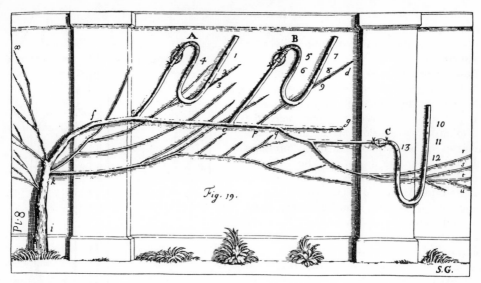

Fig. 3. U-tubes used by Stephen Hales in 1727 to measure the sap pressure in trees (15); this preceded and led to his measurement of arterial blood pressure in horses in 1733 (14).

very attractive way of beginning an inquiry into blood pressure in man—so Hales's discovery was surely not clinically oriented.

Poiseuille, in 1828, made Hales's 9-foot tube practical by using a U-tube filled with mercury (to reduce the height of the apparatus by a factor of 13.6). Why did Poiseuille want to measure blood pressure? Because physiologists (except for Poiseuille) believed that arterial blood pressure fell linearly from the beginning of the aorta to the smallest arteriole. Poiseuille, using his new manometer, made precise measurements from the ascending aorta down to the finest branch that he could cannulate; he proved that there was little decrease in pressure between the beginning and end of the arterial system and that the main drop (and therefore greatest resistance to flow) was in small arterioles (16). He then went on to his classic study of the flow of liquids through small tubes, now summarized in Poiseuille's law (17). Clinically oriented? No, actual measurements of blood pressure in man (as opposed to estimation of "hardness" of the pulse) waited until the end of his century.

Incidentally, Poiseuille didn't invent the U-tube. Hales's 1727 volume (*Vegetable Staticks*) shows U-tubes at various locations in trees, measuring sap pressure (figure 3) (15).

Strain gauge. This is now the standard transducer used to translate intra-arterial blood pressure into continuous, visible records.

Neither Tomlinson, nor Lambert and Wood almost a century later, devised the strain wire or gauge to solve a clinical problem. Tomlinson, who in 1876 recorded in the *Proceedings of the Royal Society of London* that "the temporary increase per centimeter of resistance of a wire when stretched in the same direction as the line of flow of the current is exactly proportional to the stretching force" (18), was then a Demonstrator in Natural Philosophy at King's College, London, and pretty far removed from clinical medicine. Lambert and Wood (19), who in 1947 first reported the use of strain wires to measure intra-arterial blood pressure, were not clinically motivated. As part of the war effort, they had built a human centrifuge at the Mayo Foundation and were measuring the response of man's cardiovascular system to increased gravitational forces. Because Lambert and Wood had to record at a distance from the subject, they could not use the Hamilton manometer because it had to be rigidly fixed close to its recording apparatus. This meant that they had to translate blood pressure into electrical signals and send these over wires to the central pole of the centrifuge and then to another room. The answer was the strain gauge manometer.

References

1. Comroe, J. H., Jr., and Dripps, R. D.: Ben Franklin and open heart surgery, Circ Res, 1974,

35, 661–669.

2. Comroe, J. H., Jr., and Dripps, R. D.: Scientific basis for the support of biomedical science, Science, 1976, *192*, 105-111.

3. This volume:
   a. The inside story, pp. 7-11.
   b. Feet on the ground?, pp. 24-26.
   c. Lags, pp. 106-109.
   d. Tell it like it was, pp. 89-98.
   e. Harnessing carbon monoxide, pp. 27-30.
   f. EITHER-OR? (Why not both?), pp. 31-34.

4. Howell, W. H.: The coagulation of blood, Harvey Lect, Series XII, 1916–1917, pp. 272–323.

5. Howell, W. H., and Holt, E.: Two new factors in blood coagulation—Heparin and pro-antithrombin, Am J Physiol, 1918, *47*, 328–341.

6. Charles, A. F., and Scott, D. A.: Studies on heparin, J Biol Chem, 1933, *102*, 425–448.

7. Abel, J. J., Rowntree, L. G., and Turner, B. B.: On the removal of diffusible substances from the circulating blood of living animals by dialysis, J Pharmacol Exp Ther, 1913, *5*, 275–316.

8. Cournand, A.: Cardiac catheterization. Development of the technique, its contributions to clinical medicine and its initial applications in man, Acta Med Scand [Suppl], 1975, *579*, 1-32.

9. Bernard, C.: Leçons sur la Chaleur Animale, Baillière, Paris, 1876, pp. 42, 78, 80, 81.

10. Chauveau, A., and Marey, J.: Détermination graphique des rapports du choc du coeur avec les mouvements des oreillettes et des ventricles; expérience faite à l'aide d'un appareil enregistreur (sphygmographe), C R Acad Sci (Paris), 1861, *53*, 622–625.

11. Swan, H. J. C., Ganz, W., Forrester, J., Marcus, H., Diamond, G., and Chonette, D.: Catheterization of the heart in man with use of a flow-directed balloon-tipped catheter, N Engl J Med, 1970, *283*, 447–451.

12. Lategola, M., and Rahn, H.: A self-guiding catheter for cardiac and pulmonary arterial catheterization and occlusion, Proc Soc Exp Biol Med, 1953, *84*, 667–668.

13. Head, H.: On the regulation of respiration, J Physiol, 1889, *10*, 1–70.

14. Hales, S.: Statical Essays: Containing Haemastaticks, vol. 2, Innys and Manby, London, 1733, 361 pp.

15. Hales, S.: Vegetable Staticks, Innys and Woodward, London, 1727, 376 pp.

16. Poiseuille, J. L. M.: Recherches sur la Force du Coeur Aortique, Thèse No. 166, Didot, Paris, 1828.

17. Poiseuille, J. L. M.: Recherches expérimentales sur le mouvement des liquides dans les tubes de très petits diamètres, C R Acad Sci (Paris), 1840, *11*, 961–967, 1041–1048.

18. Tomlinson, H.: On the increase in resistance to the passage of an electric current produced on wires by stretching, Proc R Soc Lond, 1876, *25*, 451–453.

19. Lambert, E. H., and Wood, E. H.: The use of a resistance wire, strain gauge manometer to measure intraarterial pressure, Proc Soc Exp Biol Med, 1947, *64*, 186–190.

Whodunit (And Why)

Part II

In Part I of "Whodunit," I asked a question, whose answer is critical to a national biomedical science policy, "How many of these key studies [crucial to clinical advances in cardiovascular and pulmonary medicine and surgery] were done to solve a specific clinical problem related to the prevention, diagnosis or treatment of a specific [human] disease; how many were done simply to learn something, completely unrelated to clinical medicine or surgery or to the genesis or course of a disease?" And because the number of such studies was very large (41% of all key articles), I believed it important to list some of these for you. Part II continues this annotated list.

Blood pumps. Everyone knows that a pump is an essential component of a heart-lung machine. Galletti and Brecher (20) devote three chapters of their *Heart-Lung Bypass* to pumps. One of the early blood pumps was the roller pump that DeBakey used in 1934 for transfusing blood—obviously a clinically oriented effort (21). However, two years before DeBakey, Van Allen described a similar pump in *JAMA* and even then disclaimed any originality for his device (22). And four years before Van Allen, two English physiologists, Bayliss and Müller, described the same roller pump, which they turned over to C. F. Palmer, Ltd., for manufacture (23). Bayliss was a cardiovascular physiologist who used his pump for laboratory experiments and not for transfusions in man. Curiously, there are no references in any of these three papers to the earlier papers in the series or to Issekutz, who used a roller pump to perfuse the liver of animals in 1927, or to Kelly, who received U.S. Patent 314851 for one in 1885!

The Potts clamp for aorta-pulmonary artery anastomosis. In the early days of the Blalock-Taussig "blue baby" operation, which created an end-to-side shunt between a branch of the aorta (such as the subclavian) and the right or left pulmonary artery, Potts devised a clamp that permitted direct side-to-side anastomosis between the aorta and pulmonary artery without sacrificing a subclavian artery. The key to the Potts operation was permitting blood flow to continue through both vessels while they were being joined; this required devising a new clamp that closed one side of the aorta (where the anastomosis was to be performed) but left an open channel for blood flow through the other side (24). Definitely a clinically oriented effort, to solve a specific surgical problem. But in the same journal (*JAMA*), only 36 years earlier, one of America's leading physiologists, G. N. Stewart (of indicator-dilution fame) described the same device "to clamp off temporarily a longitudinal portion at one side of a blood vessel while the circulation is allowed to go on through the remainder of the lumen" (25) (figure 4). Although he was a physiologist and devised the clamp for physiologic experiments (such as partial occlusion of an artery), he speculated on its possible clinical uses such as using it during lateral anastomoses of blood vessels when it is undesirable to occlude completely either vessel (the 1946 Potts operation, see page 100). Photographs of Stewart's clamp appeared in the two leading texts of experimental surgery of that era: Guthrie's in English in 1912 (26) and Jeger's in German in 1913 (27). A recurring phenomenon in many papers recording the great cardiovascular surgical triumphs of the 1940s and 1950s was the failure to mention previous work in the field. Was this piracy, or disinclination to use the library? And which was worse?

Preservation of blood and tissues. Carrel preserved arteries and veins for future use as grafts in his experimental work in 1912 (28). In 1919 Guthrie preserved vessels in formaldehyde and found that they served as scaffolding for the ingrowth of a new lining (29). Rous and Turner developed a method for preserving red blood cells in 1916 (30), although preserved blood appears not to have found its way to World War I battlefields in 1917 or 1918; for the most part, physicians used 6 per cent gum arabic in 0.9 per cent sodium chloride.

A fascinating discovery of the early 1900s was freeze drying of tissues by Shackell (31) while he was a chemist working in the Missouri Agricultural Experiment Station. His initial goal was to develop a quick and precise method to measure water content of various materials such as soil, cornchop, feces, milk, honey, levulose, butter, cheese, vinegar, and soap. This he accomplished by an improved method of vacuum desiccation. He then turned his attention to measuring the concentration of liver glycogen and found his values varied from day to day because of rapid postmortem hydrolysis of glycogen. How could he maintain premortem concentrations while drying tissue post mortem? The answer was to freeze the liver first and then subject it to vacuum desiccation.

Shackell then moved from the Agricultural Station to the Department of Physiology of the University of Missouri's School of Medicine and soon realized that his freeze-dry method had medical applications. He found that complement was preserved in freeze-dried guinea pig serum, that the coagulation factors remained intact in freeze-dried dog's blood, and that the fixed virus of rabies survived freeze-drying of rabbit brains.

In 1935, Elser, Thomas and Steffen (32) improved on Shackell's technique and used it to preserve antisera and antigens. During World War II, Flosdorf and associates first freeze-dried human plasma on a large scale and then did the same for penicillin (33, 34); thus, they solved the two urgent problems of how to store plasma for wartime needs and how to preserve penicillin, notoriously unstable in solution. Since then, freeze drying has had many medical applications and even more industrial uses (e.g., the burgeoning business of freeze-dried coffee).

Cathode ray oscilloscope. This is now standard equipment in intensive care units for monitoring blood pressure, the electrocardiogram and electroencephalogram, end-tidal CO_2 tension, and other cardiovascular and respiratory variables. The original "cathode ray indicator tube" was devised in 1897 by Braun for

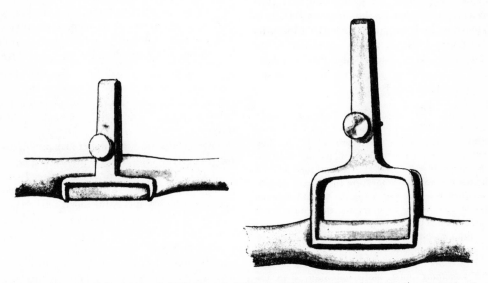

Fig. 4. Two clamps devised by G. N. Stewart in 1910 to occlude part of an artery (to be operated on) while blood flow continued through an open channel (26, 27).

the visual study of oscillatory and transient phenomena in electric circuits; for this achievement, Braun received the 1909 Nobel Prize in Physics (jointly with Marconi). The first biologic use of the cathode ray oscilloscope was in the field of basic neurophysiology. Gasser and Erlanger (35) were trying to record the true form of the action potential in nerve fibers but found that the string galvanometer was too sluggish. They needed an inertia-free system and found it in 1922 in Western Electric's modified Braun tube; this was a gas-focused cathode ray tube that operated on low voltages with simple auxiliary circuits. The Western Electric Company refused to sell their tube to Gasser and Erlanger, presumably because the company feared the possibility of infringement of its patents. So the neurophysiologists simply made their own using a distillation flask (36). The cathode ray oscilloscope became indispensible in neurophysiologic studies, came into widespread laboratory use as a monitoring device, and eventually "went clinical."

Blood oxygen tension. The name of Leland Clark is rightly associated with the development of the oxygen electrode, but several important basic investigations preceded his work. One was Danneel's finding in 1897 that, during the electrolysis of water using platinum electrodes, there was an approximate proportionality between the current and the concentration of dissolved O_2 when the e.m.f. applied was 0.02 volt. Another came 25 years later, when Professor Kučera at Prague suggested to his young associate, Jaroslav Heyrovský, that he should study certain irregularities in connection with the capillarity of mercury. This led to the invention of the polarograph (37) and to a Nobel Prize in Chemistry. In presenting the Prize to Heyrovsky, Professor Ölander said:

This [the study of irregularities in the capillarity of mercury] was one of the innumerable small problems constituting science. Heyrovský let the mercury flow through a glass capillary and weighed the drops. It was a slow and tedious method, and he resolved instead to measure the electric current obtained when he put a tension [e.m.f.] between the mercury in the capillary and that collecting at the bottom. The glass capillary does not terminate in the air, but in a solution, through which the current now will flow.

Heyrovský found that this device could be used for something much more important than the original problem. It could be used for ascertaining very small quantities of the most diverse substances dissolved in the water, and moreover, to measure their percentages.

Important new discoveries are found where they are not expected.... Discoveries are made by some scientist who noticed something strange, possibly by two [scientists], independently and in different countries. Then it is important that future team leaders and authorities granting funds do not keep him too strictly to attend his job, but give him a chance to pick up the unexpected new things, in spite of the chance of finding them being diminutive (38).

The polarograph could measure, among other things, the concentration of oxygen dissolved in liquids and it stimulated interest in measurement of oxygen tension in tissues. The first use of the platinum electrode to measure oxygen tension in animal tissues appears to be that of Davies and Brink (39). Clinically oriented? No, Davies and Brink were biophysicists interested in measuring the oxygen consumption of resting and active nerve tissue. When they placed nerve tissue in a small, saline-filled, closed chamber, they could run saline slowly through the chamber and measure the oxygen tension in the inflowing and outflowing fluid; from these values, they calculated the oxygen removed by tissue. They also used a platinum electrode to measure the oxygen tension of the surface of the brain. However, during research in aviation physiology, they decided to put a platinum electrode in the plunger of a syringe and measure the oxygen tension of blood. They ran into the problem that whole blood "poisoned" the bare tip of the wire; to protect the tip they covered it with a collodion membrane that allowed oxygen, but not blood or plasma, to diffuse to the platinum electrode (see their "Note added in proof," p. 533 [39]). In 1950 Brink, no longer working on blood oxygen electrodes, noted that the time was ripe for someone to develop a practical method for measuring blood oxygen tension *in situ*. And he added, "those interested must decide whether such [an intensive program of] development is justified" (40).

In 1953, Clark decided. He had already made a major contribution to open-heart surgery by devising a highly successful blood oxygenator — one that didn't convert blood into foam. But, to know how effective the gas exchanger was, he needed to know continuously the oxygen tension of blood after passage through the oxygenator, and for this he had to develop the oxygen electrode and make it dependable and accurate (41).

Chromatography. One of the most powerful and versatile analytic methods used in clinical medicine is chromatography. But its first use was in pure science. Michael Tswett, a Russian botanist, devised it as a way to separate and identify the constituents of green leaves; he extracted them with petrol ether and poured the mixture over a vertical column of calcium carbonate. The main constituents, in this case pigments (green chlorophyll and yellow carotenoids), migrated at different rates and separated as distinct color bands; hence the term chromatogram. In 1906, Tswett wrote:

Like light rays in the spectrum, so the different components of a pigment mixture are resolved on the calcium carbonate column according to a law and can be estimated on it qualitatively and also quantitatively. Such a preparation I term a chromatogram and the corresponding method, the chromatographic method.

It is self-evident that the adsorption phenomena described are not restricted to the chlorophyll pigments, and one must assume that all kinds of colored and colorless chemical compounds are subject to the same laws. I have so far investigated lecithin, alkannin, prodigiosin, sudan, cyanin, solanorubin, and acid derivatives of the chlorophyllins with positive success (42).

The term chromatogram is no longer wholly appropriate because it is used to separate colorless compounds (as Tswett predicted) and gases, but it is useful to remind us of its origin—the study of the pigments in green leaves.

Beta receptors. From our knowledge of β-receptors (properly termed β-adrenoreceptors) have come many clinically useful drugs, those that stimulate (e.g., isoproterenol) and those that block (e.g., propranolol) these receptors. How did the idea of β-receptors come about? First there had to be the notion that drugs acted on specific parts of a cell (receptor substances) and not on the cell as a whole. Then there had to be the concept and experimental proof of humoral transmission of nerve impulses, that nerve impulses did not leap as sparks from preganglionic fibers to ganglion cells or from postganglionic fibers to muscle or glands, but continued across anatomic gaps by liberation of highly specific chemical substances (acetylcholine or norepinephrine), formed locally within nerve endings. Walter Cannon was pretty sure in 1937 that epinephrine came in two forms, E for excitatory and I for inhibitory; the evidence was based in part on the effect of blocking agents. For example, Dale knew in 1906 that ergotoxine blocked

some of the actions of epinephrine but left others intact; ergotoxine not only blocked the characteristic increase in blood pressure from an injection of epinephrine, but reversed it (epinephrine, given after ergotoxine, actually lowered blood pressure).

In 1948, Ahlquist realized that the classification of epinephrine effects into excitatory and inhibitory was holding up progress in this field (43). After all, norepinephrine was "excitatory" because it constricted smooth muscle of systemic arterioles, but it also inhibited smooth muscle in the gut; isoproterenol was "inhibitory" because it dilated blood vessels and bronchioles, but it also excited the heart. He therefore proposed that there were two types of adrenoreceptors—alpha and beta—and that drugs be classified on the basis of whether they stimulated or blocked α- or β-receptors (exclusively, strongly, weakly, or not at all). Dibenamine (never useful clinically) served to block β-receptors and dichloro-isoproterenol (also never useful clinically) served to block β-receptors. The stage was now set for a meaningful and systematic search for highly specific stimulant and blocking agents and soon important new drugs were synthesized (e.g., propranolol).

To date, six scientists who have worked in this field have received Nobel Prizes: Dale and Loewi in 1936, Katz, von Euler, and Axelrod in 1970, and Sutherland in 1971, all for basic research that eventually led to important advances in therapeutics.

Dicumarol. The story of the first oral anticoagulant began in 1922 when Schofield reported on a new disease that occurred exclusively in cattle fed on mouldy sweet clover hay, and was characterized by subcutaneous swellings caused by hemorrhages, followed by sudden death. In all cases there was acute anemia and a greatly diminished amount of plasma prothrombin (44). Schofield established that the disease was not due to microorganisms that cause hemorrhagic septicemia (he could find none), that it was not due to poor nutrition (all of the cattle were well fed), and that it must be due to something in sweet clover that became mouldy during storage in silos because the disease vanished when the cattle munched on other fodder instead.

The next chapter in the story was by Roderick of the North Dakota Agricultural Experiment Station. He confirmed that the disease was associated with progressive decrease in plasma prothrombin but found no pathologic evidence of serious liver damage (understandable now that we know that the hepatic lesion is a specific one limited to prothrombin formation) (45).

In 1940-41, Campbell and Link (46), also working in an Agricultural Experimental Station, in Wisconsin, decided to extract and concentrate material from spoiled sweet clover hay; they soon isolated dicumarol in a pure state ($C_{19}H_{12}O_6$). From this point on, dicumarol moved in two directions: (1) One of its congeners, warfarin, was used deliberately to kill animals—this time rodents instead of cattle—but by the same mechanism (decrease in prothrombin concentration, spontaneous hemorrhages, and death); it had a huge market as a rodenticide. (The name "warfarin" was not derived from "warfare on rats" but from Wisconsin Alumni Research Foundation, which received profits from the patents.) (2)As dicumarol, it entered clinical medicine after some of Link's biochemists tried it out on themselves and concluded that "in view of the prothrombin-reducing or inactivating properties of this dicoumarin, the spread between the detectable and lethal dose, together with the relative ease with which it may be prepared and administered, it would appear that its anticoagulant properties merit consideration by the physiologist and hematologist."

Para-aminosalicylic acid (PAS) therapy of pulmonary tuberculosis. In 1940, Bernheim wrote a note to *Science* on the metabolism of tubercle bacilli (47). These bacilli, when placed in the Warburg apparatus, did not readily oxidize substances such as carbohydrates, amino acids, or hydroxy acids, but Bernheim found that when he fed them sodium salicylate, their uptake of O_2 more than doubled. Because the increase in O_2 uptake was proportional to the concentration of salicylate, Bernheim suggested that the bacilli oxidized salicylate as a substrate and that possibly it was one of their normal foods.

This observation might have gone unnoticed except that in 1931 Quastel and Wheatley (48) had discovered the principle of "competitive inhibition" when they demonstrated that malonic acid inhibited the oxidation of succinic acid by bacteria, brain and muscle, and in 1940 Woods (49) had applied this principle to explain the antibacterial action of sulfanilamide (that para-aminobenzene-sulfonamide competed with an essential bacterial metabolite, para-aminobenzoic acid, and so prevented growth of streptococci.) Because salicylate is ortho-hydroxybenzoate, Bernheim's observation, coupled with

Wood's findings, might be important for tubercle bacilli.

In 1946, Lehmann followed up Bernheim's work but found no increase in oxygen consumption when salicylates were added to tubercle bacilli. Lehmann might have given up at this point but suddenly realized that he had been using nonpathogenic tubercle bacilli and Bernheim had worked with pathogenic strains. Lehmann then found an essential metabolic difference between pathogenic and nonpathogenic tubercle bacilli: The former showed a positive salicylate effect, the latter did not (50). Lehmann stated, "the differences found seem to open up new pathways for studying the pathogenicity of the tubercle bacillus." He really meant *old* pathways because he went the competitive-inhibition route of Quastel and Wheatley (48) and Woods (49); he studied more than 50 derivatives of salicylates to learn which might inhibit growth of tubercle bacilli, presumably by fooling the bacilli to accept it instead of salicylate and so slowing or halting bacterial growth. He found PAS to be the most effective inhibitor; so began chemotherapy for tuberculosis.

ANECDOTES?

In this two-part Retrospectroscope I've related how 42 discoveries that had no relevance to clinical medicine at the time they were made have been important, or essential, to 24 important advances in clinical medicine and surgery. Some of the nonclinically oriented discoveries have come from physics, chemistry, botany, agriculture, microbiology, physiology, pharmacology, and biochemistry; some have been made by a research surgeon, a veterinarian, a photographer, even by a clergyman. Some have led to important new diagnostic tests, some to whole new fields of surgery, some to new drugs, including chemotherapeutic agents.

At the beginning of Part 1, I said that our analysis of 529 key articles showed that 41 per cent (217) reported work that, at the time it was done, had no relation whatever to the disease it later helped to prevent, diagnose, treat, or alleviate. I also said that it was time for scientists to stop the anecdotal, "let-me-give-you-an-example" approach to influencing national biomedical science policy. By recounting for you only 42 of the 217 key articles classified as "*not* clinically oriented," have I slipped into the anecdotage that I have criticized in others? I think not; 42 examples, coming from diverse fields, should be enough to convince you of the importance of supporting nondirected research (research not clinically oriented).

Other matters of course deserve "equal time," such as the role of purely clinical observations, of engineering, and of development in advancing medicine and surgery—and learning how often clinical observations led to important new research in basic science that in turn led to new clinical advances.

References

20. Galletti, P. M., and Brecher, G. A.: Heart-Lung Bypass, Grune and Stratton, New York, 1962.
21. DeBakey, M.: A continuous-flow blood transfusion instrument, New Orleans Med Surg J, 1934–1935, 87, 386-389.
22. Van Allen, C. M.: A pump for clinical and laboratory purposes which employs the milking principle, JAMA, 1932, 98, 1805-1806.
23. Bayliss, L. E., and Müller, E. A.: A simple, high-speed rotary pump, J Sci Instrum, 1928, 5, 278-279.
24. Potts, W. J., Smith, S., and Gibson, S.: Anastomosis of the aorta to a pulmonary artery, JAMA, 1946, 132, 627-631.
25. Stewart, G. N.: A clamp for isolating a portion of the lumen of a blood vessel without stopping the circulation through the vessel, JAMA, 1910, 55, 647-649.
26. Guthrie, C. C.: Blood Vessel Surgery and Its Application, Arnold, London, 1912, p. 68.
27. Jeger, E.: Die Chirurgie der Blutgefasse und des Herzens, Hirschwald, Berlin, 1913, p. 69.
28. Carrel, A.: The preservation of tissues and its applications in surgery, JAMA, 1912, 59, 523-527.
29. Guthrie, C. C.: End-results of arterial restitution with devitalized tissue, JAMA, 1919, 73, 186-187.
30. Rous, P., and Turner, J. P.: The preservation of living red blood cells in vitro. I. Methods of preservation, J Exp Med, 1916, 23, 219-237.
31. Shackell, L. F.: An improved method of desiccation, with some applications to biological problems, Am J Physiol, 1909, 24, 325-340.
32. Elser, W. J., Thomas, R. A., and Steffen, G. I.: The desiccation of sera and other biological products (including microorganisms) in the frozen state with the preservation of the original qualities of products so treated, J Immunol, 1935, 28, 433-473.
33. Flosdorf, E. W., Stokes, F. J., and Mudd, S.: The desivac process for drying from the frozen state, JAMA, 1940, 115, 1095-1097.
34. Flosdorf, E. W.: Drying penicillin by sublimation in the United States and Canada, Br Med J, 1945, 1, 216-218.
35. Gasser, H. S., and Erlanger, J.: A study of the action currents of nerve with the cathode ray oscilloscope, Am J Physiology, 1922, 59, 496-524.
36. Erlanger, J.: A physiologist reminisces, Annu Rev Physiol, 1961, 26, 1-14.
37. Heyrovský, J.: Elektrolysa so rtutovou kapkovou katkodou, Chem Listy, 1922, 16, 256-264.
38. Ölander, A.: Presentation speech (Nobel Prize in Chemistry, 1959, to J. Heyrovský), in Nobel Lectures, Chemistry, 1942-1962, Elsevier, Amsterdam, 1964, pp. 561-563.
39. Davies, P. W., and Brink, F.: Microelectrodes for measuring local oxygen tension in animal tissues, Rev Sci Instrum, 1942, 13, 524-533.
40. Brink, F., Jr.: Comment (pp. 175–177), in Brown, L. M., and Comroe, J. H., Jr.: Blood pO_2 derived from measurements of O_2 physically dissolved in blood, Methods Med Res, 1950, 2, 169-178.
41. Clark, C., Wolf, R., Granger, D., and Taylor, Z.: Continuous recording of blood oxygen tensions by polarography, J Appl Physiol, 1953, 6, 189-193.
42. Zechmeister, L.: History, scope and methods of chromatography, Ann NY Acad Sci, 1948, 49, 145-160.
43. Ahlquist, R. P.: A study of the adrenotropic receptors, Am J Physiol, 1948, 153, 586-600.
44. Schofield, F. W.: A brief account of a disease in cattle simulating hemorrhagic septicemia due to feeding sweet clover, Can Vet Rec, 1922, 3, 74-78.
45. Roderick, L. M.: The pathology of sweet clover disease in cattle, J Am Vet Med Assoc, 1929, 74, 314-325.
46. Campbell, H. A., and Link, K. P.: Studies on the hemorrhagic sweet clover disease. IV. The isolation and crystallization of the hemorrhagic agent, J Biol Chem, 1941, 138, 21-33.
47. Bernheim, F.: The effect of salicylate on the oxygen uptake of the tubercle bacillus, Science, 1940, 92, 204.
48. Quastel, J. H., and Wheatley, A. H. M.: XVI. Biological oxidations in the succinic acid series, Biochem J, 1931, 25, 1171-28.
49. Woods, D. D.: The relation of p-aminobenzoic acid to the mechanism of the action of sulphanilamide, Br J Exp Pathol, 1940, 21, 74-90.
50. Lehmann, J.: Determination of pathogenicity of tubercle bacilli by their intermediate metabolism, Lancet, 1946, 1, 14-15.

Feet on the Ground??

How a nation decides how much and what kind of biomedical research it wants to support is of great importance to the health of its people, because even the best physician cannot "deliver" new knowledge about prevention, early diagnosis, or cure until research has uncovered it. At present, "how much" research is mostly left up to Congress and "what kind" is left to specific granting agencies and their review panels, study sections, and advisory councils, who either approve or disapprove projects initiated by scientists, or sometimes propose programs of their own.

To the present array of reviewing bodies, Congress now proposes to add another: Congress. "The House of Representatives [in 1975] voted that Congress should have a veto power over all of the 14,000 grants which NSF awards each year. To accomplish this, NSF would have to submit a list of all proposed research grant awards to Congress every 30 days, as well as justifications for them. Either house could veto the award of any grant ... The provision would put Congress in the position of effectively approving research grants in every area of NSF support, from education to basic science" (1).

Why? It appears that one of the "fun games" for some Congressmen is scanning titles of approved research grants in the social and biomedical sciences and then holding up to public ridicule those that sound (to them) odd, esoteric, irrelevant, ludicrous, farcical, or absurd. The problem is that these Congressmen have not looked into the Retrospectroscope; perhaps they should, lest their public statements on what constitutes nonsensical research today form the basis for new "fun games" 10 to 20 years from now.

Let's look at a few research projects that would cause some Congressmen to roll in the aisles with laughter. A sure-fire one would have been a proposal in December 1895 if an American scientist had applied for government money to invent a machine to look at the insides of people. By 1895, science fiction writers had "invented" airplanes, submarines, and electric ray guns, and had even "created" a man reassem-

bled from assorted bits and pieces of cadavers—but none had been brash enough to conceive of a ray that would photograph bones and heart and lungs right through the skin. Yet late in December 1895, Wilhelm Roentgen in Würzberg accomplished just that. I suspect Congress would have been embarrassed when, having vetoed this absurd (hypothetical) proposal just before adjourning for the Christmas vacation in 1895, they picked up a newspaper on New Year's Day and read on the front page of a scientific discovery by a German physicist that swept the world and revolutionized the practice of medicine.

The "look-inside-people" proposal would have caused good-natured belly laughs. But if Eadweard Muybridge had applied for a grant in 1872, his proposal would have caused indignation and outrage at the waste of the public's money on a frivolous project, by someone who wasn't even a scientist and had no scientific degree and no laboratory. Here, in Muybridge's words, is what he wanted to do; these might have served as an introduction and justification for his project:

> In the spring of 1872 ... there was revived in the city of San Francisco a controversy in regard to animal locomotion ... the principal subject of dispute was the possibility of a horse, while trotting —even at the height of his speed—having all four of his feet, at any portion of his stride, simultaneously free from contact with the ground (2).

Muybridge resolved to settle the controversy. It occurred to him that a series of photographic images made in rapid succession at predetermined intervals of time would answer the question. There were no motion pictures in 1872 and most still photographs were made on glass plates prepared by the photographer. Muybridge set up several banks of 12 to 24 stereoscopic cameras arranged parallel to the track on which the horse would trot at a predicted speed. When the horse reached position 1, which was opposite camera 1, Muybridge pressed a button that clicked the shutter of camera 1 and, by a "programmed" electric motor with 11 or 23 additional contacts, exposed successively, at the proper time, the photographic plates of cameras # 2 to # 12 or # 2 to # 24. A result is shown in Figure 1 for 6 consecutive plates. Muybridge then mounted his glass plates on discs; when he rotated these, he had a very satisfactory reproduction of a miniature horse trotting along. (By mounting plates made by his stereoscopic cameras on 2 discs and rotating them at equal speeds, he could also produce 3-dimensional effects.) These apparently were the first motion pictures and, even if you don't believe that motion pictures produced in Hollywood or television studios represent an advance in civilization, motion pictures *have* been an invaluable tool in medicine and biology.

If Muybridge had written a grant application to NSF in 1872, some Congressmen would have vetoed it as frivolous. Fortunately, Leland Stanford provided an out-of-doors laboratory for Muybridge at his Palo Alto farm and later Provost William Pepper, along with trustees and friends of the University of Pennsylvania, raised funds for Muybridge to continue and publish his work on man, land animals, and birds in motion. In 1882, a French physiologist, Marey, improved Muybridge's multiple camera system by using a single camera, a strip of photographic film, and a succession of moving figures; in 1893 Edison used a moving strip and a lantern for projection, patented these, and became known as the "inventor" of motion pictures.

In 1936, J. Z. Young, if he had been an American and there had been an NSF or NIH,

might well have submitted a proposal to study nerve fibers in cephalopods, particularly in *Loligo* or squid (3). Since this is a creature that can suddenly move backward by jet propulsion of an ink-like material, some Congressmen could have had a field day likening scientists to squids—continuously moving backward while emitting large quantities of ink—and vetoed the project as irrelevant and ludicrous. In 1936, the justification written for Congress would not have predicted the impact of Young's study.

Because the squid contains giant nerve fibers up to 1 mm in diameter—50 to 1,000 times thicker than nerve fibers previously available for study—it permitted two crucial experiments: (*1*) one or more fine wire electrodes could be placed inside the nerve tube to permit scientists to measure the difference in electrical potential between the inside of the fiber and its outer surface; (*2*) the contents of the giant axone could be squeezed out, much as one rolls toothpaste from its tube, and the contents of the nerve cell and the amount of each could be measured precisely. This led to a revolution in neurophysiology and to electrophysiology in general. Electrophysiology includes electrocardiography; soon a micropipette was devised with a tip so small (0.0005 mm or less in diameter) that it could be put in heart muscle and into cells in each part of its special conducting system. Much of what we now know about the genesis of serious cardiac arrhythmias and how to evaluate proposed therapy has come from measurement of cardiac transmembrane potentials.

The studies on squid axones also led to a

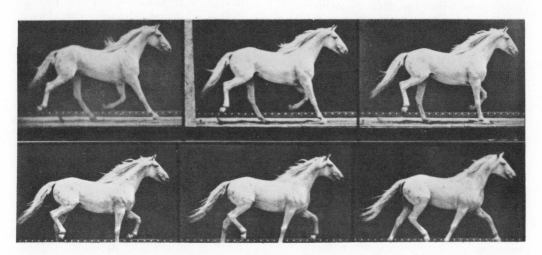

Fig. 1. Top three frames followed by bottom three frames are six consecutive photographs of a running horse, taken in rapid succession by Muybridge (2).

new science of active transport across cell membranes—how cells maintain quite different concentrations of salt inside compared to outside. Research on active transport has extended to many organ systems of the body; recently it has led to an understanding of the mechanism that causes secretion in the gastrointestinal tract and permits patients with cholera to lose huge, even fatal, amounts of intestinal fluid secretions.

I can give more examples of projects that would evoke rude sounds from some Congressmen: (a) On the causes of the torpidity of the tenrec. (b) The effect of chemical substances on the rate of beating of cilia in oyster gills. (c) Sex attractants for insects. (d) Mechanism by which a bat in utter darkness catches a tiny insect flying at top speed (4-7).

(a) provided proof that even an animal living in the tropics could be made to hibernate in its winter months by relatively small decreases in body temperature and paved the way for hypothermia of patients during cardiac surgery.

(b) may serve as a test for blood-borne substances that inhibit ciliary activity in patients, such as those with cystic fibrosis.

(c) may well enable control of specific insect pests in certain areas without creating problems of air, water, or soil pollution.

(d) demonstrated the ultrasonic echolocation mechanism by which bats, flying in pitch-black caves, can catch prey but avoid other obstacles. It could have been the lead to sonar and radar in World War II, but Griffin's studies (7) were independent of radar and were not published until 1940, when radar had just been put to military use. Griffin asks, "Had biologists understood a few decades earlier the methods by which bats orient themselves, might not the invention of radar and sonar have come sooner? Or might we not already be in a position to perfect acoustic means for self guidance for the blind? . . . Granted that in this case the engineers anticipated the biologists, one may speculate whether

this sequence is inevitable." I wonder how much Griffin's studies on echolocation in bats and birds hastened the development of the echocardiogram, a powerful new diagnostic tool in cardiology, developed in the 1950s.

I hope that scientists don't begin to submit research applications with phony titles just to escape Congressional scrutiny. Much good can come from Congress taking a serious look at approved research grants. For when members of Congress question titles that seem "irrelevant," they may learn much about the nature of scientific discovery, and this may lead them to formulate, at last, a sound national policy for basic biomedical research. And an imaginative T.V. producer might read the *Congressional Record* and find it fascinating to educate the general public with a spell-binding series on "The Usefulness of the Absurd."

Wishful thinking? Not necessarily—some "absolutely impossible" things have happened in science!

References

1. Shapley, D.: Congress: House votes veto power on all NSF research grants, Science, 1975, *188*, 338–341. [Later voted down by U.S. Senate]
2. Muybridge, E.: Animals in Motion, 1898, reprinted by Dover Publications, New York, 1957.
3. Young, J. Z.: Structure of nerve fibers and synapses in some invertebrates, Cold Spring Harbor Symp, 1936, *4*, 1–6.
4. Brown-Sequard, E.: On the causes of the torpidity of the tenrec, The Medical Examiner, 1852, *93*, 549–550.
5. Bowman, B. H., McCombs, M. L., and Lockhard, L. H.: Cystic fibrosis: Characterization of the inhibitor to ciliary action in oyster gills, Science, 1970, *167*, 871–873.
6. Jacobson, M., Beroza, M., and Jones, W. A.: Isolation, identification and synthesis of the sex attractant of gypsy moth, Science, 1960, *132*, 1011.
7. Griffin, D. R.: The navigation of bats, Sci Am, 1950, *183*, 52–55.

Harnessing Carbon Monoxide

The brief inhalation of low, nontoxic concentrations of carbon monoxide is now a standard procedure in pulmonary function laboratories to measure the rate of diffusion of gas across the alveolar-capillary membranes of ventilated, perfused alveoli, to estimate pulmonary capillary blood volume, and to provide an index of the area and thickness of the alveolar-capillary membranes and of the number of capillaries participating in gas exchange. Some now believe that a low DL_{CO} may be a very early sign of pulmonary emphysema; if so, the CO test may be used widely for early diagnosis of this disease.

Who first thought of using a toxic gas for the safe measurement of an important function of the lung—and why? How did the clinical test originate? The story is divided into two parts, separated by a period of 35 years. Part one began in the 1890's when Christian Bohr, the distinguished Danish physiologist, believed that oxygen passed from alveolar gas to pulmonary capillary blood by active secretion as well as by passive diffusion (1). And J. S. Haldane, Oxford's great respiratory physiologist, was equally convinced that lungs secreted oxygen. In 1897, Haldane and Smith (2) wrote:

In the animals investigated the normal oxygen tension in the arterial blood is always higher than in the alveolar air, and in some animals even much higher than in the inspired air. The absorption of oxygen by the lungs thus cannot be explained by diffusion alone.

August Krogh disagreed, even though Krogh had been a student of Bohr's and was Bohr's assistant from 1899 till 1908. In a series of experiments that required devising the Krogh spirometer, the Krogh microtonometer for measuring the tension of gases in arterial blood, and the Krogh bicycle ergometer, August and his wife, Marie Krogh, systematically disproved the theory of oxygen secretion. A. Krogh's 1910 experiments led him to the unqualified conclusion that "The absorption of oxygen and the elimination of carbon dioxide in the lungs takes place by diffusion and diffusion alone. There is no trustworthy evidence of any regulation of this process on the part of the organism" (3). But

Marie Krogh still believed it necessary to prove that diffusion alone was also sufficient to account for the *maximal* transfer of oxygen during severe muscular exercise and for the transfer of oxygen when alveolar Po_2 was low. This she did in her 1914 M.D. thesis, published in 1915 (4). She started with the assumption that "an essentially indifferent gas, like carbon monoxide, must pass through the alveolar epithelium by diffusion alone—an assumption which has never been questioned by anybody." She then improved her earlier technic (5) and described a single-breath test in which the subject first expired to residual air, then inspired deeply from a spirometer containing 1 per cent CO in air, then expired part way, held his breath for 6 seconds, and then completed the expiration. She sampled alveolar gas twice during the two-stage expiration (at the beginning and end of the breath-holding period) and measured the concentration of CO in each sample. From these and other measurements, she calculated the uptake of CO. It seems certain that Marie Krogh devised this first quantitative measurement of pulmonary diffusing capacity in man only to settle a controversy over a basic physiologic mechanism: does oxygen pass from alveolar gas to blood by secretion or only by diffusion? In her 1915 paper, she *did* measure diffusing capacity in 22 subjects and in 8 patients with asthma, emphysema, bronchitis, tuberculosis, or previous pneumonia, but apparently never used the test seriously for clinical diagnosis.

The Kroghs clearly showed that two great physiologists were wrong in their theory of O_2 secretion. But even so, each of the two played an important role in developing Marie Krogh's CO test (in addition to provoking her to devise the test to prove conclusively that they were wrong!); each provided tools and knowledge that M. Krogh needed. Haldane had done important work on CO, had determined that hemoglobin had a very high affinity for CO compared to O_2, and that CO (apart from combining with hemoglobin) was a physiologically indifferent gas that did not enter into chemical reactions with tissues and could move through tissues only by diffusion. And Haldane (with Priestley) had developed a technic to sample alveolar gas, and M. Krogh had to obtain and analyze alveolar gas to calculate the amount of CO transferred during the 6-second breath-holding period.

As for Bohr—Lilienthal and Riley (6) credit him with laying the foundation for all methods that measure pulmonary diffusing capacity, whether for O_2 or for CO. Gas diffuses from alveoli to blood in pulmonary capillaries only when the partial pressure of the gas is higher in alveolar gas than that in blood. And the magnitude of the *difference* determines the rate of diffusion of gas; therefore, the rate slows when the Po_2 or Pco in alveolar gas decreases or when the Po_2 or Pco of pulmonary capillary blood increases. Since diffusing capacity is defined as the amount of gas transferred each minute for a difference of one-millimeter mercury in partial pressure across the membranes, it is essential that the pressure difference be measured accurately. Bohr (7) had developed the principles for calculating the *mean* partial pressure of O_2 in pulmonary capillary blood (which is *not* the average of the Po_2 in pulmonary artery blood entering the capillary and of the Po_2 in pulmonary vein blood leaving the capillary); Bohr's "integration technic" later (1946) formed the basis for Lilienthal and Riley's O_2 method (8). But Bohr also recognized that, because of the remarkable affinity of hemoglobin for CO, measurable quantities of CO could leave alveolar gas and combine with hemoglobin in capillary blood and all the while plasma Pco remained so low that it did not significantly decrease the difference between Pco in alveolar gas and in plasma and hence did not hinder the inward diffusion of CO; this formed the basis for M. Krogh's CO method because it permitted her to calculate CO uptake, without the need to sample mixed venous blood (impossible in 1914), and to measure its Pco.

August Krogh, in his article that disproved pulmonary secretion of O_2 (3), paid this tribute to Bohr, a year before Bohr died in 1911:

I shall be obliged in the following pages to combat the views of my teacher Prof. Bohr on certain essential points and also to criticise a few of his experimental results. I wish here not only to acknowledge the debt of gratitude which I, personally, owe to him, but also to emphasize the fact, patent to everybody, who is familiar with the problems here discussed, that the real progress, made during the last twenty years in the knowledge of the processes in the lungs, is mainly due to his labours and to that refinement of methods, which he has introduced. The theory of the lung as a gland has justified its existence and done excellent service in bringing forward facts, which will survive any theoretical construction, which has been put or shall hereafter be put upon them.

Part two of this story began 35 years later. Except for a few isolated uses of Krogh's CO test by Barcroft (9) and Harrop and Heath (10), her method was essentially forgotten or unused until 1950. In that year, I was asked to be Editor of a "methods volume" on Pulmonary Function Tests (11). I designated one chapter "Gas-Blood Diffusion." Why, if Krogh's work had really been forgotten? Entirely because of a new approach by Lilienthal, Riley, and their associates at the Naval Air Station in Pensacola during World War II. In their work on aviation physiology, they had devised direct technics for measuring Po_2 and Pco_2 of blood and a new method for determining effective alveolar pressures of these gases. With these, they set out to determine whether an appreciable difference in Po_2 occurs between alveolar gas and arterial blood when man exercises at high altitude. From this research came their elegant 1946 paper (8) reporting on their brilliant, intellectually exciting use of physiologic principles to measure pulmonary diffusing capacity for O_2 (DLo_2) in man.

So it *was* necessary in 1950 to have a "methods section" on Gas-Blood Diffusion and I prevailed upon Seymour Kety to write it. Some perhaps thought this was an inappropriate selection of author, because Kety was best known for his newly developed method for measuring cerebral blood flow in man—pretty far removed from the lungs. But Kety's method required that his subjects inhale nitrous oxide and he was in the process of writing a scholarly analysis of gas exchange at the lungs and other tissues for *Pharmacological Reviews* (12). Kety studied all previous work on pulmonary diffusion of O_2 and CO and in his 1950 article (13) concluded:

. . . the necessity for obtaining samples of mixed venous blood makes it appear doubtful that the determination of Do_2 by means of the Bohr equation will ever achieve clinical usefulness . . . [My note: Lilienthal and Riley's 1946 paper *assumed* values for Po_2 in mixed venous blood; the new technic of cardiac catheterization made it possible to obtain samples of such blood and replace assumed values with measured values.]

Marie Krogh brilliantly side-stepped the difficulties inherent in the Bohr equation and measured the diffusion coefficient of the lungs by means of CO ... It appears that the determination of Do_2 by Krogh's method [My note: by measuring Dco and calculating Do_2 from it] would constitute a practicable and clinically useful technique for defining the diffusion characteristics of the alveolar membrane in health and disease.

That same year, Robert Forster joined our staff and at once set to work mastering the new infrared meter for rapid analysis of CO and our new mass spectrometer for rapid analysis of helium. Within a relatively short time, he, with Fowler and Bates, had modified Krogh's technic and developed a rapid and clinically useful single-breath technic (14–16). In the same year, Filley independently reported on his steady state CO method (17).

What have we learned from this account of the development of a clinical test? Certainly we've learned that eminent scientists can be wrong occasionally but that their being wrong sometimes provides the stimulus for an important discovery. We've learned that research on a fundamental physiologic problem can provide the basis for a practical clinical test. We've learned that putting good scientists into research laboratories in wartime can produce exciting basic advances and we've learned the value of asking a brilliant, disinterested scientist to be an "ombudsman" and indicate the directions for future work.

What we have *not* learned from this account is why there was a 35-year lag between Krogh's work and the development of a clinical test of Dco, which, being non-invasive, did not have to wait for cardiac catheterization in man. It would be simple to say that pathology dominated clinical science until the 1940's and few clinicians had been trained to think physiologically. However, A. Krogh and Lindhard (18), working in the same department as M. Krogh, had measured pulmonary blood flow (cardiac output) two years earlier using essentially the same non-invasive technic (measuring uptake of a soluble "inert" gas, nitrous oxide, as determined by its disappearance from alveolar gas)—and their test, modified in several ways, *was* used in the 1920's, 1930's, and 1940's until it was replaced by the direct Fick method.

It seems that something inherent in pulmo-nary medicine between 1915 and 1945 inhibited the development of tests of pulmonary function. Was it because pulmonary medicine in the first half of the twentieth century was really tuberculosis medicine that required largely roentgenograms and bacteriologic tests for diagnosis? All of us with a deep interest in pulmonary medicine should ponder on the reasons for the long quiet period in the early twentieth century because "Those who cannot remember the past are condemned to repeat it."

Addendum

Forster believes that the rapid progress made in the 1950's owed much to the development and use of the rapid infra-red carbon monoxide analyzer that took the place of laborious and time-consuming methods used in the 1910's by the Kroghs. True, but Max Liston, who devised our infra-red analyzer, tells me that Lord Kelvin reported to the Royal Society in the 1800's that, using a rotating shutter between a mantle lamp and a cylindrical chamber with a small hole, Kelvin could hear sounds when "mine damp methane" was placed in the apparatus; Kelvin proposed its use to test for safety of air in mines. And many physicists published infrared spectra for gases in the 1930's. But there was still no rapid CO analyzer for clinical use until after World War II.

References

1. Bohr, C.: Ueber die Lungenathmung, Skand Arch Physiol, 1891, *2*, 236-268.
2. Haldane, J., and Smith, J. L.: The absorption of oxygen by the lungs, J Physiol, 1897-98, *22*, 231–258.
3. Krogh, A.: On the mechanism of gas-exchange in the lungs, Skand Arch Physiol, 1910, *23*, 248–278.
4. Krogh, M.: The diffusion of gases through the lungs of man, J Physiol (London), 1915, *49*, 271–300.
5. Krogh, A., and Krogh, M.: On the rate of diffusion of carbonic oxide into the lungs of man, Skand Arch Physiol, 1910, *23*, 236–247.
6. Lilienthal, J. L., and Riley, R. L.: Diseases of the respiratory system. Circulation through the lungs and diffusion of gases, Ann Rev Med, 1954, *5*, 237–284.

30

7. Bohr, C.: Ueber die Spezifische Tätigkeit der Lungen bei der respiratorischen Gasaufnahme und ihr Verhalten zu der durch die Alveolarwand stattfindenden Gasdiffusion, Skand Arch Physiol, 1909, 22, 221–280.

8. Lilienthal, J. L., Riley, R. L., Proemmel, D. D., and Franke, R. E.: An experimental analysis in man of the oxygen pressure gradient from alveolar air to arterial blood during rest and exercise at sea level and at altitude, Am J Physiol, 1946, 147, 199–216.

9. Barcroft, J., Binger, C. A., Bock, A. V., Doggart, J. H., Forbes, W. S., Harrop, G., Meakins, J. C., and Redfield, A. C.: Observations upon the effect of high altitude on the physiological processes of the human body carried out in the Peruvian Andes, chiefly at Cerro De Pasco, Trans R Soc London B, 1923, 221, 351–480.

10. Harrop, G. A., Jr., and Heath, E. H.: Pulmonary gas diffusion in polycythemia vera, J Clin Invest, 1927, 4, 53–70.

11. Comroe, J. H., Jr.: Pulmonary Function Tests, in Methods in Medical Research, vol. 2, J. H. Comroe, Jr., ed., Year Book Publishers, Chicago, 1950, pp. 74–244.

12. Kety, S. S.: The theory and applications of the exchange of inert gas at the lungs and tissues, Pharmacol Rev, 1951, 3, 1–32.

13. Kety, S. S.: Pulmonary diffusion coefficient, in Methods in Medical Research, vol. 2, J. H. Comroe, Jr., ed., Year Book Publishers, Chicago, 1950, pp. 234–248.

14. Forster, R. E., Fowler, W. S., Bates, D. V., and Van Lingen, B.: The absorption of carbon monoxide by the lungs during breathholding, J Clin Invest, 1954, 33, 1135–1145.

15. Forster, R. E., Cohn, J. E., Briscoe, W. A., Blakemore, W. S., and Riley, R. L.: A modification of the Krogh carbon monoxide breathholding technique for estimating the diffusing capacity of the lungs; a comparison with three other methods, J Clin Invest, 1955, 34, 1417–1426.

16. Ogilvie, C. M., Forster, R. E., Blakemore, W. S., and Morton, J. W.: A standardized breathholding technique for the clinical measurement of the diffusing capacity of the lungs for carbon monoxide, J Clin Invest, 1957, 36, 1–17.

17. Filley, G. F., MacIntosh, D. J., and Wright, G. W.: Carbon monoxide uptake and pulmonary diffusing capacity in normal subjects at rest and during exercise, J Clin Invest, 1954, 33, 530–539.

18. Krogh, A., and Lindhard, J.: Measurements of the blood flow through the lungs of man, Skand Arch Physiol, 1912, 27, 100–125.

EITHER–OR? (Why Not Both?)

• Humphry Davy in 1800 prepared his own hydrogen, put a measured amount of it in a spirometer, breathed it back and forth 7 times, and then, from the initial and final concentrations of H_2 in the spirometer, measured his own lung volume.

• John Hutchinson in 1840 measured vital capacity and its subdivisions in several thousand normal subjects, proposed normal values for men and women of different height, weight, and age, and devised a test to measure maximal voluntary inspiratory and expiratory effort. He also used his tests to diagnose pulmonary disease before it could be detected by other means.

• Luigi Luciani in 1877 estimated intrapleural pressure in animals from measurements of their intraesophageal pressure, obtained from a balloon-catheter placed in the esophagus.

• Marie Krogh in 1915 published details of her single-breath carbon monoxide test to measure pulmonary diffusing capacity in man.

• Hürter in 1912 punctured the radial artery of man to obtain blood samples, and Stadie in 1919 used this technic to measure arterial O_2 saturation of patients with pneumonia. Van Slyke and Neill developed their manometric method for measuring blood O_2 and CO_2 in 1924.

• Fleisch devised his meter for measuring instantaneous rate of air flow in 1925.

Despite these pioneering studies stretching back 140 years, in 1940 only a few clinical physiologists in a few countries—and practically no physicians—had an interest in measuring pulmonary function in man. Indeed, in 1940 no textbook of physiology included even a paragraph on pulmonary function (apart from vital capacity). But only six years later the golden age of clinical pulmonary physiology began.

What happened between 1940 and 1946? These, of course, were the years in which we first prepared for and then participated in World War II. But we had also participated in World War I in 1917–1918 and no special benefits accrued to pulmonary physiology.

Why "yes" in 1940–46 and "no" in 1917–18? I believe several factors were responsible. President Roosevelt decided in 1940 to organize a National Defense Research Committee (NDRC) to coordinate research in developing military weapons—followed in July 1941 by a second decision, to form an Office of Scientific Research and Development (OSRD). The OSRD (headed by Vannevar Bush) had two divisions—the existing NDRC and a new Committee on Medical Research (headed by an eminent renal physiologist, A. N. Richards, later to become President of the National Academy of Sciences). Roosevelt, Bush, and Richards believed that solution of certain physiologic problems would help the over-all war effort and that their solution required (1) support of biomedical research by government (Army, Navy, Air Force, and the new OSRD); (2) full use of government and university laboratories; (3) the building of new research facilities for both government and universities when needed; (4) the recruiting of well-trained scientists, in and out of uniform, to work in them, with at least some freedom to investigate basic as well as targeted problems.

Another important factor was that the time was ripe for the solution of certain physiologic problems. What were these problems and who worked on them? The Air Force had fighter planes with open cockpits (pressurized cabins weighed more and reduced speed and maneuverability). It was easier to increase pressure only in the pilot's alveoli than in the whole cabin—but no one knew whether pilots could tolerate increased alveolar pressure and, if they did, whether it would improve oxygenation of their arterial blood and permit them to climb to higher altitudes and gain tactical advantage over enemy planes. The OSRD and then the Air Force asked Wallace Fenn to work on pressure breathing, and soon the team of Fenn, Otis, and Rahn, working at the University of Rochester, had completed their classic studies on the pressure-volume relations of the lungs and thorax and the work of breathing, and the modern era of pulmonary mechanics had begun. Pressure breathing was not new in 1942 but Fenn, Otis, and Rahn *were* new, both to respiratory physiology and to human physiology, and fresh minds looking at an old problem made a big difference.

The Air Force had another problem—how to identify when and where inward leaks of air occurred in oxygen masks when a fighter pilot moved his head quickly up and down and side to side. John Lilly, in his first postdoctoral year in Detlev Bronk's Johnson Foundation for Medical Physics at the University of Pennsylvania drew on his engineering background at California Institute of Technology to devise an instrument (now known as a nitrogen meter or analyzer) that recorded continuously and almost instantaneously the nitrogen concentration in an extremely small sample of air. This instrument a few years later became the keystone in single-breath analysis of uneven distribution of inspired air to alveoli and is now widely used to measure "closing" volume. Leak detection was not new in 1942, but John Lilly was and again it made a big difference.

The Air Force also needed to know how fully arterial blood was saturated with oxygen. One way was to draw arterial blood and analyze it. But, in 1942, arterial puncture was far from an accepted procedure. The needs of aviation medicine widened its use by clinical investigators, and then, as fears about its dangers faded, they introduced it into clinical medicine. I did my first arterial puncture on Bob Dripps in 1942 and, since he survived, he then did his first on me. At the end of the war, it became a standard procedure in pulmonary function laboratories.

But the Air Force also wanted to measure arterial O_2 saturation *continuously* in subjects during simulated flight conditions. Glenn Millikan was ready with the answer. Millikan had worked in Barcroft's laboratory at Cambridge in the 1930s, had used the Hartridge-Roughton

continuous flow apparatus (for measuring rapid chemical reactions) to study the velocity of the O_2–myoglobin reaction, and had modified this apparatus to make it rugged, compact, and portable. Millikan joined the staff of the Johnson Foundation in 1939, about the time Germany went to war with England. Because of his strong ties with England, Millikan wanted to do something to help in its war effort. He knew that it would be important to pilots to know their arterial O_2 saturation (he himself was a mountain climber and his father-in-law, Mallory, was an early climber of Mt. Everest); toward this end he developed the first ear oximeter. It was widely used in aviation laboratories in wartime and then, with improvements, in physiologic investigation in peacetime.

Riley and Lilienthal began their classic studies on pulmonary diffusing capacity for O_2 (Do_2) while they were assigned to the Pensacola Naval Air Station. They wondered why normal subjects at high altitude became more cyanotic during exercise and specifically whether the deepening cyanosis was caused by failure of Po_2 in blood and gas to come to near-equilibrium when alveolar Po_2 was low. Although their Do_2 method is not widely used now, it reopened the field of pulmonary diffusing capacity and led to their own comprehensive examination of ventilation-blood flow relationships in the lung.

At the University of Southern California low pressure chamber, two physiologists, Drs. Scott and Drury, were studying the effects on man of different types of pressure breathing—increased pressure only during inspiration, only during expiration, or during both. This required separating the inspiratory and expiratory lines; the simplest way was to use a large-bore 3-way aluminum stopcock and turn it manually from the inspiratory to the expiratory line during each breath. One day an engineer visited their laboratory. The physiologists wondered if this tedious manual task could be done by electrically operated valves. The engineer thought the task could be done better with a mechanical valve. His name was Ray Bennett; in a short time, he developed the first "flow-sensitive" (now called "Bennett") valve, the forerunner of many subsequent automatically controlled valves for intermittent positive pressure breathing.

Linus Pauling wrote in 1946, "On October 3, 1940, at a meeting in Washington, called by Division B of the National Defense Research Committee, mention was made of the need for an instrument which could measure and indicate the partial pressure of oxygen in a gas. During the next few days we devised and constructed a simple and effective instrument for this purpose." This was the Pauling oxygen meter that capitalized on existing knowledge that the magnetic susceptibility of oxygen was considerably greater than that of other gases.

The Medical Division of the Chemical Corps at Edgewood, Maryland, also had biologic problems to solve. One was to determine the cause of death of occupants of nearly closed, poorly ventilated pill boxes when flame throwers were used to clear them out. Was it heat alone? Or anoxia (due to exhaustion of O_2 by flame)? Or increased concentrations of CO or CO_2 (caused by incomplete or complete combustion)? The answer required portable, rapidly responding gas analyzers to measure gas concentrations continuously within the pill boxes. Infrared absorption spectra of gases were well known and Fastie and Pfund had already constructed infrared analyzers. These were quickly modified for field use. Pulmonary physiologists were there and remembered to use them constructively when peace came.

Edgewood arsenal also housed pilot plants that manufactured war gases such as phosgene. Occasional accidents there exposed workers to inhalation of phosgene. Some of these workers developed tachypnea and dyspnea and Morton Galdston and I were assigned the job of measuring their lung function. The first tests of pulmonary function that I participated in were on these workers in a laboratory at nearby Johns Hopkins Hospital. This led directly toward my later interest both in pulmonary function and in the causes of dyspnea.

Cardiac catheterization had been used in man long before 1940. Forssmann had catheterized his own heart in 1929 and radiologists had used the technic in the 1930s to inject radiopaque materials in the right heart to improve pulmonary arteriography. And in 1941 Cournand, with Ranges, had written about right atrial catheterization to obtain samples of mixed venous blood. But it was the investigation of traumatic shock in man in wartime that brought together Cournand, Riley, Gregerson, Bradley, and Richards (among others) to study a large number of patients by many technics, one of which was measurement of right atrial pressure. World War II did not discover either arterial puncture or cardiac catheterization, but it did much to speed

their acceptance into clinical investigation and then into clinical medicine in the post-war period.

I'm sure that other new devices and concepts originated in the 1940–46 period or that their development or acceptance was speeded during this time. I've mentioned some that I believe redirected a number of scientists into new types of research once the war was over—and whose new activities then paid off handsomely in pulmonary physiology. One example in my own laboratory was Ward Fowler, my first post-war, postdoctoral fellow in 1946. I asked him what he wanted to study. He thought a bit and answered that almost everyone was measuring physiologic changes *discontinuously* and that he'd like to measure something continuously. I replied along these lines: "Here's Millikan's ear oximeter that estimates arterial O_2 saturation continuously, and Lilly's meter that measures the N_2 concentration of a gas continuously and a flow meter that measures air flow continuously." Fowler put them together and ushered in the era of rapid, single-breath analysis of pulmonary function.

Something that had no direct connection with pulmonary physiology also helped to keep the new crop of scientists working on lungs and respiration and to attract many more—and that something was the new science of chemotherapy, greatly accelerated by the needs of wartime. When chemotherapy of tuberculosis arrived in 1946 and when antibiotics could be counted on to keep alive patients who formerly succumbed to a wide variety of chronic pulmonary diseases, pulmonary medicine became a different kind of specialty with broad interests in the diagnosis, prevention, and management of all types of pulmonary diseases and respiratory problems. At last it became a challenging specialty to those who previously had passed it by.

This look into the retrospectroscope gives us a glimpse into the golden era of *applied* pulmonary physiology. Does this glimpse argue for the support of applied, mission-oriented, targeted research? Indeed it does! And this brings us back to the title of this note: "EITHER—OR?" I have little patience with basic scientists who argue that only fundamental research is worthy of support and equally little patience with engineers and clinicians who argue that mission-oriented research is all that we need. This is the EITHER one OR the other approach—one that in a few years predictably leads to a marked decline in the quality of science. The BOTH approach makes more sense, although it raises more problems. The BOTH approach requires that someone must decide *how much of each*. And someone must decide *if, when,* and *why* support for one should be increased and *for how long* without detriment to the other. It requires genius to answer these questions. Someone had it in World War II; who but a genius (or a lucky gambler) could have assigned Fenn (who had never done research on man), Rahn (a youngster investigating why rattlesnakes changed color), and Otis (another youngster interested in grasshopper eggs and in the oyster heart) to work on pressure breathing in man and have it pay off? Not all applied research pays off; someone less than a genius had assigned Fenn in World War *I* to study the effect of changing the hydrogen ion concentration on the viscosity of dough! The recent, very costly space program has widely publicized its "spin-off" for science,

but it had no demonstrable effect on pulmonary medicine. It produced a bit of miniaturization here and there but little else. Among the highly touted accomplishments· of the space program were telemetry and the mass spectrometer. But Einthoven had written a paper on telemetry in 1907, 60 years before the space age, and pulmonary physiologists were using mass spectrometers in the early 1950s (borrowed from researchers in the oil industry who used them long before then).

World War II put good scientists into intimate contact with fascinating problems ready for solution and their enthusiasm carried over into new, rewarding post-war careers. And it had a tremendous spin-off—its success led in a few years to a new type of peacetime research organization—the National Institutes of Health!

Out of the Mouth of Babes

I've always believed that a main responsibility of a faculty member is to be a talent scout—to determine the special abilities of his medical students in clinical care, in teaching, or in research, and then to encourage them to be the very best they can in their field of unusual competence. One field, of course, is research. I see no way for faculty to determine this special talent of their students unless students have contact with research while they are still in medical school. Now I know that even a whispered suggestion that students be involved in research will call forth cries of anguish from those who believe that too many medical students now opt for research and too few for taking care of sick people. So before you write a letter of protest to Congress, let me state pretty strongly that, as one who lately has been a patient in and out of hospitals, I'm all in favor of doctors (and nurses) who genuinely *care for* sick people and know how to go about it. Let me also state, again as a recent patient, that I'm equally in favor of research that would have prevented me from being a patient in the first place!

Providing a little bit of research experience for medical students helps both ways. Of course it helps to identify those with unusual originality and unique talents for a career in research (more of this later). But it also makes a better physician of one with no desire to do research. How? Lots of ways. It teaches him to read scientific articles critically and to look objectively at data published in journals. There is no course labelled "Critical Evaluation of Data" in any medical school catalogue and yet the most important job of the school's faculty is to encourage and teach students to continue their own scientific education for the 40 years after they've flown the nest, when they must now judge for themselves what's good and bad, what to adopt and what to shun. A little research also teaches the medical student the importance of controlled studies, especially when he must evaluate new modes of therapy. It teaches him a systematic approach to problem-solving, and once in practice, he'll realize that almost every patient presents a new problem to him. And it teaches him that numbers are better than guesses when it comes to diagnosis, prognosis, and evaluation of treatment. If I were dean of a medical school and had complete dictatorial powers, I would substitute some months of research (laboratory or clinical) for cook-book laboratory experiments—not as a device to recruit researchers but as a device to produce better future physicians.

Some congressmen would of course ask, "Where's the direct, immediate pay-off?" The answer is that from early to modern times, some very remarkable discoveries have been made by youngsters who were still medical students. Let me give you a few examples:

Humphry Davy was still a 19-year-old student in Dr. Beddoes's "Pneumatic Institution" in Bristol when he prepared and inhaled large quantities of nitrous oxide and discovered its marked analgesic effect. Near the end of July 1799, Davy wrote:

> In one instance, when I had headache from indigestion, it was immediately removed by the effects of a large dose of the gas, though it afterwards returned, but with much less violence. In a second instance, a slighter degree of headache was wholly removed by two doses of gas.
>
> The power of the immediate operation of the gas in removing intense physical pain, I had a very good opportunity of ascertaining.
>
> In cutting one of the unlucky teeth called *dentes sapientiae*, I experienced an extensive inflammation of the gum, accompanied with great pain, which equally destroyed the power of repose, and of consistent action.
>
> On the day when the inflammation was most troublesome, I breathed three large doses of nitrous oxide. The pain always diminished after the first four or five inspirations. (1)

Later, in the Conclusion to Section III of the same work, Davy wrote, "As nitrous oxide in its extensive operation appears capable of destroying physical pain, it may probably be used with advantage during surgical operations in which no great effusion of blood takes place." Gibson (2) surmised, "Unfortunately no one read as far as page 556, or understood this proclamation of the surgical anesthetic value of nitrous oxide," for it was not until 1844 that Wells in America put this observation to practical use.

William Morton, although already practicing dentistry, entered Harvard for medical training. It was in 1846 (as a medical student-dentist) that he demonstrated the first use of ether as a surgical anesthetic agent (3, 4). So as a reminder of Humphry Davy and of William Morton, as each congressman is wheeled into an operating room for whatever, I would inform him, "You will be free of pain during this operation because of discoveries by two medical students."

Incidentally, practically every article about Morton speaks of him as a dentist and only a few mention that he was a medical student. However, the Catalogue of Students Attending Medical Lectures at Harvard University in Boston 1845-46 does list "Morton, William Thomas Green, Boston; Charles T. Jackson, lecturer." (Jackson was not listed as a regular faculty member but did teach chemistry.) But the records of the medical department of Harvard between 1845-86 do not list Morton as a graduate. Of equal interest is that no one has been able to confirm that he received a dental degree at the Baltimore College of Dental Surgery (now the University of Maryland), or even matriculated there, although he did study dentistry in Horace Well's office in Farmington, Connecticut. (Wells was the first to use nitrous oxide for producing anesthesia.) Although Morton never earned a degree in either medicine or dentistry, he later received honorary degrees in both.

J.-L.-M. Poiseuille devised the mercury manometer for measuring arterial blood pressure when he was only 29 years old and still a medical student (5). In addition, he measured intra-arterial pressure starting with the ascending aorta and ending with the smallest artery into which he could insert a cannula and proved that intra-arterial pressure fell but little in these main conduits. Some years later, he did his classic measurements on resistance to flow in small tubes and established Poiseuille's Law (6).

Lysle Peterson received his M.D. degree in 1950 but in 1949 published the first successful method for accurate and continuous recording of arterial blood pressure in man (7). He stated:

A small plastic catheter, inserted into an artery through a needle, is left in the artery when the needle is withdrawn. Attached to a capacitance manometer, this technique permits recording for long periods of time without discomfort and allows relatively free mobility of the subject. The record, received by an ink-writing oscillograph, permits continuous knowledge of blood pressure and provides an opportunity for observation of any changes in the contour of the pulse wave which may develop. The apparatus is compact, mobile, and flexible.

By comparing the contour of the pulse waves in the same subject under different conditions, one can obtain information concerning changes in stroke volume, vasoconstriction, or distensibility of the arterial system.

This method, as modified by Seldinger and others, is now used universally in intensive care units and recovery rooms.

Eugene Landis, later Professor of Physiology at Harvard, did his direct measurements on arteriolar, capillary, and venular blood pressure while a medical student at the University of Pennsylvania (1922-26). Figure 7 of his report, received for publication in 1925 (8), has been reprinted in its original or modified form in practically every textbook of physiology since then; it demonstrates unequivocally that the main site of resistance to blood flow is in the arterioles.

Paul Langerhans found the special pancreatic cells (later named the "islets of Langerhans" and still later discovered to be the source of insulin) in 1868 while he was a medical student at the University of Berlin (9). Before this important discovery, he had already published one study of cutaneous nerves and another on tactile corpuscles in the skin.

Charles Best was a medical student at the University of Toronto when Banting wheedled the use of a laboratory from Professor Macleod for the summer of 1921. Banting also asked for ten dogs and a research assistant. The assistant assigned was medical student Best. Within several months Banting and Best had discovered insulin (10).

Jay McLean had been accepted by Johns Hopkins Medical School as a second year student but had to wait a year before he could be admitted. During that year, he did research in Professor William Howell's physiology department "to determine if I could solve a problem by myself." He did. He discovered heparin (11), to the amazement and disbelief of his professor, a longtime leader in research on blood coagulation.

Walter Cannon entered Harvard Medical School in 1896, the year after Roentgen's discovery of x-rays. He at once went to work using the new technique to study gastrointestinal motility in conscious animals by giving them bismuth to swallow and studying gastric contractions by roentgenogram. He gave his first account before the American Physiological Society in May 1897; his classic paper on the influence of emotions on gastric motility was published a year later (12a). Incidentally, another medical student, Albert Moser, worked with Cannon that same year on esophageal motility (12b). He died of tuberculosis only five years later.

John Fulton wrote his first paper in 1920, a year before he received his B.S. degree and a Rhodes Scholarship. Between then and the end of 1927 (when he received his M.D. degree), he had 40 publications, including his classic 644-page monograph, "Muscular Contraction and the Reflex Control of Movement," published in 1926 (13).

Josef Breuer began his medical training at the age of 17 and completed his requirements for qualification at age 25. One of his clinical teachers offered him an assistantship that allowed him time to work in Hering's physiology laboratory. That year Breuer discovered the Hering-Breuer (or Breuer-Hering) reflex (14) and presented his work early in 1868 to the Vienna Academy of Science. Shortly thereafter, Breuer entered the private practice of medicine but found time for research on the semicircular canals. Yet Breuer's greatest achievement was to lay the groundwork for Freud's study of psychoanalysis. Breuer's biographer wrote:

> Between 1880 and 1882 Breuer treated a hysterical patient, Miss Anna O. His handling of this famous case started a scientific revolution. He had been the first physician in Vienna to make therapeutic use of hypnosis, and he used it in this case. Proceeding entirely empirically, Breuer and his patient discovered with surprise that a symptom would disappear and never return if he could bring her to relate the exact circumstances in which the symptom had appeared for the first time and to give expression to her feelings on that occasion. The patient's name for the procedure was "talking cure." Breuer later termed it "catharsis."

> Breuer first met Freud in . . . the late eighteen-seventies. . . . Despite their close friendship at the time Freud did not hear about the case of Miss Anna O. until the treatment had ended in 1882. It took Freud another twelve years to persuade Breuer to publish a detailed report of the case. . . .

> But he [Breuer] was aware of what he had started. Towards the end of his *Curriculum* he says: "This book was at first rather unfavourably received, but appeared in its fourth edition last year. For Freud it was the seed from which psychoanalysis grew." (15)

Maurice Raynaud in 1862 first described the syndrome of symmetrical ischemia of the extremities that now bears his name (16). He was then a medical student and his thesis won him the M.D. degree. He wrote, in part, about his patient:

> Under the influence of very moderate cold, and even at the height of summer, she sees her fingers become ex-sanguine, completely insensible, and of a whitish yellow colour. . . . The feet, more impressionable even than the hands, are regularly attacked at meal times and whilst digestion is going on. . . . The complete disappearance of attacks of local syncope has always been noted by this lady as the first index of a commencing pregnancy.

Ivar Sandström entered medical school at the University of Uppsala in 1872 and received his preclinical degree in 1878. In 1877, he discovered the parathyroid glands; he wrote, in part:

> About three years ago [1877] I found on the thyroid gland of a dog a small organ, hardly as big as a hemp seed, which was enclosed in the same connective tissue capsule as the thyroid, but could be distinguished therefrom by a lighter color. A superficial examination revealed an organ of a totally different structure from that of the thyroid, and with a very rich vascularity. . . . The existence of a hitherto unknown gland in animals that have so often been a subject of anatomical examination called for a thorough approach to the region around the thyroid gland even in man. Although the probability of finding something hitherto unrecognized seemed so small that it was exclusively with the purpose of completing the investigations rather than with the hope of finding something new that I began a careful examination of this region. So much the greater was my astonishment therefore when in the first individual examined I found on

both sides at the inferior border of the thyroid gland an organ of the size of a small pea, which, judging from its exterior, did not appear to be a lymph gland, nor an accessory thyroid gland, and upon histological examination showed a rather peculiar structure. After several examinations not only was I convinced of the constancy of its appearance but I was also able to show that two such glands in most cases occur on each side. (17)

Paul Ehrlich's first paper, published in 1877 when he was a medical student aged 23, had tremendous impact on the new science of bacteriology since his was the first *analytic* study of staining methods (18). In it, and in his 1878 thesis based on it, he criticized the histologists because they cared little for the *theory* of staining despite the fact that improvements in the practice of technical dyeing might well be expected to result from a correct theory. Sir Henry Dale has commented that in it are already

> the lines of the theoretical approach to medical and biological problems, even the germs of some of the detailed conceptions, which were so largely to dominate Ehrlich's ways of thought and plans for experiment, during all the rest of his scientific career.
>
> Ehrlich's immediate and most direct application, of the interests and the principles which he had developed so precociously in this Thesis, was to the differential staining of the white cells of the blood and the tissues, showing that the granules in the protoplasm of different types could be recognized as oxyphile, basophile or neutrophile, according to their respective affinities for dyes, of which the tinctorial components were acidic or basic in nature, or combinations of both. In these studies, and in others which he made, in this early period, on the nature of the red blood corpuscles and their pathological variations, can be found the basis for a large part of modern haematology. Clear descriptions will be found, for example, at this early date, of the presence, in the blood from certain cases of anaemia, of immature red cells, of the type so familiar in more recent years as "reticulocytes", and of their characteristic staining with certain dyes. (19)

But far more important was the concept of the "magic bullet"—that specific chemicals could be synthesized to attach to specific receptors on cells—the basis for his later discovery of Salvarsan and of much of modern chemotherapy.

Adam Thebesius undoubtedly discovered the channels connecting the cavities of the heart with the coronary vessels in the myocardium (20), connections known today as Thebesian vessels, and undoubtedly he discovered them while he was a medical student at Leyden. The fact that Vieussens, two years earlier, found the same openings into the cardiac cavities does not diminish the value of Thebesius's careful injection techniques. Actually, Vieussens and Thebesius found the same small openings connected to the coronary circulation, although Vieussens performed forward injections through the coronary arteries, and Thebesius performed retrograde injections through the coronary sinus and veins.

Joseph Black began his medical studies in 1744 at the University of Glasgow and concurrently began his investigation of alkalies then in use for treating patients with stones in the kidney and bladder. In 1752 he moved to Edinburgh where he took additional medical courses and continued his research, which culminated in the discovery of CO_2 and the beginning of quantitative chemistry. On heating limestone or chalk, Black (who believed in *weighing* things and not merely observing) found it became lighter, presumably because it lost "air"; limestone lost an equivalent amount of air when added acid caused effervescence. But the gas released was not air because it extinguished both flame and life (21). Black had rediscovered CO_2 (originally discovered in 1662 by Van Helmont) and begun the "chemical revolution" of the 18th century.

Lorenzo Bellini, 19 years old and a medical student at Pisa, changed the standard picture of the kidney from a hard, solid, fleshy organ (22). Bellini found that

> the state of affairs is otherwise, for the substance of the kidneys is nothing else than an aggregate of an infinite number of vessels of a kind peculiar to itself. Having cut through any part of the kidney, certain fibres or filaments extending from the outer surface to the hollow or pelvis are quite plainly visible. . .
>
> If therefore you compress these filaments from their further end, that is, with respect to the pelvis, and examine them, you will find water welling up everywhere. If you are not afraid to present this to your tongue, you will discover a certain saltiness and in some the taste of urine. You can test this also if you cut across the body of the kidney, for then you may also see this same juice arise from the renal ducts severed in this way and you may clearly observe its quality and nature. You may observe this much more easily if you apply a glass lens to your eye for then, when the tubules are compressed, the

urine is very clearly seen welling out as if gushing forth from so many little water pipes.

From these things we can confidently infer that the substance of the kidney, even though they have called it parenchyma, is nothing else than . . . a mass of canaliculae and capillary spaces through which the urine flows into the pelvis. . . .

From medical student to professor! The next year, at age 20, Bellini was appointed professor of philosophy and theoretical medicine at Pisa.

Thomas Young, one of the most eminent of British scientists, solved the riddle of visual accommodation while a 20-year-old medical student; a year later he was elected a Fellow of the Royal Society of London to honor this achievement. Scientists before Young knew that vision could be sharp and clear whether a person was looking at a near or far object. The favorite explanation was that the eyeball itself shortened or lengthened and so appropriately changed the distance between the lens and the retina. Young (23) showed instead that the intraocular ciliary muscles contracted (because of nerve stimulation) or relaxed (with none) and the change in thickness of the ciliary muscle effected a thinning or thickening of the lens, which had elastic properties.

Paul Bert is famous today for his 1,178-page volume, "La Pression Baromètrique," but during his lifetime in France he was best known for his work on skin grafting, which he published in 1863 while he was a student in medicine and an assistant to Claude Bernard (24); it was responsible for fostering the specialty of skin grafting during the war of 1870. His obituary in the *Lancet* (November 20, 1886) speaks only of his pioneer work on skin grafting and fails to mention his definitive work on high altitude hypoxia and hyperbaric environments, or even that he was a great physiologist (25)! It is interesting that Bert himself did not regard his studies on skin grafting as experimental surgery but as a technique for learning how transplanted tissues live in a new environment. It was in a sense a stepping stone from his Professor's study on the internal environment to Bert's later studies on how changing the external environment (high and low pressures and high and low oxygen tensions) affects body function.

Martin Flack had just completed his preclinical work at Oxford when he became involved in the search for the sinoauricular node (26). As Gibson (27) relates the story:

The village of Borden [in Kent, where Flack lived] was agog when in 1903 the celebrated anatomist Sir Arthur Keith took up week-end residence there. With some sixth sense he learned that the butcher's boy [Flack] had just completed his preclinical work at Oxford and was about to select a teaching hospital in London for his clinical studies. In a twinkling the student found himself admitted to the London Hospital and scheduled for week-end research in Borden with Keith.

The drudgery of cutting serial sections of 130 moles' hearts, staining them, and studying them under the microscope was relieved by daily games of golf, learned from James Braid's manual. One evening Sir Arthur came back from cycling to be told by Flack that he had spotted a new structure in the right auricle. It appeared consistently in all other hearts examined as something resembling an electrical conducting system. Thus was discovered the sinoauricular node or cardiac pacemaker [also known as the Keith-Flack node].

Jan Swammerdam was not the first to see capillaries and objects floating in them but he was the first to recognize these floaters as blood corpuscles, probably in the year 1665 while he was still a medical student (28). Harvey had to postulate the presence of capillaries if blood really went around in a circle, because he never saw them. Malpighi, with the aid of a microscope, described pulmonary capillaries in a frog in 1661; Malpighi also saw bodies floating in them but believed them to be fat globules. Swammerdam, however, identified them as red blood cells:

I saw a serum in the blood, in which were a vast number of orbicular particles, in shape like flat ovals, but very regular. These particles also seemed to contain another fluid, but when I viewed them sideways they resembled crystalline clubs, and several other figures also, according as they were turned about in various directions in the serum of the blood. I further observed that the more these objects were magnified with a microscope, the fainter their colour appeared to become.

This was not his first discovery as a medical student. A year earlier he had discovered the valves in lymphatic vessels and in 1667 he discovered that the lungs of newborn float if respiration has already occurred before death.

Kenneth Evelyn, more than two years before he received his M.D. degree at McGill University, devised a photoelectric colorimeter that at least for several decades was the best instrument of its type. In 1936 anyone who was in pulmonary research and was lucky enough to have a little money bought a spirometer, a Van Slyke manometric apparatus, and an Evelyn photoelectric colorimeter; if he had the third of these, he had a stream of visitors to his laboratory bench to use it.

Evelyn summarized its advantages in his 1936 paper (29):

> exceptional stability is secured by using a lamp of such low power requirement that it may be operated by a storage battery.
>
> High illuminating efficiency obtained by the use of a reflector and smooth control of light intensity over a wide range permit the use of color filters of very high selectivity, thus greatly extending the scope of the apparatus.
>
> . . . simplicity and convenience of operation have been improved by using standard test-tubes in place of conventional absorption cells.
>
> Complete mechanical rigidity, absence of moving parts, and a large safety factor in all important components eliminate the usual causes of unsatisfactory performance.

William MacCallum and **Eugene Opie** were members of the first class of the Johns Hopkins University School of Medicine, which entered in 1893 and was graduated in 1897. While still medical students, they made important contributions to knowledge of parasitic infections of red blood cells of birds (30, 31). Laveran had discovered the malarial parasite in 1880 and European scientists in 1885 had found that some birds harbored a similar parasite, a hematozoan. Malaria was still a scourge at that time. Of the British Army in India, 76,000 of 178,000 men were admitted to hospitals for malarial fever in 1897; there were 15,000 deaths annually in Italy and there was much malaria in the United States. Knowledge of the life cycle of the parasite in man was incomplete and the theory that the parasite was transmitted by a mosquito was only a conjecture. It was not until 1897 that Ross found, in the stomach of a mosquito, bodies that were probably an evolutionary stage of the human malarial parasite, and he continued and confirmed his work on malarial parasites in birds.

Ross, in his Nobel lecture on researches on malaria, delivered December 12, 1902, wrote:

> I am happy to be able to begin this part of the narrative with a brief account of the brilliant and important discovery of MacCallum. It will be remembered that Manson had thought the motile filaments to be flagellated spores; that I had studied them much without being able to learn anything new about them. . . .

In 1897 MacCallum undertook a study of the motile filaments. Working with the *Halteridium* of birds he noticed first that the gametocytes seemed to be of two kinds, namely one kind which produced the motile filaments, and another kind which did not do so. On watching two of these cells, one of each kind in the same field of the microscope, he observed (July 1897) that the filaments escaped from one as usual; that it moved about actively for a time; and then approaching the other gametocyte actually entered it. Other observations of MacCallum and Opie, made both on *Halteridium* and on the crescentic gametocytes of the aestivo-autumnal parasite of man, confirmed this beautiful discovery. The fact, as previously shown by Sacharoff, that the filaments contain chromatin was now explained; and also the facts that they escape and move about in the blood. They are, indeed, sperms which are emitted from the one kind of gametocytes, the males, and which fertilize the other kind, the females. Thus these minute parasites, among the lowest of creatures, have their sexes, and a form of sexual reproduction precisely like that of the highest animals.

More than this, MacCallum observed in the case of *Halteridium* of the crow that the female cell, motionless before fertilization, afterwards becomes elongated and vigorous, and moves across the field *in vitro*. This motile form had apparently long been seen by Danilewski and had been called by him a *vermicule*. (32)

Some years later, Ross (then Sir Ronald) said about this discovery by two young medical students: "I have ever since felt disgraced as a man of science!" (for Ross had erroneously interpreted the sperm cell wriggling *into* the penetrated female cell as a flagellated spore trying to escape *from* it!) (33)

Alfred Vogl was a third-year medical student when, in 1919, an emaciated young girl with congenital syphilis and juvenile tabes was admitted to the Wenckebach Clinic in Vienna. His chief asked Vogl to inject 1 ml of salicylate of mercury (an antisyphilitic drug) every other day. By chance, a retired Austrian army surgeon, brushing up on civilian medicine, told Vogl, "I received this sample in the mail this morning; it's a mercurial antisyphilitic, Novasurol. Maybe you can use it." He did. Fortunately, the nurses of the Wenckebach Clinic collected urine daily and regularly measured and charted its volume. The patient's urine volume went from 500 to 1,200 to 1,400 to 2,000 ml on consecutive days;

four days later when Vogl began the injections again, tall columns again appeared on the chart of urine volumes (34). Vogl then injected Novasurol into a patient with advanced congestive heart failure in whom customary diuretics failed to increase his meager urine output. Within 24 hours the patient had urinated more than 10 liters! And so, mercurial diuretics (of which Novasurol was the first) were discovered; they remained the most effective diuretic until 1957, when Beyer came up with chlorothiazide. You won't find the name of Vogl, the medical student, on Saxl's 1920 paper, or on Saxl and Heilig's 1920 article, but that is how a so-so antisyphilitic drug became a powerful diuretic.

Guillaume Lamy and **Sydney Rowland,** two other medical students, had an important influence on medicine without doing research.

Lamy decided to study medicine at the Faculty of Paris about 1667. Lower had performed the first transfusion of blood from dog to dog in England in 1665 (reported in 1666 in the Philosophical Transactions) and on November 23, 1667, had transfused blood from a docile animal (a sheep) to change the character of a man whose brain was considered "a little too warm" (the concept that a man's personality was determined by his blood was still deeply rooted in the 17th century). However, Jean-Baptiste Denis, physician to Louis XIV, performed four transfusions of blood from sheep or calf to man in Paris, the first of which was in mid-June 1667 (and probably the first recorded transfusion of animal blood to man). His fourth patient died from a transfusion reaction. Denis was tried for manslaughter but was exonerated. In 1667 Lamy wrote a "Letter to M. Moreau" (35) (published in 1668) excoriating the practice of transfusion. Lamy cautioned against diseases produced by impurities in the blood and warned of the danger of coagulation. His letter influenced Moreau and the newly formed Académie des Sciences to forbid transfusion in Paris without permission (36); a few years later the French Parliament prohibited transfusion of blood to human beings throughout France. The Royal Society of England then deprecated transfusion and it was forbidden by Rome. This put an end to blood transfusion for almost 150 years and justifiably so, because the essential knowledge of blood groups and incompatibility of blood from two sources did not surface until 1900, and a safe anticoagulant was not available until 1914.

Rowland was a medical student when Roentgen discovered x-rays in December 1895. Obviously one with remarkable prescience and initiative, he founded the *Archives of Clinical Skiagraphy* in 1896, "a series of collotype illustrations with descriptive text, illustrative applications of the new photography to Medicine and Surgery." The preface to the first number is dated April 2, 1896; in it, Sydney Rowland, B.A. Camb., expressed the hope that the new publication "might take a permanent place in Medical literature." It became the *Archives of Skiagraphy* in April 1897, then the *Archives of the Roentgen Ray* in July 1897, edited by W. S. Hedley and Sydney Rowland, M.A., M.R.C.S., and eventually the *British Journal of Radiology* (1928).

CONCLUDING REMARKS

I believe that if, without digging further, we simply accept as the immediate "pay-off" of medical student research the discovery of carbon dioxide, ether, nitrous oxide, insulin, heparin, mercurial diuretics, and the parathyroid glands; the proof that human emotions can profoundly affect body function; invention of the mercury manometer for measuring blood pressure; the concept that special chemicals specifically combine with special components of cells (basic to most chemotherapy); learning how to go about skin grafting and how to eliminate malaria—research by medical students has paid off handsomely. But we must add a slightly delayed "pay-off": it converted some hesitant medical school researchers into sure-fire, brilliant career investigators. And, most important to a skeptic who is willing to wait a little longer for the "pay-off" (when he himself gets sick and wants the best there is in diagnosis and treatment), a bit of medical student research experience may well provide him with a physician who early on learned to read critically, evaluate data objectively, and know when new knowledge gained in laboratory research is ready to save human lives.

In 1970, I received a letter from a Swiss physician who had been a research fellow in the early 1950s. It reads in part:

Some of your Research Fellows may end up in private practice as I did and the teaching expended on them may appear to be lost. However, my conviction is that although scientific thinking alone is not enough to advance the art of medicine, there will be no advance at all without its rigorous application in everyday medicine such as I practice very happily.

Note: I wish to express my appreciation to Horace Davenport for his account of Albert Moser; to Leroy Vandam for verifying the academic status of Morton; and to William C. Gibson, Professor of Medical History at the University of British Columbia, who has kindly called to my attention some of the examples included in this *Retrospectroscope;* for other instances of research accomplished by young men and women, see references (27), (36), and especially Gibson's monograph, "Young Endeavour" (2).

I have merely scratched the surface of biomedical research performed by young investigators because I decided to include only those who would today be considered medical students by U. S. definitions. This of course excluded many young British and European physicians who had completed all requirements to practice medicine and then engaged in some very remarkable research leading to a thesis and an M.D. degree. It also excludes all of those who did their research while serving as interns or residents (such as Alvin Coburn, who wrote his classic monograph on rheumatic fever on the basis of observations made while he was a resident, and Carl Koller, who discovered the local anesthetic properties of cocaine while he was an intern). Further, I decided to include only truly outstanding research done by medical students that has stood the test of decades; this means that I have not even delved into the work of thousands of medical student researchers since 1950 when NIH training grants permitted many medical students to have a summer research experience or even a "drop-out" year.

References

1. Davy, H.: Researches, Chemical and Philosophical; Chiefly Concerning Nitrous Oxide, or Dephlogisticated Nitrous Air, J. Johnson, London, 1800.
2. Gibson, W. C.: Young Endeavour. Contributions to Science by Medical Students of the Past Four Centuries, Charles C Thomas, Springfield, Illinois, 1958.
3. Bigelow, H. J.: Insensibility during surgical operations produced by inhalation, Boston Med Surg J, 1846, *35*, 309-317.
4. Morton, W. T. G.: Comparative value of sulphuric ether and chloroform, Boston Med Surg J, 1850, *43*, 109-119.
5. Poiseuille, J.-L.-M.: Recherches sur la Force du Coeur Aortique, Thèse No. 166, Didot, Paris, 1828.
6. Poiseuille, J.-L.-M.: Recherches expérimentales sur le mouvement des liquides dans les tubes de très petits diamètres, C R Acad Sci Paris, 1840, *11*,
961-967, 1041-1048.
7. Peterson, L. H., Dripps, R. D., and Risman, G. C.: A method for recording the arterial pressure pulse and blood pressure in man, Am Heart J, 1949, *37*, 771-782.
8. Landis, E. M.: The capillary pressure in frog mesentery as determined by micro-injection methods, Am J Physiol, 1926, *75*, 548-570.
9. Langerhans, P.: Beiträge zur mikroskopischen Anatomie der Bauchspeicheldrüse, Inaugural Dissertation, University of Berlin, 1869.
10. Banting, F. G., Best, C. H., Collip, J. B., Macleod, J. J. R., and Noble, E. C.: The effect of pancreatic extract (insulin) on normal rabbits, Am J Physiol, 1922, *62*, 162-176.
11. McLean, J.: The thromboplastic action of cephalin, Am J Physiol, 1916, *41*, 250-257.
12a. Cannon, W. B.: The movements of the stomach studied by means of the roentgen rays, Am J Physiol, 1898, *1*, 359-382.
12b. Cannon, W. B., and Moser, A.: The movements of the food in the esophagus, *Ibid.*, 434-444.
13. Fulton, J. F.: Muscular Contraction and the Reflex Control of Movement, Williams and Wilkins, Baltimore, 1926.
14. Breuer, J.: Die Selbsteuerung der Athmung durch den Nervus vagus, Sitzungsber Akad Wissen Wien, 1868, *58*, 909-937.
15. Ullmann, E.: About Hering and Breuer, in *Breathing: Hering-Breuer Centenary Symposium,* Ciba Foundation Symposium, R. Porter, ed., J. & A. Churchill, London, 1970, pp. 3-15.
16. Raynaud, M.: De l'Asphyxie Locale et de la Gangrène Symètrique des Extrémités, Rignoux, Paris, 1862.
17. Sandström, I. V.: Om en ny körtel hos menniskan och åtskilliga däggdjur, Upsala Lakaref Förh, 1880, *15*, 441-471.
18. Ehrlich, P.: Beiträge zur Kenntnis der Anilinfärbungen und ihrer Verwendung in der mikroskopischen Technik, Arch Mikrosk Anat, 1877, *13*, 263-277.
19. Dale, H. H.: Introduction, in *The Collected Papers of Paul Ehrlich,* F. Himmelweit, ed, Pergamon, London, 1956.
20. Thebesius, A. C.: Disputatio Medica Inauguralis de Circulo Sanguinis in Corde, A. Elzevier, Leyden, 1708.
21. Black, J.: Experiments upon Magnesia Alba, Quicklime and some other Alcaline Substances, William Creech, Edinburgh, 1796.
22. Bellini, L.: Exercitatio Anatomica de Structura et Usu Renum, Stella, Florence, 1662.
23. Young, T.: Observations on vision, Philos Trans R Soc Lond, 1793, *83*, 169-181.
24. Bert, P.: De la Greffe Animale, No. 118, J.-B. Baillière et fils, Paris, 1863.
25. Fulton, J. F.: Foreword, in Bert, P.: *Barometric Pressure,* M. A. Hitchcock and F. A. Hitchcock, trans., College Book Co., Columbus, Ohio, 1943.

26. Keith, A., and Flack, M.: The form and nature of the muscular connections between the primary divisions of the vertebrate heart, J Anat Physiol, 1907, *41*, 172-189.

27. Gibson, W. C.: Student discoveries in the pulmonary and cardiovascular systems, Chest, 1972, *61*, 283-286.

28. Swammerdam, J.: Biblia Naturae, sive Historia Insectorum, H. Boerhaave, ed., van der Aa and van der Aa, Leyden, 1737-38, Vol. II, pp. 832-833.

29. Evelyn, K. A.: A stabilized photoelectric colorimeter with light filters, J Biol Chem, 1936, *115*, 63-75.

30. MacCallum, W. G.: Notes on the pathological changes in the organs of birds infected with haemocytozoa, J Exp Med, 1898, *3*, 103-116.

31. Opie, E. L.: On the haemocytozoa of birds, J Exp Med, 1898, *3*, 79-101.

32. Ross, R.: Researches on malaria, Nobel lecture, December 12, 1902, in *Nobel Lectures, Physiology or Medicine, 1901-1921*, Elsevier, Amsterdam, 1967, pp. 65-67.

33. Harvey, A. M.: Medical students on the march: Brown, MacCallum and Opie, Johns Hopkins Med J, 1974, *134*, 330-345.

34. Vogl, A.: The discovery of the organic mercurial diuretics, Am Heart J, 1950, *39*, 1-4.

35. Lamy, G.: Lettre à M. Moreau contre les prétendues utilités de la transfusion, Paris, 1668.

36. Gibson, W. C.: Student medical researchers and their contributions, N Engl J Med, 1961, *264*, 802-810.

How To Make Hasenpfeffer

In July 1974, Congress amended the Public Health Service Act to establish National Research Service Awards. In this 1974 "National Research Act," Congress declared that "the success and continued viability of the Federal biomedical and behavioral research effort depends on the availability of excellent scientists and a network of institutions of excellence capable of producing superior research personnel." In short, Congress re-established NIH Research Fellowships and Research Training Programs. But with an important change—it asked the National Academy of Sciences to determine, year by year, the nation's over-all need for biomedical personnel, the subject areas in which research personnel are needed, and the number of personnel needed in each area. Congress also instructed the Secretary of HEW to make Fellowship and Training Awards to fill only these documented needs.

This seems to make sense. Until 1975, the number of Research Fellowships and Traineeships was determined by the law of supply and demand: *supply* for the most part meant how much money Congress appropriated and the National Institutes of Health allocated for training awards (and for research of newly trained scientists), and *demand* meant how many young men and women wanted a full-time or part-time career in medical research. Now the number trained will be determined by national need. For example, what needs to be decided for the lungs is what problems remain to be solved, the urgency of each, and how many scientists with what special training are needed to solve them. Then Congress will appropriate enough dollars to train the precise number of the right kinds of scientists, and the right kinds of young men and women will apply, be selected for research training, enter the training pipelines, come out in three to five years, and start turning out the right answers.

Now of course it isn't this simple. Every branch of medicine will want all of its problems solved all at once and there won't be enough dollars for trainee stipends or enough qualified candidates, enough trainers for the trainees, enough laboratories for them to work in, or enough research dollars in three or four years to pay for their research once they are established, independent scientists! And anyone who's been in the research business very long knows that not every trainee who looks good in the interview ought to do research at the end of his or her traineeship; indeed, one of the main purposes of putting people to work as research trainees is to see who's likely to succeed and who's not. So that means feeding more trainees into training programs than will be suited for research careers and likely to survive in the competition for research dollars. And the selection of the right number of trainees also depends on how many who are now in the research business retire, or die, or become deans.

I suppose all these problems that relate to numbers can be fed into computers and solved. But how do we get the right people to work on the right problems? Here the Retrospectroscope should tell us how to go about it. All we need to do is to identify 500 or 1,000 scientists who are already accepted as "superior research personnel," look into our Scope and see how they connected with the "right" field, i.e., that in which they made their important contribution. I've just completed step one of a pilot run. My plan couldn't be simpler: I said, "I'll collect the list of publications of some scientists who are highly regarded for their contributions to pulmonary or respiratory science and see how they entered scientific research. The easiest way to learn how they began is to read the first published scientific paper of each; I'll then know how to start the next generation on the right track." In table 1, I've collected the titles of the first articles published by 43 scientists. In Table 2, their names are listed alphabetically* (along with a few words identifying each with one or more fields of pulmonary or respiratory research).

---

* This list is not intended to represent my Roll of Honor or Hall of Fame since this would include **a**

TABLE 1

TITLES OF THE FIRST PUBLISHED SCIENTIFIC ARTICLE OF FORTY-THREE
SCIENTISTS WHOSE NAMES APPEAR ALPHABETICALLY IN TABLE 2

1. Hereditary elliptocytosis associated with increased hemolysis.
2. The gaseous metabolism of the submaxillary gland.
3. Intrapulmonary mixing of helium in health and in emphysema.
4. The action of ouabain (G-strophanthin) on the circulation in man, and a comparison with digoxin.
5. Factors promoting venous return from the arm in man.
6. Blood coagulation in haemorrhagic diseases.
7. The effect of testosterone proprionate on the arginase content of the liver, kidney and intestine.
8. Metabolism of leucocytes taken from peripheral blood of leukemic patients.
9. Les variations du sucre sanguin à la suite de l'injection intraveineuse de novarsénobenzol.
10. The respiratory rate and ventilation in the newborn baby.
11. The vaso-dilator action of potassium.
12. Syndrome de Looser, ostéopathie de famine et ostéomalacie.
13. Experimental studies on heteroplastic bone formation.
14. Fatty acid components in the unfertilized egg of arbacia punctulata.
15. Ueber die Bildung von Oxyden mehrwertiger Metalle aus ihren Hydroxyden.
16. Gas stores of the body and the unsteady state.
17. Salt antagonism in gelatine.
18. The medical use of thiocyanates in the treatment of arterial hypertension.
19. The measurement of intraesophageal pressure and its relationship to intrathoracic pressure.
20. The relation of philosophy to science.
21. On the morphology and mitosis of *Trichomonas buccalis*.
22. Pathogenesis of so-called diffuse vascular or collagen disease.
23. A propos d'un nouveau filtre sanguin à grand débit.
24. Influence de la teneur en calcium et en potassium du liquide céphalo-rachidien sur le système vasomoteur.
25. A note on the papillary adenoma of the corpus uteri.
26. The inhibition of frostbite wheals by the iontophoresis of anti-histaminic agents.
27. *Klebsiella* in respiratory disease.
28. Effect of certain drugs and ions on the oyster heart.
29. The surface tension of aqueous solutions of dipolar ions.
30. Demonstration of apparatus for recording muscle and nerve action potentials.
31. Histochemical studies on the lens following radiation injury.
32. Effect of cyanide on respiration of the protozoan, *Colpidium Campylum*.
33. Endobronchial tuberculosis.
34. Structure and function of placenta and corpus luteum in viviparous snakes.
35. Diet determinations. A graphic method.
36. Sulfapyridine therapy in pneumonia: Discussion of apparent failures and complications.
37. The reaction of vitamin A with Lieberman-Burchard reagent.
38. Calcium determination by flame photometry; method for serum, urine and other fluids.
39. Demonstration of anatomy of giant fiber system of squid by microinjection.
40. Observations on the physiology of the Lepidopteran heart, with special reference to reversal of the beat.
41. Zur Kenntnis der Differenzierungsvorgänge im Epithel des Ductus cochlearis.
42. Measurements of the ventilation-perfusion ratio inequality in the lung by the analysis of a single expirate.
43. Ligation of inferior vena cava.

Let's look at the titles in table 1. Only seven of the 43 titles really deal with respiration or the lungs—nine if we consider respiration in the very broadest sense. But even more astonishing is that in only five instances does the title of the first published article deal with the research area in

hundred or more names. My list does, however, include a broad sample: it contains some internists, pediatricians, anesthetists, anatomists, pathologists, physiologists, pharmacologists, biophysicists, bioengineers, four deans, three Nobel laureates (and some others who also deserved to be), the NHLI Director for Lung Diseases, and a few presidents of the American Thoracic Society. Regardless of the category, each has done superior research.

which the scientist eventually made his important contributions! I estimate that a National Committee charged with selecting appropriate research topics for pulmonary or respiratory fellows going into the 1975 training pipeline (to meet 1978 national needs) would reject 35 of the 43 areas of research. And I believe that a 1975 Congress would be concerned if the NHLI awarded a future pulmonary scientist a traineeship to study arbacia eggs, the oyster heart, viviparous snakes, the squid, or the lepidopteran heart. But since we're looking at the genesis of successful pulmonary scientists, there must be a lesson here.

The lesson seems to be that the first step in

46

recruiting a talented, creative scientist is to get him involved in science, in any science, in any field. (As Professor Carl Schmidt used to say: "In making hasenpfeffer, the first step is to catch the rabbit!") In their first paper, only seven scientists dealt with lungs or pulmonary ventilation. Four more entered the field with their second paper, an additional ten by their fifth paper, another six by their tenth paper, five more by their fifteenth, and another four by their twentieth. The other seven came aboard after twenty or more publications in other fields. Fenn had already distinguished himself in two other fields (muscle contraction and potassium metabolism) before he became a pulmonary physiologist.

To make manpower planning in specific areas even more complex, only about half of those on my list limited their research to the lungs and respiration once they entered the field. The other half occasionally, or often, worked in other areas and some left the field completely. Fry now works largely on experimental atherosclerosis. Pitts, after his classic studies on the respiratory centers, gained greater fame as a renal physiologist. U. S. von Euler, after his very important

TABLE 2

ALPHABETICAL LIST OF SCIENTISTS; THE TITLE OF THE FIRST PUBLISHED
ARTICLE OF EACH APPEARS SOMEWHERE IN TABLE 1

(Phrases in parentheses refer to area of best-known pulmonary or respiratory research of each scientist.)

1. Mary Ellen AVERY (Respiratory distress syndrome; lung metabolism)
2. Joseph BARCROFT (Oxygen and hemoglobin)
3. David V. BATES (Clinical pulmonary physiology)
4. William A. BRISCOE (Distribution of pulmonary ventilation and perfusion)
5. E. J. Moran CAMPBELL (Dyspnea; mechanical factors in breathing)
6. Ronald V. CHRISTIE (Emphysema; elastic properties of lungs; pulmonary function)
7. Leland C. CLARK (PO$_2$ electrode; artificial heart-lung; artificial blood)
8. John A. CLEMENTS (Pulmonary surfactant; respiratory distress syndrome)
9. André COURNAND (Intrapulmonary gas mixing; ventilation/perfusion ratios; clinical pulmonary physiology)
10. Kenneth W. CROSS (Respiration in newborn babies)
11. Geoffrey S. DAWES (Fetal and neonatal respiration and circulation; chemoreflexes)
12. Pierre DEJOURS (Chemoreflexes; regulation of breathing; exercise)
13. William DOCK (Ventilation and blood flow to lung apices)
14. Arthur B. DuBOIS (Body plethysmograph; pulmonary blood flow; clinical pulmonary physiology)
15. U. S. von EULER (Hypoxia and pulmonary arteriolar constriction; regulation of breathing)
16. Leon E. FARHI (Pulmonary and tissue gas exchange)
17. Wallace O. FENN (Pressure-volume curve; O$_2$ – CO$_2$ diagram)
18. Robert E. FORSTER (Pulmonary diffusing capacity; rapid reactions of hemoglobin)
19. Donald L. FRY (Pressure-volume-air flow relationships)
20. John S. HALDANE (Carbon dioxide and regulation of breathing)
21. H. Corwin HINSHAW (Chemotherapy of tuberculosis)
22. Jerome I. KLEINERMAN (Experimental pathology of pulmonary disease; emphysema)
23. Claude J. M. LENFANT (Comparative respiratory physiology; regulation of Hb - O$_2$ affinity)
24. Isidoor R. LEUSEN (Cerebrospinal fluid and regulation of breathing)
25. Averill A. LIEBOW (Pulmonary and bronchial circulations; lung pathology)
26. Jere MEAD (Mechanics of breathing)
27. Jay A. NADEL (Mechanisms of airway constriction; tantalum bronchograms)
28. Arthur B. OTIS (Work of breathing; hypoxia; comparative physiology)
29. John R. PAPPENHEIMER (Cerebrospinal fluid and regulation of breathing)
30. Richard E. PATTLE (Alveolar lining layer and surfactant)
31. Solbert PERMUTT (Mechanics of ventilation and of pulmonary blood flow)
32. Robert F. PITTS (Organization of the respiratory centers)
33. Donald F. PROCTOR (Upper and lower airways; air flow; pleural pressure)
34. Hermann RAHN (Gas exchange; inert gases; environmental physiology)
35. Dickinson W. RICHARDS (Pulmonary function; uneven alveolar ventilation; clinical pulmonary physiology)
36. Richard L. RILEY (Diffusing capacity; ventilation-perfusion ratios; airborne infection)
37. Eugene D. ROBIN (Intracellular acid-base metabolism and gas exchange; regulation of breathing; pulmonary embolism)
38. John W. SEVERINGHAUS (PCO$_2$ electrode; regulation of respiration; high altitude physiology)
39. Norman C. STAUB (Pulmonary capillaries, lymph and edema; pulmonary structure-function)
40. S. Marsh TENNEY (Adaptations to high altitude; regulation of breathing)
41. Ewald R. WEIBEL (Morphometry of the lung)
42. John B. WEST (Uneven distribution of gas and blood; gas exchange)
43. James L. WHITTENBERGER (Artificial respiration; mechanics of breathing)

work on regulation of breathing and the effects of hypoxia on the pulmonary circulation, won the Nobel Prize for his studies on norepinephrine and then went on to work on prostaglandins. Dickinson Richards was one of the giants in pulmonary physiology well before he (with Cournand) won the Nobel Prize for cardiovascular studies using the cardiac catheter. Einthoven (not on my list) did important work on the mechanics of breathing in 1892 before he invented the electrocardiogram.

My pilot study is open to many criticisms: It has looked at only those in the forefront of their field and not at those equally needed in science to confirm and extend the new discoveries and tie up the loose ends; it has looked only at those who entered scientific careers in an earlier era; it has *not* looked at those who tried their hand at research and decided that it was not for them. But even more important, this study gives no inkling of why each of the 43 gave science a try in the first place, who and what made it possible for him or her to stay in science, and why each initially or much later decided to work on pulmonary and respiratory problems. I know the answers to these why's, who's, and what's for my own career (see addendum # 2) but not for the 43 scientists in table 2—even for those whom I've known well for many years. Factors influencing career decisions and directions are usually quite complex.

What can we learn by this look into the Retro-spectroscope? First, that it is essential to get creative young men and women actually involved in research. *Any* research? Probably yes, because it seems that the first research project is for most young scientists a time for deciding whether research is the right career choice. Second, the young scientist should be encouraged to learn broadly in science, in anticipation of a change, sooner or later, in his research interests. And third, a field looking for research recruits will have no trouble attracting them if there are exciting and challenging problems to be solved.

Addenda

1. Sorry—I forgot to tell you which scientist in table 2 wrote which article whose title is in table 1. The order is the same in both tables: Avery wrote #1, Barcroft #2 and so on down to Whittenberger and #43. The journal reference for each is given in the references.

2. The title of *my* first paper had nothing to do with respiration or the lungs. It was "Further studies on the pharmacology of acetyl β-methyl choline and the ethyl ether of β-methyl choline." I did the work in the summer vacation between my second and third years of medical school, instead of spending the summer as usual playing tennis in my hometown of York, Pennsylvania. Why? Because I was engaged to marry a Philadelphia girl and I wanted to stay in Philadelphia. Simple enough. The answer to "Why did I stay in science?" is more complex, as indeed I suspect it is with most of us.

References

1. Pediatrics, 1955, *16*, 741-752.
2. J Physiol, 1900, *25*, 265-282.
3. Clin Sci, 1950, *9*, 17-29.
4. Clin Sci, 1950, *9*, 1-16.
5. Lancet, 1945, *1*, 460-461.
6. Q J Med, 1927, *20*, 471-480.
7. J Biol Chem, 1942, *143*, 795-796.
8. Cancer, 1951, *4*, 1009-1014.
9. C R Soc Biol, 1922, *86*, 714-717.
10. J Physiol, 1949, *109*, 459-574.
11. J Physiol, 1941, *99*, 224-238.
12. Rev Rhum, 1944, *11*, 134-142.
13. J Exp Med, 1920, *32*, 745-766.
14. Biol Bull, 1940, *79*, 354-355.
15. Z Anorg Allg Chem, 1922, *124*, 70-80.
16. J Appl Physiol, 1955, *7*, 472-484.
17. Proc Natl Acad Sci USA, 1916, *2*, 534-538.
18. Am J Med Sci, 1943, *206*, 668-686.
19. J Lab Clin Med, 1952, *40*, 664-673.
20. Essays in Philosophical Criticism, London, Longmans, 1883.
21. U Calif Publ Zool, 1926, *29*, 159-174.
22. Arch Int Med, 1949, *89*, 1-26.
23. Presse Méd, 1956, *64*, 382-383.
24. Arch Int Pharmacodyn, 1948, *75*, 422-424.
25. Yale J Biol Med, 1936, *8*, 353-356.
26. J Clin Invest, 1949, *28*, 564-566.
27. Ann Int Med, 1956, *45*, 1010-1026.
28. Physiol Zool, 1942, *15*, 418-435.
29. J Am Chem Soc, 1936, *58*, 1851-1855.
30. Proc R Soc Med, 1941, *35*, 78-79.
31. Arch Pathol, 1953, *55*, 20-30.
32. Proc Soc Exp Biol Med, 1932, *29*, 542-544.
33. Am Rev Tuberc, 1942, *45*, 477-483.
34. Proc Soc Exp Biol Med, 1939, *40*, 381-382.
35. Arch Int Med, 1927, *39*, 93-97.
36. Ann Int Med, 1940, *14*, 1032-1041.
37. Science, 1945, *102*, p. 17.
38. J Biol Chem, 1950, *187*, 621-630.
39. Proc Soc Exp Biol Med, 1954, *85*, 854-855.
40. Physiol Comp Oecol, 1953, *3*, 286-306.
41. Acta Anat, 1957, *29*, 53-90.
42. Clin Sci, 1957, *16*, 529-547.
43. Arch Surg, 1940, *41*, 1334-1343.

48

Roast Pig and Scientific Discovery

Part I

"Mankind, says a Chinese manuscript, for the first seventy thousand ages ate their meat raw, clawing or biting it from the living animal.... The manuscript goes on to say that the art of roasting, or rather broiling (which I take to be the elder brother) was accidentally discovered in the manner following. The swine-herd, Ho-ti, having gone out into the woods one morning, as his manner was, to collect mast for his hogs, left his cottage in the care of his eldest son Bo-bo, a great lubberly boy, who being fond of playing with fire, as younkers of his age commonly are, let some sparks escape into a bundle of straw, which kindling quickly, spread the conflagration over every part of their poor mansion, till it was reduced to ashes. Together with the cottage . . . what was of much more importance, a fine litter of new-farrowed pigs, no less than nine in number perished. . . . Bobo was in utmost consternation, as you may think, not so much for the sake of the tenement, which his father and he could easily build up again with a few dry branches, and the labour of an hour or two, at any time, as for the loss of the pigs. While he was thinking what he should say to his father, and wringing his hands over the smoking remnants of one of those untimely sufferers, an odor assailed his nostrils, unlike any scent which he had before experienced. What could it proceed from?—not from the burnt cottage—he had smelt that smell before—indeed this was by no means the first accident of the kind which had occurred through the negligence of this unlucky young firebrand. Much less did it resemble that of any known herb, weed, or flower. A premonitory moistening at the same time overflowed his nether lip. He knew not what to think. He next stooped down to feel the pig, if there were any signs of life in it. He burnt his fingers, and to cool them he applied them in his booby fashion to his mouth. Some of the crumbs of the scorched skin had come away with his fingers, and for the first time in his life (in the world's life, indeed, for before him no man had known it) he tasted—*crackling*! Again he felt and fumbled at the pig. It did not burn him so much now, still he licked his fingers from a sort of habit. The truth at length broke into his slow

understanding, that it was the pig that smelt so, and the pig that tasted so delicious; and surrendering himself up to the newborn pleasure, he fell to tearing up whole handfuls of the scorched skin with the flesh next it, and was cramming it down his throat in his beastly fashion, when his sire entered amid the smoking rafters, armed with retributory cudgel, and finding how affairs stood, began to rain blows upon the young rogue's shoulders, as thick as hailstones, which Bo-bo heeded not any more than if they had been flies. The tickling pleasure which he experienced in his lower regions had rendered him quite callous to any inconveniences he might feel in those remote quarters. His father might lay on, but he could not beat him from his pig, till he had fairly made an end of it, when, becoming a little more sensible of his situation, something like the following dialogue ensued.

"You graceless whelp, what have you got there devouring? Is it not enough that you have burnt me down three houses with your dog's tricks, and be hanged to you! but you must be eating fire, and I know not what—what have you got there, I say?"

"O, father, the pig, the pig! do come and taste how nice the burnt pig eats."

Bo-bo, whose scent was wonderfully sharpened since morning, soon raked out another pig, and fairly rending it asunder, thrust the lesser half by main force into the fists of Ho-ti, still shouting out "Eat, eat, eat the burnt pig, father, only taste—O Lord!"—with such-like barbarous ejaculations, cramming all the while as if he would choke. . . .

In conclusion (for the manuscript here is a little tedious), both father and son fairly sat down to the mess, and never left off till they had despatched all that remained of the litter." (1)

Charles Lamb, in his "Dissertation upon Roast Pig" then continues his narration: Ho-ti's cottage was from that time on quickly rebuilt and just as quickly burnt down, until soon father and son were haled into court along with the atrocious evidence (burnt pig). Within a few days after the trial (during which the jury acquitted both father and son) the judge's and jury's houses were a-burning and "there was nothing to be seen but fires in every direction. . . . Eventually, a sage arose who made a discovery that the flesh of swine, or indeed of any other animal, might be cooked (*burnt,* as they called it) without consuming a whole house."

This is one of the earliest accounts of the important role of *Chance* in scientific discovery and the wondrous benefits to mankind that accrue from it. Some like to call it "serendipity"— a word coined by Horace Walpole in 1754, based on the title of a fairytale, "The Three Princes of Serendip," (the former name of Ceylon) the heroes of which were always making discoveries, by accidents and sagacity, of things they were not in quest of—the faculty of making happy and unexpected discoveries. The definition comes from the *Oxford English Dictionary;* some wag's more recent definition is that serendipity is looking for a needle in a haystack but coming up with the farmer's daughter. (I accept the latter only if modified to read—"but coming up with an ugly toad which the finder recognizes as the farmer's beautiful daughter and miraculously converts toad to daughter.")

So many have written on *Chance* or *Serendipity* in science that, in writing once more, I should do more than entertain you with the same or additional stories. Because the main purpose of my peering into a retrospectroscope is to examine the past to learn a lesson or two that will help us in the present and future, this look should lead to some useful, or at least controversial, recommendations. It will, but I have put these at the end of Part II. First, I want to give examples of two types of discoveries in which chance played an important role: (A) some in which chance helped a scientist to reach his committed goal or get to it more quickly and (B) those in which chance changed his goals and set him in a new direction.

A. CHANCE SPEEDED OR COMPLETED A SCIENTIST'S ONGOING WORK

The Cholecystogram
Everyone in medicine and surgery knows that Evarts Graham was a leader of pulmonary surgery in this country. But he was more than that. In 1909, Abel and Rowntree had shown that chlorinated phenolphthaleins were excreted al-

most entirely in the bile and it occurred to Graham and his associates that if they could substitute a radiopaque element for chlorine, they should be able to get a roentgenographic shadow of the contents and contours of the gall bladder. The element they selected was iodine, and the compound sodium tetraiodophenolphthalein. Warren Cole, then a resident in surgery, did the injections.

Six dogs were injected intravenously, and x-ray photographs were made of the gall bladder regions in all of them at frequent intervals after the injection. In five of the dogs no shadow was obtained, but fortunately a faint shadow was obtained in the sixth one. At first we were at a loss to understand why we had obtained a faint shadow in one dog but none at all in the other five animals. The idea then occurred to us that the reason for the failure was probably due to the fact that the animals were not fasting and that, therefore, the injected substance was not staying in the gall bladder for a long enough time to be concentrated and, therefore, to make a shadow. From the standpoint of the future development of cholecystography we often feel grateful to that one dog which cast a shadow, probably because he was accidentally given no food. If we had failed to get a shadow in all of these animals we probably should have abandoned the whole idea as a fruitless one. It is curious on how fragile a thread the destiny of some events hangs. When we came to investigate the matter we found that, as a matter of fact, through some mishap the animal keeper during the time of the experiment had for some reason neglected to feed the one dog on the morning of the injection but he had fed all of the others. Greater efficiency on the part of the animal keeper would doubtless have resulted in a complete failure of our experiment and, therefore, we would have given up the whole idea. Sometimes efficiency can be a curse. (2)

Staining of Tubercle Bacilli
On March 24, 1882, Robert Koch lectured to the Physiological Society of Berlin on the etiology of tuberculosis. After pointing out that one seventh of all people die of tuberculosis and that the mortality rate is especially high (one-third or more) for those in their potentially productive middle age years, he then described his method for staining tubercle bacilli in sputum and tissue (3). In the audience was Paul Ehrlich, whose 1878 doctoral thesis dealt with the affinity of dyes for specific tissues. After the lecture, Ehrlich went to his laboratory and set up slides covered with tuberculous sputum. He

stained these according to Koch's directions and left them overnight on the cold laboratory stove. In the morning the charwoman in the laboratory started the fire, which speeded the staining by its effect on the waxy-coated bacteria so that when Ehrlich arrived, the tubercle bacilli were everywhere to be seen. On communicating this information and on showing the slides to Robert Koch, the latter became so impressed that he turned his investigations toward the causes underlying the disease rather than to mere descriptions of the effects of tuberculosis (4). Koch said, "We owe it to this circumstance alone that it has become a general custom to search for the bacillus in sputum" (5).

Gram Stain

Beveridge (5) recounts the origin of this stain:

A Danish physician, while staining bacteria, inadvertently took the wrong bottle from the rack and poured Lugol's iodine on a smear which he had been staining with gentian violet. Thinking his preparation had been spoilt, he tried to wash out the stain with alcohol so that he could start again. But when he examined the smear to see if he had decolourised it he found that many of the bacteria retained a deep purple colour. There is no need to tell readers who are bacteriologists that the name of the Dane was Gram, for the staining technique he developed as a result of this "accident" has made his name a familiar word in every bacteriological laboratory.

Positive Pressure Respiration

Alvan Barach devoted his medical lifetime to scientific and clinical pulmonary medicine and is especially known for his pioneering work on oxygen, helium-oxygen therapy, pressure breathing, and the equalizing-pressure chamber. He decided to be a pulmonary physician when he was five years old (that was in 1900) and watched his family physican terminate a severe attack of laryngeal dyspnea in his mother. His "one aim, one business, one desire" was to study breathing difficulties, as he put it years later (6).

Some years ago, he gave me this account of what he had learned from a patient. He was examining a patient with severe asthma (or emphysema) and noted that on every expiration, the patient pursed his lips and breathed out against this additional resistance. Barach thought this to be an unnecessarily tiring experience for his patient and said, "Look here. Watch how I breathe in and out—slowly and fully, with my mouth open—never through pursed lips. Now

you do it." The good patient tried to emulate Barach's pattern and soon turned blue. Barach immediately realized the importance of the patient's pattern in maintaining a positive airway pressure during expiration and preventing early collapse of diseased airways. Barach "told it like it was" in 1938 (7), when he gave this as his explanation of why patients with asthma and emphysema so frequently pursed their lips during expiration and arbitrarily increased the resistance to the egress of air:

This mechanism, developed by the patients themselves, appeared to have the physiological advantage of keeping open bronchiolar passageways, thereby producing a more efficient emptying of the alveolar air. It was suggested that the expiratory grunt in lobar pneumonia was a similar protective mechanism. Furthermore, it was found that patients with more or less continuous asthma of moderate degree will frequently obtain marked relief of their wheezing when they follow the instruction to breathe through partially closed lips for 3 to 10 minutes. The râles in expiration will at times clear up immediately, apparently due to distending the bronchioles through internal pressure. This observation provided an additional stimulus to employ positive pressure respiration in the treatment of acute pulmonary edema; we reported in a preliminary communication three cases in which a swift clearance of the moist râles in the chest took place, even in the presence of advanced circulatory deficiency. (7)

Coarctation of the Aorta

Successful closure of the ductus arteriosus in children in 1938 emboldened cardio-thoracic surgeons to eye repair of aortic coarctation as the next target. However, this operation required clamping the thoracic aorta above and below the aortic constriction long enough to perform an end-to-end anastomosis of the aorta, and the fear of ischemic paralysis in the lower half of the body held back a rush to deal with coarctation. However, in the early 1940s, Clarence Crafoord in Stockholm had a bad day in operating on a patient with a patent ductus arteriosus. The patient's ductus tore loose, leaving a gaping hole in the aorta. Crafoord had no choice but to clamp the aorta until he could sew the hole in it. The aorta was clamped almost 30 minutes but the patient recovered with no sign of paralysis of the lower extremities (8). Crafoord reasoned that, because patients with coarctation of the aorta usually have well-developed collateral circulation between the upper and the lower part of the body, he would have sufficient additional time in these patients to repair their constricted aorta. He decided it was time to go ahead, and performed two successful operations in October 1944 (9).

It was the combination of the accidental experience with the ductus and clear reasoning that led Crafoord to perform resection of the coarcted segment and end-to-end anastomosis in the successful treatment of coarctation of the aorta.

Sulfapyridine

Sulfapyridine is no longer an official drug (its only indication now is to treat dermatitis herpetiformis), but in the years 1938 to 1945, when sulfanilamide did not cure pneumococcal pneumonia and penicillin (which did) was not readily available, sulfapyridine was life saving in patients with pneumonia. I will never forget the excitement in Philadelphia in 1938 when Flippin and Pepper (10) published the first report on the use of sulfapyridine in the United States in case after case of pneumococcal pneumonia, both of whom recovered.

It was Lionel Whitby (later Sir Lionel) in England who did the first laboratory and clinical studies of the effectiveness of sulfapyridine against pneumococcal pneumonia. He was in the midst of testing the new drug in mice:

Mice inoculated with pneumococci were being dosed throughout the day, but were not treated during the night. Sir Lionel had been out to a dinner party and before returning home visited the laboratory to see how the mice were getting on, and while there light heartedly gave the mice a further dose of the drug. These mice resisted the pneumococci better than any mice had ever done before. Not till about a week later did Sir Lionel realize that it was the extra dose at midnight which had been responsible for the excellent results. From that time, both mice and men were dosed day and night when under sulfonamide treatment and they benefited much more than under the old routine. (5)

Experimental Hypophysectomy

In a personal communication to W. I. B. Beveridge (5), Dr. A. V. Nalbandov told the following intriguing story of how he discovered the simple method of keeping chickens alive after the surgical removal of the pituitary gland (hypophysectomy):

In 1940 I became interested in the effects of hypophysectomy of chickens. After I had mastered the surgical technique my birds continued to die and within a few weeks after the operation none remained alive. Neither replacement therapy nor any other precautions taken helped and I was about ready to agree with A. S. Parkes and R. T. Hill who had done similar operations in England, that hypophysectomized chickens simply cannot live. I resigned myself to doing a few short-term experiments and dropping the whole project when suddenly 98% of a group of hypophysectomized birds survived for 3 weeks and a great many lived for as long as 6 months. The only explanation I could find was that my surgical technique had improved with practice. At about this time, and when I was ready to start a long-term experiment, the birds again started dying and within a week both recently operated birds and those which had lived for several months, were dead. This, of course, argued against surgical proficiency. I continued with the project since I now knew that they could live under some circumstances which, however, eluded me completely. At about this time I had a second successful period during which mortality was very low. But, despite careful analysis of records (the possibility of disease and many other factors were considered and eliminated) no explanation was apparent. You can imagine how frustrating it was to be unable to take advantage of something that was obviously having a profound effect on the ability of these animals to withstand the operation. Late one night I was driving home from a party via a road which passes the laboratory. Even though it was 2 A.M. lights were burning in the animal rooms. I thought that a careless student had left them on so I stopped to turn them off. A few nights later I noted again that lights had been left on all night. Upon enquiry it turned out that a substitute janitor, whose job it was to make sure at midnight that all the windows were closed and doors locked, preferred to leave on the lights in the animal room in order to be able to find the exit door (the light switches not being near the door). Further checking showed that the two survival periods coincided with the times when the substitute janitor was on the job. Controlled experiments soon showed that hypophysectomized chickens kept in darkness all died while chickens lighted for 2 one-hour periods nightly lived indefinitely. The explanation was that birds in the dark do not eat and develop hypoglycaemia from which they cannot recover, while birds which are lighted eat enough to prevent hypoglycaemia. Since that time we no longer experience any trouble in maintaining hypophysectomized birds for as long as we wish.

Experimental Poliomyelitis

Landsteiner discovered poliovirus in 1909 and reported the experimental transmission of poliomyelitis to monkeys. However, a satisfactory vaccine against polio was not developed until the 1950s and early 1960s. Part of this long delay was due to a conviction that poliomyelitis could be transmitted only to monkeys and chimpanzees, and, in pre-NIH days, this limited research on experimental polio to a few well-endowed research centers that could afford to pay for monkeys. A discovery that enabled both poor and rich to work on experimentally produced polio was the finding of Armstrong in 1939 that polio could be transmitted to the cotton rat (*Sigmodon hispidus hispidus*) and from it to the white mouse (11).

Paul, in his *History of Poliomyelitis* (12), tells about Armstrong's discovery:

I have many times tried to extract the reasons from . . . Charles Armstrong which prompted him to attempt to adapt poliovirus to cotton rats instead of to mice. Rats would seem to have been a singularly unfavorable species of rodent, particularly since many a trial had shown that they are quite resistant to the commoner viral infections that attack man. . . .

The only satisfactory answer I could ever obtain from Dr. Armstrong was that there was currently at the NIH a colony of various species of rats being used in investigations on Weil's disease, a spirochaetal infection transmitted to man by rats. Apparently an excess supply of these rodents, including a specimen of the cotton rat (*Sigmodon hispidus hispidus*), was turned over to Dr. Armstrong, who promptly tested its susceptibility to the Lansing strain of poliovirus.

Armstrong's first experiments were begun in November 1937. Luck was with him on two counts: in his choice of the particular species of rat as the test animal; and in his choice of the Lansing strain, eventually identified as belonging to Type II poliovirus, which, as it turned out later, was the type most amenable to this sort of adaptation. He began by inoculating the 19th monkey passage of Lansing virus into several species of rodents, including one cotton rat. This lone animal remained well until the 25th day, when it developed a disease resembling experimental poliomyelitis, and lo and behold, when it was sacrificed the pathological report confirmed the diagnosis. . . .

This discovery, soon confirmed by others, meant that at last a strain of poliovirus was available that could be used to study the experimental disease in a far cheaper animal than the monkey. It meant neutralization tests could be done by using this strain with a sufficient number of animals to yield statistically significant results. Infinitely more important, instead of there being only a few laboratories which could afford to work with polioviruses, many could now join in the attack. In fact, Armstrong's discovery turned out to be one of those tremendously significant ones that have occasionally punctuated the history of poliomyelitis and turned it in a new direction. It suddenly accelerated progress that had only been inching along during the previous decade. A new era had begun. . . .

Charles Armstrong's discovery in 1939 suddenly shed a completely new light on the behavior of poliovirus, with implications which neither he nor anyone else had appreciated or even contemplated. Not only could mice replace monkeys as the test animal in many studies of experimental poliomyelitis, but investigators could start considering the possibility that they might, after all, manipulate strains of poliovirus so as to change their virulence for humans without altering their antigenicity. As a result, such strains might be used as immunizing agents in man.

B. CHANCE CHANGED A SCIENTIST'S GOAL

Penicillin

Almost everyone knows the story of the penicillium mold that floated in the breeze through an open window onto an open culture plate in Alexander Fleming's laboratory. In accepting the Nobel award in 1945, Fleming said (13):

In my first publication I might have claimed that I had come to the conclusion, as a result of serious study of the literature and deep thought, that valuable antibacterial substances were made by moulds and that I set out to investigate the problem. That would have been untrue and I preferred to tell the truth that penicillin started as a chance observation.

And on another occasion Fleming said:

There are thousands of different molds, and there are thousands of different bacteria, and that chance put that mold in the right spot at the right time was like winning the Irish Sweepstakes. (14)

Actually, practically the same incident happened in Tyndall's laboratory in 1877, when penicillium mold and airborne bacteria alighted on the same spot on Tyndall's culture plates and the mold mopped up the bacteria. But Tyndall was a physicist interested in, among other things, scattering of light by unseen particles floating in air; although he helped Pasteur in winning his fight against the theory of spontaneous generation, it was by using his new physical methods to identify air that was "optically pure" and air that was not.

Fleming never proved that penicillin was an antibiotic in animals or man and never purified the substance. That fell to Florey, Chain, and the Oxford group. Chance also favored them in three ways. First, they did not begin their study in the hope of finding a clinically useful antibiotic; second, they elected, for no known reason, to infect mice and not guinea pigs (they were indeed lucky because penicillin is nontoxic to mice and quite toxic to guinea pigs); and third, although they believed their stable extract to be pure penicillin, 99 per cent of the extract consisted of impurities and only 1 per cent was penicillin. (Had the combined effect of the impurities been toxic—it was *not*—it would have masked completely the safety of penicillin and might have delayed further attempts for some years [15]).

Percussion and Auscultation

Another oft-quoted example of chance is that three factors led Auenbrugger to use the technic of percussion in medicine. (*1*) His father was an innkeeper who regularly tapped on his barrels to learn how much was liquid and how much was air. (*2*) Auenbrugger was an accomplished musician with an excellent ear for pitch. (*3*) He chose medicine for his career instead of music or innkeeping. And two factors led Laennec to devise his stethoscope. In the introduction to the second part ("Diagnosis") of his *Treatise,* Laennec wrote:

In 1816, I was consulted by a young woman labouring under general symptoms of diseased heart, and in whose case percussion and the application of the hand were of little avail on account of the great degree of fatness. The other method just mentioned being rendered inadmissable by the age and sex of the patient, I happened to recollect a simple and well-known fact in acoustics, and fancied at the same time, that it might be turned to some use on the present occasion. The fact I allude to is the augmented impression of sound when conveyed through certain solid bodies, as when we hear the scratch of a pin at one end of a piece of wood, on applying our ear to the other. Immediately, on this suggestion, I rolled a quire of paper into a sort of cylinder and applied one end of it to the region of the heart and the other to my ear, and was not a little surprised and pleased, to find that I could thereby perceive the action of the heart in a manner much more clear and distinct than I had ever been able to do by the immediate application of the ear. From this moment I imagined that the circumstance might furnish means for enabling us to ascertain the character, not only of the action of the heart, but of every species of sound produced by the motion of all thoracic viscera. (16)

The Pancreas and Diabetes Mellitus

Von Mering and Minkowski, professors at the University of Strasbourg, were engaged in 1889 in studying the external secretion of the pancreas and particularly its role in digestion. As part of their research, they learned to remove the pancreas completely from dogs. A laboratory assistant noted that large numbers of flies swarmed about the urine of a dog whose pancreas had been removed and called this observation to the professors' attention. Minkowski analyzed the urine and found it loaded with sugar. It was this chance finding that led to the certain knowledge that the pancreas had multiple functions, one of which was to regulate the concentration of blood glucose.

Ergotoxine-Epinephrine Interaction

Although at first glance, this observation seemed to be only a pharmacologic curiosity, it led first to the knowledge that epinephrine had two types of actions, then to their separation by the ability of certain drugs to block what we now call α-receptors and finally to finding β-receptors and drugs that stimulate and block those. Sir Henry Dale tells how it came about (17):

In 1904, however, at the age of 29, faced with what then seemed a rather bleak academic prospect, I accepted a research post in the Wellcome Physiological Research Laboratories, then at Herne Hill. These laboratories did a number of important services to the business of Burroughs Wellcome & Co., but they were also rather a pet project of the sole proprietor of that business, Mr. (later Sir) Henry S. Wellcome, who told me that it was his wish that research of permanent value to science might be done there. . . . When I accepted the appointment, Mr. Wellcome said to me that, when I could find an opportunity for it without interfering with plans of my own, it would give him a special satisfaction if I would make an attempt to clear up the problem of ergot, the pharmacy, pharmacology and therapeutics of that drug being then in a state of obvious confusion. Pharmacological research was for me a complete novelty, and I was, frankly, not at all attracted by the prospect of making my first excursion into it on the ergot morass. . . . Barger . . . had already prepared from ergot a number of the substances which then figured in the pharmacological literature, with claims made for each to be ergot's "active principle." I thought that I might make a beginning by testing some of these, for the kind of pharmacological activity which was within reach of my limited technical competence. So I began with their effects on the arterial blood-pressure of the anaesthetized, or, more commonly, the spinal cat.

54

... By one of my greatest strokes of good fortune, however, it was to give me an immediate opportunity of making a mistake of my own—a really shocking "howler." I was finishing one of these experiments on a spinal cat, to which I had given successive doses of one of Barger's ergot preparations, when a sample of dried suprarenal gland substance was delivered to me from the Burroughs Wellcome factory, with a request that I would test it for the presence of a normal proportion of adrenaline. The moment seemed opportune; a boiled extract was easily prepared, and there was a cat most suitable, as it seemed, for the required test. Successive injections of the extract elicited, to my surprise, only falls of the arterial pressure, and, with the confidence of inexperience, I condemned the sample without hesitation. And then, by another and almost incredibly fortunate coincidence, the same sequence of events was repeated in detail a week later. Again I was finishing an experiment on a spinal cat, which again had been heavily dosed with an ergot preparation, when a sample of suprarenal gland substance was again delivered for testing. Quite possibly it was from the same batch again, sent to control not only the quality of the material, but also the competence of the new young pharmacologist; but that was never revealed to me. The result was, of course, the same as on the earlier occasion; but reference to my notes now raised the question whether the cat's response to adrenaline might have been so altered, by the heavy doses of ergot given in both cases, that the normal, pressor action had been reversed. It seemed unlikely, but control tests showed promptly that, in an animal not thus treated with ergot, both samples of the suprarenal material had the usual pressor action, representing a normal content of adrenaline, and then that treatment with ergot reversed this action of pure adrenaline itself.

Epinephrine and Ephedrine

The striking effects of each of these on blood pressure and on the sympathetic nervous system were first noted by chance. Sir Henry Dale (18) tells the story of how Oliver and Schäfer discovered the action of an extract from the adrenal medulla:

Dr. George Oliver, a physician of Harrogate, employed his winter leisure in experiments on his family, using apparatus of his own devising for clinical measurements. In one such experiment he was applying an instrument for measuring the thickness of the radial artery; and, having given his young son, who deserves a special memorial, an injection of an extract of the suprarenal gland, prepared from material supplied by the local butcher, Oliver thought that he detected a contraction or, according to some who have trans-

mitted the story, an expansion of the radial artery. Whichever it was, he went up to London to tell Professor Schäfer what he thought he had observed, and found him engaged in an experiment in which the blood pressure of a dog was being recorded; found him, not unnaturally, incredulous about Oliver's story and very impatient at the interruption. But Oliver was in no hurry, and urged only that a dose of his suprarenal extract, which he produced from his pocket, should be injected into a vein when Schäfer's own experiment was finished. And so, just to convince Oliver that it was all nonsense, Schäfer gave the injection, and then stood amazed to see the mercury mounting in the arterial manometer till the recording float was lifted almost out of the distal limb.

Ephedrine was an old Chinese herbal remedy unknown to Western medicine. In 1922–24, Carl Schmidt, then an instructor in pharmacology at the University of Pennsylvania, went to China for two years to be an associate in pharmacology at Peking Union Medical College where he worked with K. K. Chen, who had just received a Ph.D. in Physiology at Wisconsin. Although their goal was to uncover active drugs from a huge number of remedies listed in Chinese *Materia Medica*, they were both skeptical, to the point of baiting a Chinese druggist with the question, "Is there a really potent drug in this whole group of native herbs?" The druggist responded by giving them a sample of Ma Huang. The two pharmacologists put it on a shelf and went about their other studies. In 1923 they remembered the Ma Huang, made a decoction from it and injected it intravenously in an anesthetized dog still alive at the end of a student experiment. Like Schäfer some years before with adrenaline, they were amazed to observe a tremendous, long-lasting rise in systemic arterial blood pressure (19). The Chinese druggist's Ma Huang put Chen into a long and productive career of pharmacology and for 34 years he directed pharmacological research at Eli Lilly & Co.

References

1. Lamb, Charles: A dissertation upon roast pig, in *The Essays of Elia*, orig. ed. 1823, reprinted 1892, Little, Brown Co., Boston.
2. Graham, E. A.: The story of the development of cholecystography, Am J Surg, 1931, *12*, 330–335.
3. Koch, R.: Die Aetiologie der Tuberculose, Berlin Klin Wochenschr, 1882, *19*, 221–230. En-

glish translation, deRouville, W., Med Classics, 1937–1938, *2*, 853–880.

4. Gibson, W. C.: Young Endeavour. Contributions to Science by Medical Students of the Past Four Centuries, Charles C Thomas, Springfield, Ill., 1958.

5. Beveridge, W. I. B.: The Art of Scientific Investigation, Random House, New York, 1950.

6. Barach, A. L., in *Who's Who in America, 1974–1975*, ed. 38, vol. 1. p. 152.

7. Barach, A. L., Martin, J., and Eckman, M.: Positive pressure respiration and its application to the treatment of acute pulmonary edema, Ann Intern Med, 1938, *12*, 754–795.

8. Johnson, S. L.: The History of Cardiac Surgery 1896–1955, Johns Hopkins Press, Baltimore, Md., 1970.

9. Crafoord, C., and Nylin, G.: Congenital coarctation of the aorta and its surgical treatment, J Thorac Surg, 1945, *14*, 347–361.

10. Flippin, H. F., and Pepper, D. S.: The use of 2 (*p*-aminobenzenesulphonamido) pyridine in the treatment of pneumonia. A preliminary report, Am J Med Sci, N. S., 1938, *196*, 509–513.

11. Paul, J. R.: A History of Poliomyelitis, Yale University Press, New Haven, Conn., 1971.

12. Armstrong, C.: The experimental transmission of poliomyelitis to the eastern cotton rat, *Sigmodon hispidus hispidus*, USPHS Pub Health Rep. 1939, *54*, 1719–1721.

13. Fleming, A.: Penicillin, in *Nobel Lectures, Physiology or Medicine, 1942–1962*, Elsevier, Amsterdam, 1964.

14. Austin, J. H.: The roots of serendipity, Sat Rev World, November 1974, pp. 60–64.

15. Taton, R.: Reason and Chance in Scientific Discovery, A. J. Pomerans, trans., Hutchinson Scientific and Technical, London, 1957.

16. Willius, F. A., and Keys, T. E.: Classics of Cardiology, vol. 1, Dover Publications, New York, 1941, p. 326.

17. Dale, H. H.: Adventures in Physiology with Excursions into Autopharmacology, Pergamon Press, London, 1953.

18. Dale, H.: Accident and opportunism in medical research, Br Med J, 1948, *2*, 451–455.

19. Chen, K. K., and Schmidt, C. F.: The action of ephedrine, the active principle of the Chinese drug, Ma Huang, J Pharmacol Exp Ther, 1924, *24*, 339–357.

Roast Pig and Scientific Discovery

Part II

In Part I,I gave a classic instance of Chance, or Serendipity, related by Charles Lamb in his "Dissertation upon Roast Pig." In this essay, Lamb tells how many centuries ago Bo-Bo, the Chinese swineherd's son, stumbled upon the delicacy of roast pork when he accidentally burned down his father's house and barn and in the process roasted ("burnt") nine newly farrowed pigs. I then gave (A) eight examples in which chance speeded or completed a scientist's ongoing work and (B) five examples in which chance changed the direction of a scientist's work and pointed him toward a new goal. In Part II, I will give more examples of a change in direction of a scientist's work that resulted from chance, and speculate on the role of chance in speeding the advance of science.

Anaphylaxis

"Phylaxis," a word seldom used, comes from the Greek, meaning "protection." "Anaphylaxis" means, strictly speaking, *"without protection"* and, therefore, hypersensitive; in its usual context, it means that the first injection of a substance, instead of conferring protection against a second injection, makes the organism hypersensitive. Charles Richet, Nobel Laureate in Physiology, 1913, tells how he discovered the phenomenon (20):

These are the circumstances under which I first observed this phenomenon. You will allow me to go into some details on the origins. You will find that it is by no means the result of profound thought but a simple observation, almost a fortuitous one; so that my merit has only been in letting myself see the facts which were plain before me.

In tropical waters, Coelenterata are to be found floating on the surface, also known as Physalia (Portuguese galleys). The basic structure of these creatures is a pocket filled with air so that they can float like a bladder. A bucco-anal cavity is subjoined to this pocket, with very long tentacles which hang in the water. These feelers sometimes run to two or three meters long and are equipped with small devices which adhere like sucking cups to objects encountered. Within each of these innumerable suction-cups is a pin-point which drives into the foreign body that is being touched. At the same time, this pin-point causes penetration of a subtle but strong poison, which is contained in the tentacles, so that contact with a feeler of the Physalia is tantamount to a multiple injection of poison. On touching a Physalia an acute sensation of pain is felt immediately, due to the penetration of this liquid venom. This is similar in relative intensity to a swimmer's mishap when he bumps into a jelly-fish in the water.

During a cruise on the yacht of Prince Albert of Monaco, the Prince advised me to study Physalia poison, together with our friends Georges Richard and Paul Portier. We found that it is easily dissolved in glycerol and that by injecting this glycerol solution, the symptoms of Physalia poisoning are reproduced.

When I came back to France and had no more Physalia to study, I hit upon the idea of making a comparative study of the tentacles of the Actinia (*Actinia equina, Anemone sulcata*) which can be obtained in large quantities, for Actinia abound on all the rocky shores of Europe.

Now Actinia tentacles, treated with glycerol, give off their poison into the glycerol and the extract is toxic. I therefore set about finding how toxic it was, with Portier. This was quite difficult to do, as it is a slowly acting poison and three or four days must elapse before it can be known if the dose be fatal or not. I was using a solution of one kilo of glycerol to one kilo of tentacles. The lethal dose was of the order of 0.1 liquid per kilo live weight of subject.

But certain of the dogs survived, either because the dose was not strong enough or for some other reason. At the end of two, three or four weeks, as they seemed normal, I made use of them for a new experiment (italics added).

An unexpected phenomenon arose, which we thought extraordinary. A dog when injected previously even with the smallest dose, say of 0.005 liquid per kilo, immediately showed serious symptoms: vomiting, blood diarrhoea, syncope, unconsciousness, asphyxia and death. This basic experiment was repeated at various times and by 1902 we were able to state three main factors which are the corner-stone of the history of anaphylaxis: (1) a subject that had a previous injection is far more sensitive than a new subject; (2) that the symptoms characteristic of the second injection, namely swift and total depression of the nervous system, do not in any way resemble the symptoms characterizing the first injection; (3) a three or four week period must elapse before the anaphylactic state results. This is the period of incubation.

It is said that lightning never strikes twice in the same place, but read how Sir Henry Dale discovered in 1913 that anaphylactic contraction of smooth muscle resulted from the formation of cell-fixed antibodies (21):

Then I had another stroke of luck. I was studying a rather weak activity of a similar kind which fresh blood serum exhibited when it was applied to strips of involuntary muscle taken from a dead guinea-pig, and I suddenly encountered a strip of this tissue from one particular guinea-pig which responded with a contraction of peculiar violence when it was treated with a mere trace of horse serum, though it behaved quite normally in the presence of blood serum from other animals—cat, dog, rabbit, sheep, or man. And it occurred to me that many guinea-pigs in that laboratory were used for testing the strength of antitoxic horse serum, and that an economically minded colleague might have provided me with a survivor from such a test. The verification of that suspicion gave us a new idea about the meaning of the anaphylactic or allergic condition.

Because Dale worked in the days before there were large-scale grants, he and other scientists often used an animal that survived one experiment as the subject of another, a necessary but risky practice; in this case the twice-used guinea pig received horse serum each time—first to standardize an antitoxin and second to test responses of 'normal' uterine smooth muscle to horse serum.

The Function of the Carotid Body

Although DeCastro, on the basis of his brilliant neuro-histologic studies, deduced in 1928 that the carotid body must be a chemoreceptor organ (one that "tastes" the blood and reports on its chemical composition to the brain), it remained for Heymans and his associates to demonstrate this concept experimentally. Eric Neil, a close associate of Heymans, states that although DeCastro wrote in French and Heymans was a French-speaking Belgian, Heymans made his 1930-31 discovery without knowing of DeCastro's 1928 work. This is how Heymans made his discovery, according to Neil (22):

At the end of a long experimental day in which he had been examining the effects of drugs on *baroreceptor* reflexes, the dog was still in good experimental condition, with one carotid bifurcation denervated and the other bifurcation still innervated by its sinus nerve. He remembered a saying of his father, which, paraphrased, was "At the end of a good experiment which has given clear results, if the animal is in satisfactory experimental condition, try an imaginative or even a facetious experiment." He decided to test the effect of injection of sodium cyanide into the carotid artery on each side. The drug was known to cause hyperpnoea and was believed to stimulate the medullary respiratory centres directly. On injecting cyanide into the carotid which supplied the innervated bifurcation the usual hyperpnoea resulted, but when the injection was made on the denervated side no respiratory response occurred. Repeating the dual procedure several times he obtained the same results. He and his colleagues realized that they had proved that sodium cyanide provoked a chemical reflex and that the old hypothesis of a central action was wrong. The subsequent days were spent in repeating the experiment in newly-prepared animals and confirming their findings. The first demonstration of the carotid chemoreflex aroused by histotoxic anoxia was made in this manner. Important though it was, the full development of our understanding of a possible *physiological* role of the carotid chemoreflexes in monitoring or in affecting the breathing could hardly have occurred so quickly if Heymans had not already been armed with the formidable technique required for perfusing the carotid bifurcation (using either a donor dog or a Dale-Schuster pump) with blood of altered chemical composition [as Heymans had done before in testing for chemosensitivity in the "cardio-aortic" regions].

Development of Collateral Circulation

John Kobler, in his biography of John Hunter (23), tells how, in 1785, that remarkable man discovered the concept and fact of collateral circulation:

Most varieties of stag shed their antlers and grow a new pair every year. Among the pending investigations on John's crowded agenda was the mode of this growth. Through what channels did the new cartilage derive its nutriment? Probably, John speculated, through the two carotid arteries running up the sides of the animal's neck.

Richmond Park, a crown property of almost twenty-five hundred acres lying on the south bank of the Thames, seven miles from the center of London, had originally been enclosed by Charles I as a deer-hunting preserve, and though it had since been opened to the public, deer by the hundreds still roamed its thick groves. One of the privileges George III had accorded John was that of drawing upon the deer herds for experimental material, and in July of that year the surgeon availed himself of it. He had park wardens snare a young stag. He then laid bare one of the carotid arteries and tied it with surgical thread.

When he returned to examine the stag a few days later, it was as he expected: the antler corresponding to the ligated artery had stopped growing and felt cold to the touch. Clearly, it was receiving no nutriment. Would it be shed sooner than usual? On re-examining it a week later, after the wound around the ligature had healed, he saw, to his astonishment, that the antler was warm again and had resumed growing.

Could he have failed to ligate it securely? Was blood somehow still passing through it? He ordered the stag killed and brought to Leicester Square, where he dissected the area at the base of the antlers. He satisfied himself that he had not bungled the ligature. Yet a curious change had taken place. Some of the smaller arterial branches, above and below the ligature, were enlarged. It was through this mysteriously arisen auxiliary system, John reasoned, that blood must have been supplied to the antlers.

His swift conclusion was, in the words of Sir James Paget, one of the great pathologists of the nineteenth century, "a signal instance of the living force there is in facts when they are stored in a thoughtful mind." From the single observation of the altered blood vessels John deduced the entire principle of collateral circulation. According to this principle, the smaller, tributary arteries will, under "the stimulus of necessity," to use John's typically vitalist phrase, assume the functions of the larger. To verify this, John had Everard Home ligate the femoral artery of a dog and, later, dissect the leg. Home reported the same findings. Here was further confirmation of John's belief in the body's ability to throw up its own defenses.

Shortly thereafter, Hunter, instead of amputating the leg of a patient with a popliteal aneurysm, as was then the custom, simply ligated the artery above the aneurysm and allowed collateral circulation to provide adequate blood flow to save the limb.

Immunization

Jenner in 1798 had shown that inoculating a subject with cowpox produced a rather mild disease that then protected the individual against fatal or disfiguring smallpox. However, the idea of deliberately attenuating *virulent* bacteria and then using these to develop protection against disease and to prevent epidemics required first the discovery of the bacterial cause of many infectious diseases and then the genius of Louis Pasteur. Pasteur had been assigned the task of doing something about cholera in fowl, which was devastating the poultry farms in France. Beveridge (24) tells how Pasteur hit on the new concept:

> Pasteur's researches on fowl cholera were interrupted by the vacation, and when he resumed he encountered an unexpected obstacle. Nearly all the cultures had become sterile. He attempted to revive them by sub-inoculation into broth and injection into fowls. Most of the subcultures failed to grow and the birds were not affected, so he was about to discard everything and start afresh when he had the inspiration of re-inoculating the same fowls with a fresh culture. His colleague Duclaux relates:
>
> > "To the surprise of all, and perhaps even of Pasteur, who was not expecting such success, nearly all these fowl withstood the inoculation, although fresh fowl succumbed after the usual incubation period."

This resulted in the recognition of the principle of immunisation with attenuated pathogens.

ANTU—A Rat Poison

It was Curt Richter, Professor of Psychobiology at Johns Hopkins University, who discovered a powerful poison, selective for Norway rats, at a time when it was needed badly. What does psychobiology have to do with rat poison? Absolutely nothing. Richter was interested in studying taste and the ability of animals to select a proper diet by using their sense of taste. Dr. Richter tells how studies on taste led to a rat poison (25):

> In 1931 Dr. Herbert Fox, a research chemist at du Pont, observed that as this chemical [phenyl thiourea], in the form of fine dust, was blown through his laboratory, some fellow-workers complained of a very bitter taste while most of them denied tasting anything at all. In testing a large number of persons, Fox found that although about 85 per cent could not taste this compound, even in large amounts, about 15 per cent found it extremely bitter. . . .

In 1939 this substance became of special interest to me in relation to results of my dietary self-selection studies, which showed that the rat has an extraordinary ability to select beneficial substances and avoid harmful ones. These studies demonstrated that the rat's appetite is a good guide to its nutritional needs; that in fact it is reliable enough to use in determining nutritive values of various food-stuffs; that it helps the rat to avoid harmful or non-nutritive substances—which is of particular importance in view of its inability to vomit. Results of these studies indicated that taste of food-stuffs—natural or chemically purified—plays an important part in dietary selections, determining chiefly whether or not an animal will ingest a substance. It naturally interested me to determine the extent to which observations on the role played by taste in dietary selections in rats can be transferred to man—whether man and rats have similar taste abilities.

Thus, when I first heard that phenyl thiourea has such a bitter taste to some people while having for others no taste at all, I wondered whether likewise some rats would taste it and others not. Ability to taste it was tested in a simple experiment. A minute amount of phenyl thiourea powder—as much as can be put on the small end of a toothpick—was placed on the tongues of six rats. The rats were then watched for signs of distaste—attempts to get rid of the powder with their paws or tongues. After watching for over half an hour, I decided that even if they could taste it they did not find it very bitter. To my great surprise the next morning all six rats were dead. They were found to have died of massive pulmonary edema and pleural effusion. Their chests and lungs were filled with fluid. Later, systematic tests showed that as little as 1-2 milligrams sufficed to kill a rat, and that when phenyl thiourea was mixed in food in small amounts, 1-2 per cent, our laboratory rats ate it freely and died. Thus it was demonstrated for the first time that phenyl thiourea is highly toxic to rats, and that rats will eat it in toxic amounts.

Richter had set out to prove that nature had provided rats with taste receptors that enabled them unerringly to select the good and reject the bad—but with Norway rats, nature instead gave them receptors that allowed them to enjoy a lethal man-made poison. Richter realized the potential value of a rat poison and directed the secret wartime development and large scale testing of a derivative (alpha naphthyl thiourea: ANTU). Incidentally, he also found that chronic administration of phenyl thiourea blocked the formation of the thyroid hormone; Astwood followed up this work and discovered the clinical usefulness of antithyroid drugs in 1943 (26).

Radioimmune Assay

This new analytic procedure has permitted hospital laboratories and research scientists to make highly specific and sensitive measurements of many hormones such as insulin, growth hormone, ACTH, and parathyroid hormone. Berson and Yalow discovered it by chance (27):

About 15 years ago we were interested in evaluating whether diabetics destroyed insulin more rapidly or more slowly than normal subjects. It had been recognized that not all diabetes is associated with an absolute deficiency of insulin, and Dr. Arthur Mirsky . . . suggested that this phenomenon might be traceable to an overly active insulin-destroying enzyme, insulinase. To test this hypothesis, we injected radiolabeled insulin intravenously and determined the rates of disappearance and degradation of the tagged hormone. Surprisingly, we found that insulin did not disappear more rapidly from the circulation of the diabetics but was retained in the plasma for longer periods than in the normal subjects. However, it turned out that this slow disappearance rate was not directly related to the presence of diabetes. Rather, it was because the diabetics had anti-insulin antibodies, which complexed with the hormone in the plasma, thus preventing the insulin molecule from passing through the capillary walls. . . . During the course of these studies we found it convenient to use radio labeled insulin as a tracer, giving increasing amounts of unlabeled hormone in order to quantitate the insulin-binding capacity of the plasma antibodies. It was evident that the labeled and unlabeled insulins were competing for antibody combining sites and that the extent of this competition could serve as the basis for an assay of insulin.

Motion Sickness

Gay and Carliner were allergists at the Johns Hopkins Hospital and, naturally, in 1947, were interested in using old and new antihistaminic drugs to treat their allergic patients. That year, Searle & Co. sent them a new drug, Dramamine®, for clinical investigation of its value in controlling hay fever and hives. The allergists gave the new drug to a number of patients, one of whom incidentally had suffered all her life from car sickness. During an interview at the hospital, she volunteered the information that since she had been taking the new drug, she had no further difficulty with motion sickness. Dr. Gay immediately realized the importance of her observation and switched her back and forth between Dramamine and a placebo of sugar; after Dramamine she never had car sickness, but after the placebo, she always had severe sickness. Gay and Carliner

(28) then found other victims of car sickness and airsickness and these were, without exception, completely freed of discomfort, provided the drug was taken just before exposure to the motion that provoked the illness.

The new drug had a large-scale clinical trial by the Armed Forces because General Omar Bradley recognized the military value of such a drug in landing operations such as that in Normandy in 1945. Soon "Operation Seasick" had Dr. Gay aboard a troopship with 1,500 soldiers for 12 days in a rough North Atlantic; the study showed that drugs could be effective both in preventing and relieving motion sickness.

Catheterization of Coronary Arteries and Coronary Sinus

Physiologists had for many decades perfused the coronary arteries of animals with Ringer solution, modified Ringer solutions, or blood (even hypoxemic blood) but were apprehensive about sending a block of an unoxygenated foreign fluid through the coronary circulation for fear of inducing serious arrhythmias. Yet successful coronary arteriography required flow of a highly concentrated, radiopaque solution through the coronary circulation. How did visualization of the coronary arteries become a diagnostic test? Litwak (29) tells this story:

In 1958 an event transpired in Cleveland which was destined to have virtually unparalleled influence on medicine's understanding of coronary artery disease. F. Mason Sones, Jr. and his colleagues at the Cleveland Clinic were studying a young adult and had withdrawn their catheter from the left ventricle into the supravalvar area in preparation for an aortagram. Their equipment at that time did not allow them to precisely visualize the catheter tip immediately prior to injection of the contrast material. The usual dose of 35 ml. of a 90 per cent diatrizoate compound was injected and, to Sones' horror, the right coronary artery and its distal branches were clearly visualized. Obviously, the catheter had accidentally entered the right coronary orifice and dye injected. The patient had remained stable throughout the entire procedure. That fortuitous event taught Sones that, contrary to views held at that time concerning electrical instability of the heart, non-oxygen carrying fluid could be injected into a major coronary artery without untoward event. Secondly, Sones realized that with proper equipment he could reduce the coronary artery injectate by ten-fold and he would then be able to sequentially study the entire coronary circulation of man and visualize vessels with a dimension of 100 microns or larger.

Effler writes of this:

The . . . introduction of selective coronary arteriography in 1958 did . . . much more than improve the diagnosis of ischemic heart disease. Figuratively speaking, Sones' catheter pried open the lid of a veritable treasure chest and brought forth the present era of revascularization surgery. His technic did provide for accurate diagnosis in coronary arterial disease but, more important, it defined the needs of the individual patient. For these reasons alone, coronary arteriography was a monumental contribution . . .

The first catheterization of the coronary sinus in man was also accidental. After Cournand and Ranges introduced the technique of cardiac catheterization to cardiologists in 1941, several teams began to use the new method to measure cardiac output in man, using the Fick principle. The latter required knowing the O_2 content of samples of systemic arterial and mixed venous blood, drawn simultaneously, to determine the difference between the two. Mixed venous blood could at last be obtained from a catheter properly placed in the patient's right heart. The main problem that plagued workers in the early 1940s was that blood drawn through the catheter sometimes didn't seem to be well-mixed venous blood.

Cournand, about 1941, attempting to catheterize the right ventricle, obtained a sample of blood with a lower oxygen content than right atrial blood. Because the fluoroscopic picture showed that the catheter tip was misplaced and was probably in the coronary sinus (by mere chance), and Cournand was concerned about possible damage to the lining of the sinus, he hastily withdrew the catheter.

Stead and co-workers had trouble with 3 patients because the sample of blood from the right heart had a very low O_2 content; they concluded that the catheter must have slipped into the coronary sinus, discarded the data, and went on to study better-behaved patients (30).

Sosman, a radiologist in Boston who worked with Dexter on cardiac catheterization, listed among his "failures and errors" (31) unexpected locations of the catheter tip and published in his figure 3C a roentgenogram showing a catheter tip in the coronary venous sinus; he confirmed its location by measuring the O_2 saturation of blood drawn through it (only 25 per cent instead of the usual 75 per cent in truly mixed venous blood).

Bing and his associates wrote in 1947, "When the catheter is in the coronary sinus, it is seen curved upward toward the base of the heart. . . .

In the first five cases, intubation of these vessels was fortuitous. . . . In the remaining four cases, catheterization of the sinus was carried out deliberately. . . . The difference between the oxygen contents of peripheral arterial blood (and hence of coronary arterial blood), and of coronary venous blood varied from 11.3 to 18.7 vol %, while the total systemic arteriovenous oxygen difference varied from 2.8 to 7.3 vol %" (32a). Bing, a pioneer in using the catheter to diagnose, with precision, congenital heart lesions in children, quickly changed directions and now pioneered in the new, richly rewarding field of coronary blood flow and cardiac metabolism in man (32b).

Probenecid

The discovery of penicillin as a powerful, relatively nontoxic antimicrobial drug was made in 1941. It was difficult to produce in large quantities, and, to make matters worse, much of the penicillin administered to patients was excreted rapidly by their renal tubules and ran out in the urine so that it required huge doses of penicillin to maintain an effective concentration of it in blood. Beyer and Sprague at Sharp & Dohme hit upon the idea of using paraaminohippurate, also secreted by the renal tubules, to block the outpouring of penicillin. It worked but took large amounts. They synthesized other compounds that might be even more effective in lower doses. The first of these was carinamide, better than the hippurate, but not good enough. The next was probenecid, considerably better at blocking penicillin excretion; but now, ironically for them, there was no market for such a drug. The U.S. Office of Scientific Research and Development (OSRD) had given top priority to the mass production of penicillin, initially for the British troops in World War II and then for American soldiers as well, and soon there was enough to go around, without blocking urinary excretion of penicillin.

However, in 1950, Berliner and his associates found the renal tubular mechanism for excretion of urates in man (33), and during the next year, Bishop, Rand, and Talbott found that probenecid greatly increased uric acid secretion in normal man and in a patient with gout (34). So a drug designed to keep penicillin in the body turned out to be useful in getting uric acid out of the body and so an effective treatment for human gout.

Oral Diuretics

The first powerful oral diuretic, chlorothiazide, resulted from careful bedside observation, basic research, and chance. The careful bedside observation was that of Southworth, who noted in 1937 that patients taking then-new sufanilamide had acidosis, and that volunteers taking sulfanilamide had a marked increase in urine volume and in their excretion of sodium and potassium. The basic research was first the discovery by Roughton of a new enzyme, carbonic anhydrase, in red blood cells, that tremendously speeds the reaction: $CO_2 + H_2O \rightleftarrows H_2CO_3 \rightleftarrows H^+ + HCO_3^-$; second, Davenport's finding that this enzyme is present in stomach and kidney, both acid-producing organs; third, the work of Pitts and Alexander showing that acidification of urine in the renal tubules requires carbonic anhydrase.

Beyer, at Merck, Sharp & Dohme, had been trying, by means of drugs, to prevent loss of valuable penicillin in urine (see *Probenecid*). When the props were knocked out from under the program by mass production in the United States, he changed direction and started to devise drugs that increased renal excretion of sodium and water, instead of blocking urinary excretion of penicillin. The work of Davenport and Pitts led Beyer to investigate a large group of sulfanilamide derivatives to find a more potent and less toxic inhibitor of carbonic anhydrase, believing that it would be a more potent diuretic; chlorothiazide was the result. Chance entered this story in three ways: (1) The OSRD quickly produced penicillin in large quantities, making Beyer's conservation program unnecessary. (2) Although chlorothiazide is both a carbonic anhydrase inhibitor and a potent diuretic, its diuretic effect was found to be unrelated to its action on carbonic anhydrase. (3) Beyer wanted a diuretic to treat patients with congestive heart failure; because of a long-known association between salt and hypertension, Beyer's diuretic soon became an important antihypertensive drug. It is rare, except in chemotherapy, that one substance becomes the drug of choice in treating two important diseases (congestive heart failure and essential hypertension). Its discovery soon led to other types of oral diuretics, some of which, such as ethacrynic acid and furosemide, either do not inhibit carbonic anhydrase at all, or at most have a very weak action on the enzyme.

Triamterine, another oral diuretic, was also discovered by chance. Some years ago, Lettré noted that a particular benzo*iso*alloxazine specifically inhibited certain cancer cells *in vitro*. Haddow (35) tried to confirm this. He couldn't, but found something totally unrelated; an alloxazine compound similar to Lettré's but it colored the hair of albino rats because its alloxazine penetrated into growing hair. Haddow was curious to learn whether a naturally occurring pigment such as xanthopterin (which occurs in the wings of butterflies and is related to folic acid) could also cause a color change in the fur of albino rats; it did not.

So far the story is pretty far removed from the kidneys or oral diuretics or triamterine itself. But Haddow examined the kidneys of the rats that he treated with xanthopterin and found that they were hypertrophied, that the hypertrophy started almost at once after injection of xanthopterin, and that the growth was due to a great outburst of mitotic activity in the renal tubules. This was a most unusual effect of a drug, but one that did not lend itself to clinical use because the xanthopterin was excreted in the tubules and formed crystals there.

But now the direction of Haddow's research changed to look for a chemical with a xanthopterin-like effect on tubules, but one that didn't form crystals that blocked the tubule. The right compound, triamterine, came from an unexpected quarter—a study of agents that were carcinogenic. So an initial chance observation on cancer-inhibiting agents and an unexpected bonus in a later study of cancer-inducing agents led to a valuable oral diuretic agent.

Fetal Respiration

In 1936, Marshall and Rosenfeld at Johns Hopkins University noted that sodium cyanide was a good respiratory stimulant, acting reflexly through the newly discovered carotid chemoreceptors. However, because its action was too brief to be of much help in overcoming respiratory depression, they reasoned that a compound that liberated cyanide slowly into the bloodstream and over a long period might be worth studying. They decided to test pyruvic acid cyanohydrin. But the next step was to find a test animal—one that was completely apneic for long periods but still alive. Because everyone knew that the fetus *in utero* never breathed, they settled on fetal apnea as a good baseline for testing the effectiveness of a respiratory stimulant with a prolonged effect. To their amazement they found that full-term fetuses of rabbits, cats, and guinea pigs all made active, regular, and frequent respiratory movements. The problem then changed from the study of a new drug (cyanohydrin) to "direct observation of intrauterine respiratory movements of the fetus and the role of carbon dioxide and oxygen in their regulation" (36).

Alloxan and Experimental Diabetes

Shaw Dunn was not the first to describe acute renal failure as a sequela of crush injury, but he was the first to demonstrate that the renal injury was restricted to the ascending limbs of Henle's loops and second convoluted tubules of the kidney. He became interested in whether crush of skeletal muscles releases toxic factors, such as uric acid or phosphoric acid, that are responsible for the renal damage. In testing a series of uric acid derivatives, he found that alloxan (the ureide of mesoxalic acid) produced selective damage to the same renal tubules. However, the dose of alloxan required to produce this lesion killed many of the animals within a day or two; they had distinctive symptoms before death but they were not attributable to renal disease. At this point Dunn turned aside from the kidneys to explore the cause of these symptoms, since no one had ever studied the pharmacologic or toxic effects of alloxan. He came up with the remarkable finding that alloxan caused selective necrosis of the insulin-producing islets of Langerhans in the rabbit pancreas and left the other endocrine glands untouched (37). An investigation into the cause of renal failure in crush injury thus led Dunn to find a substance capable of producing experimental diabetes mellitus. Since then, alloxan has also been found to produce pulmonary edema in cats and dogs and so has provided a tool for studying the effects of increased pulmonary capillary permeability.

Isoniazid, an Antituberculosis Drug

In 1945, Ernest Huant had been in the habit of administering what he called "P.P. (pellagra preventing) vitamin" or nicotinamide to patients undergoing radiation therapy to lessen postradiation nausea and vomiting and to improve tolerance of the skin to x-rays. Although the radiation was directed primarily against tumors, during the course of this work Huant noted clearing of densities in the chest films of certain patients who also had pulmonary tuberculosis. "With all reservations," he cautiously described his clinical findings with nicotinamide and tuberculosis in the *Gazette des Hôpitaux*, and urged specialists in tuberculosis to test his findings and determine their utility (38). I don't believe that this observation changed the direction of Huant's studies, but it certainly changed that of physicians interested in treating tuberculosis.

That same year Vital Chorine indicated that he had been studying the influence of various vitamins on experimental leprosy. He admitted his surprise at the finding that large doses of nicotinamide protected against the disease in rats. Because of the relationship between the bacillus of leprosy and that of tuberculosis, Chorine attempted a similar experiment with a human strain of the tubercle bacillus and found that large doses of nicotinamide completely prevented development of tuberculosis in guinea pigs (39). Soon thereafter, many derivatives of nicotinamide were tested, and isoniazid was found.

Beri-Beri

Beri-beri, a severe polyneuritis, was first described more than 1,300 years ago in China. The ravages of beri-beri in the Dutch Indies in the late nineteenth century led the Dutch government to appoint a special commission to study the disease on the spot. The new science of bacteriology and the almost overnight explanation of many mysterious diseases as germ-induced led the commission to look for a specific bacterial cause of beri-beri. A disease suddenly afflicted chickens near the laboratory in Java and because in many respects it closely resembled beri-beri in man, these chickens seemed to be heaven-sent to help Eijkman find the cause of beri-beri.

Christiaan Eijkman in his Nobel Lecture in 1929 tells the story (40):

Attempts to induce the infection with material from affected birds or from birds which had died of the disease were inconclusive since all the chickens, even those kept separate as controls, were affected. No specific micro-organism or any higher parasite was found.

Then suddenly the disease cleared up and we were unable to continue our investigations. The affected chickens recovered and there were no new cases. Fortunately suspicion fell on the food, and rightly so, as it very soon turned out.

The laboratory was still housed provisionally and in a very makeshift manner at the military hospital, although it was administered by the civilian authorities. The laboratory keeper—as I afterwards discovered—had for the sake of economy fed the chickens on cooked rice which he had obtained from the hospital kitchen. Then the cook was replaced and his successor refused to allow military rice to be taken for civilian chickens. Thus, the chickens were fed on polished rice from 17th June to 27th November only. And the disease broke out on 10th July and cleared up during the last days of November.

Deliberate feeding experiments were then conducted in order to check more thoroughly whether or not the probable connection between diet and the disease actually existed. It was found for certain that the polyneuritis was due to the diet of cooked rice. The chickens were attacked by the disease after 3-4 weeks, and in many cases somewhat later, whereas the controls which were fed on unpolished rice remained healthy. In many cases, birds suffering from the disease could be cured by a suitable alteration in diet.

And so arose the concept that the disease was caused by the *absence* of something (later named a vitamin and still later, thiamin) rather than by the *presence* of of something (bacteria or their toxins).

Some Other Chance Discoveries

I shall do no more here than merely list a few chance discoveries recounted in considerably greater length elsewhere in this volume, e.g., McLean's discovery of heparin while he was looking for a *coagulant* (41); Ringer's accidental discovery of the role of Ca^{2+} and K^+ in regulating myocardial performance (41); the accidental discovery of the anesthetic effects of ether by Morton and by Long, and of nitrous oxide by Wells (42); the chance discovery of a new mercurial diuretic by Vogl, who really wanted an antisyphilitic drug (43); the circumstances that led Jacobson to use microvascular surgical technics (41); Chargaff's finding a heparin-*antagonist* while designing a compound to *prolong* its effect (41); Roentgen's discovery of x-rays (44); and Heyrovsky's turning a routine problem into the science of polarography (45).

And some chance discoveries are too well known to be repeated (e.g., Galvani's discovery of "animal electricity," Volta's creation of the "Voltaic pile" or battery, and the accidental discharge of a shotgun that gave William Beaumont the chance to study gastric physiology by direct vision in his patient, Alexis St. Martin).

The list would be longer yet if I mentioned some oft-quoted chance discoveries that sound authentic but may well be apocryphal: e.g., that a Smith, Kline and French chemist found that his precious, newly synthesized sympathomimetic crystals "vanished" when he went out to lunch and only later realized that his new compound Benzedrine®, was volatile; that the Hungarian government forced vintners to add phenolphthalein, an indicator, to their cheap white wines to distinguish them from genu-wines, until an epidemic of diarrhea followed and a new laxative was born; that a University of Illinois chemistry student discovered the cyclamate, sucaryl, when he accidentally put his cigarette first on some chemicals on a bench top and then between his lips; that copper and lime, now known as Bordeaux mixture and a commercially important fungicide for fruit trees and vines, was first sprayed on stakes in vineyards only to frighten away pilferers; and that Ramon discovered by chance that formalin can weaken or eliminate the toxicity of toxins without diminishing their antigenicity (all he wanted to do was use formalin to preserve the toxins).

COMMENTS ON CHANCE

I've not become involved in a massive research effort to determine how often chance has played an appreciable, important, or essential role in major discoveries in biomedical science. A skillful investigative reporter or private eye might know how to get the evidence, but I don't. Even a little gentle probing has taught me that most scientists don't like to be regarded as *discoverers*, but rather as *scientists* who have meticulously and logically planned each step in a direct line leading from ignorance to full knowledge. Few "tell it like it was" in their scientific writing, and editors of journals probably delete, as unscientific, most of the "chance" story that authors do put in their manuscripts. However, the Retrospectroscope shows that some scientists in their initial reports do acknowledge their indebtedness to chance and many more do so later in life when the highest honors have assured them of a place in Science's Hall of Fame. These late-in-life reports lead me to believe that chance is a pretty important element in scientific advance.

If it is, how might this affect our attitude toward the support of science and scientists? Two extreme views will surely come to some minds: (1) Since chance is an important factor in discovery and since chance is really finding things by bumbling and stumbling, science has no need for highly intelligent, superbly trained men and women who proceed carefully and doggedly step by step toward a logical goal. (2) As a corollary of the first, what science really needs is a large corps of scientists in motion who bounce from project to project (as do molecules from other molecules in random motion) and so increase tremendously the number of fortuitous observations and the likelihood of a great discovery.

I'd rather train my Retrospectroscope in several different directions. First, let's look at the word that Horace Walpole coined: serendipity. The two dictionaries on my desk have changed Walpole's definition to "an apparent aptitude for making discoveries accidentally" (Webster's New World) and "the faculty for making desirable discoveries by accident" (Random House). But that was *not* what Walpole said, which was "making discoveries, by accidents and sagacity, of things which they were not in quest of" (46). The key words (omitted in recent years) are "*and* sagacity." Webster's New World defines *sagacity* as "penetrating intelligence, keen perception and sound judgment" and Random House as "acuteness of mental discernment and soundness of judgment."

Now let's look at Pasteur, who said much the same in the mid-1800s when he wrote: "Dans les champs de l'observation, le hasard ne favorise que les esprits preparés," translated freely as "Chance favors only the prepared mind." And let's look at Joseph Henry, America's great physicist, who said the same thing some years before Pasteur when he commented, "The seeds of great discoveries are constantly floating around us, but they only take root in minds well prepared to receive them."

It seems that many discoveries, either clinical or nonclinical, are made—and then developed in different directions—by individuals who not only have prepared minds, but are willing to change the direction of their effort, not daily or weekly, but when a new observation—possibly a chance observation—appears to be far more important than the problem before them. This requires three additional qualities besides the ability to observe what chance has put before them: judgment on what is very important, less important, or trival; a prepared mind; and a flexible mind. The old adage "never change horses in midstream" may be good advice when on horseback in midstream but may be bad advice in science.

In Part I (47), I arbitrarily divided chance discoveries into (A) those in which chance speeded or completed a scientist's ongoing work, and (B) those in which chance changed a scientist's goals. Scientists have reported more instances of chance in the (B) category than in the (A). Why? Probably because an exciting *new* idea, concept, or experiment has usually been responsible for giant steps in science instead of small ones. But to capitalize fully on new concepts requires not only flexible scientists but also flexible science administrators and a flexible national science policy. What if the scientist, looking for a needle in a haystack and finding an ugly toad instead, was convinced he could convert it into a thing of beauty but hadn't the freedom to profit from serendipity?

References

20. Richet, C. R.: Anaphylaxis. Nobel Lecture, December 11, 1913. *Nobel Lectures, Physiology or Medicine, 1901-1921*, Elsevier, Amsterdam, 1967, pp. 473-490.
21. Dale, H. H.: Accident and opportunism in medical research, Br Med J, 1948, *2*, 451-455.
22. Neil, E.: An appraisal of the work of Corneille Heymans on baroreceptor and chemoreceptor reflexes, Arch Int Pharmacodyn Ther, 1973, *202* (Supplement, pp. 283-293).
23. Kobler, J.: The Reluctant Surgeon, A Biography of John Hunter, Doubleday, Garden City, N. Y., 1960.
24. Beveridge, W. I. B.: The Art of Scientific Investigation, Random House, Vintage Books, New York, 1950.
25. Richter, C.: Experiences of a reluctant rat-catcher. The common Norway rat—friend or enemy?, Proc Am Philos Soc, 1968, *112*, 403-415.
26. Astwood, E. B.: Treatment of hyperthyroidism with thiourea and thiouracil, JAMA, 1943, *122*, 78-81.
27. Berson, S. A., and Yalow, R. S.: Radioimmunoassay: A status report, Hosp Prac, 1968, *3* (11), 73-83.
28. Gay, L. N., and Carliner, P. E.: The prevention and treatment of motion sickness. I. Seasickness, Johns Hopkins Hosp Med Bull, 1949, *84*, 470-487.
29. Litwak, R.: The growth of cardiac surgery: Historical notes, Cardiovasc Clin, 1951, *3*, 5-50. (Personal communication from F. M. Sones, Jr., see p. 38.)
30. Stead, E. A., Jr., Warren, J. V., Merrill, A. J., and Brannon, E. S.: The cardiac output in male subjects as measured by the technique of right atrial catheterization. Normal values with observations on the effect of anxiety and tilting, J Clin Invest, 1945, *24*, 326-331.
31. Sosman, M. C.: Venous catheterization of the heart. I. Indications, technics, and errors, Radiology, 1947, *48*, 441-450.
32a. Bing, R. J., Vandam, L. D., Gregoire, F., Handelsman, J. C., Goodale, W. T., and Eckenhoff, J. E.: Catheterization of the coronary sinus and the middle cardiac vein in man, Proc Soc Exp Biol Med, 1947, *66*, 239-240.
32b. Bing, R. J., Hammond, M. M., Handelsman, J. C., Powers, S. R., Spencer, F. C., Eckenhoff, J. E., Goodale, W. T., Hafkenschiel, J. H., and Kety, S. S.: The measurement of coronary blood flow, oxygen consumption, and efficiency of the left ventricle in man, Am Heart J, 1949, *38*, 1-24.
33. Berliner, R. W., Hilton, J. G., Yü, T.-F., and Kennedy, T. J., Jr.: The renal mechanism for urate excretion in man, J Clin Invest, 1950, *29*, 396-401.
34. Bishop, C., Rand, R., and Talbott, J. H.: The effect of benemid (p-[di-n-propylsulfamyl]-benzoic acid) on uric acid metabolism in one normal and one gouty subject, J Clin Invest, 1951, *30*, 889-895.
35. Haddow, A.: In *CIBA Foundation Symposium on Chemistry and Biology of Pteridines*, G. E. W. Wolstenholme and M. P. Cameron, ed., Churchill, London, 1954, pp. 100-103.
36. Snyder, F. F., and Rosenfeld, M.: Direct observation of intrauterine respiratory movements of the fetus and the role of carbon dioxide and oxygen in their regulation, Am J Physiol, 1937, *119*, 153-166.
37. Dunn, J. S., Sheehan, H. L., and McLetchie, N. G. B.: Necrosis of the islets of Langerhans produced experimentally, Lancet, 1943, *1*, 484-487.
38. Huant, E.: Note sur l'action de très fortes doses d'amide nicotinique dans les lesions bacillaires, Gaz Hôp, 1945, *118*, 259-260.
39. Chorine, V.: Action de l'amide nicotinique sur les bacilles du genre *Mycobacterium*, C R Acad Sci, 1945, *220*, 150-151.
40. Eijkman, C.: Antineuritic vitamin and beriberi, in *Nobel Lectures in Physiology or Medicine, 1922-1941*, Elsevier, Amsterdam, 1965, pp. 199-207.
41. This volume, "Tell it like it was," pp. 89-98.
42. This volume, Speculation on speculation, pp. 99-105.
43. This volume, Out of the mouth of babes, pp. 35-43.
44. This volume, The inside story, pp. 7-11.
45. This volume, Whodunit (and why), Part II, pp. 18-23.
46. Lewis, W. S.: Selected Letters of Horace Walpole, Yale University Press, New Haven, 1973. (See letter to Sir Horace Mann, 28 January 1754, pp. 53-57, including a photographic reproduction of Walpole's handwritten letter on p. 56.)
47. This volume, Roast pig and scientific discovery, Part I, pp. 48-55.

Missed Opportunities

President Johnson once suggested that many important scientific discoveries were locked up in scientific laboratories and that the time had come to unlock these. I don't believe for a minute that LBJ was right. Scientists might try to publish *prematurely* (and sometimes succeed) but it's rare to find one who locks up his discoveries and keeps them hidden from the scientific public. Normal behavior of scientists is to make sure their observations and measurements are correct and then try to get them published as soon as humanly possible in the most widely read and prestigious journal in the field.

It is true, however, that researchers occasionally make important observations but don't know they've made them, or have all the information needed for a major discovery but don't make it. There's no way of telling how often it's happened and to whom but my guess is that it's an occurrence that few confess to; maybe more would after a few drinks, but rarely in writing. I call them "missed opportunities."

Sulfanilamide

Probably the most important miss here was the two-time synthesis of sulfanilamide before it was discovered a third time and finally put to clinical use. Sulfanilamide was first prepared in Vienna in 1908 by Paul Gelmo, then working for his doctoral thesis. At about the same time, Heinrich Hörlein (later to become director of the medical division of the great I. G. Farbenindustrie) went to work with the Bayer Works and centered his research work on dyes. Because sulfanilamide was an easy starting point on which to construct dyes that were particularly color-fast (presumably because of the tight combination of the sulfanilamide element with the proteins of wool and silk), he began with several dyes formed with sulfanilamide as the base. Hörlein never tested sulfanilamide for antibacterial properties, although Paul Ehrlich, a

fellow German, had discovered arsphenamine, the "magic bullet" against syphilis, in 1909.

The second synthesis of sulfanilamide was in 1915, by Jacobs and Heidelberger at the Rockefeller Institute for Medical Research in New York. They decided to synthesize and test a number of chemical agents in the hope of finding one that was more bactericidal or less toxic against pneumococcal and streptococcal infections than optochin (an early but now-forgotten bactericidal drug). In their systematic search they prepared para-aminobenzene sulfonamide (sulfanilamide), much as Gelmo had in 1908. In line with then-current dogma, they thought that in order to fight infection *in vivo,* a substance had to be directly lethal to bacteria, and they didn't think that a substance as chemically simple as sulfanilamide could kill bacteria directly.

Heidelberger wrote in 1972 (1):

Like everyone else at the time, Walter Jacobs and I thought that a substance had to be directly bactericidal in order to be useful in combatting bacterial infections. We had been successful with trypanosomiasis by applying Jacobs' idea of changing the -OH of -COOH to NH_2, as $-CONH_2$, in order to get an organic arsenical past tissue barriers. Accordingly, when we tried to get something better than optochin against pneumococcal and streptococcal infections, we started first with amides and then, by analogy, went on to $-SO_2NH_2$. *The possibility that any substance as simple as sulfanilamide could cure bacterial infections never entered our heads, nor did our microbiologist even ask to test it* [italics added]. We even improved Gelmo's method of preparation and went on to convert sulfanilamide into highly bactericidal substances which killed infected mice faster than the infections alone!

As slaves to an idea, we missed the boat in 1915, losing the chance to save many thousands of lives, and the development of the sulfonamides was delayed twenty years.

The third discovery of sulfanilamide came in 1932 when Klarer and Mietzsch, chemists at I. G. Farbenindustrie, synthesized a red dye, "Prontosil," which three years later, Domagk, a German who won the 1939 Nobel Prize, showed to be a remarkable antibacterial agent in man. However, Fourneau's group at the Pasteur Institute in Paris quickly discovered that the active component of the red dye was none other than sulfanilamide, first used by Hörlein at I. G. Farbenindustrie in 1909, and that the rest of the compound was totally unnecessary.

No one will ever know whether chemists and pharmacologists at I. G. Farbenindustrie in the 1930s synthesized and tested *sulfanilamide* first or whether they tested only Prontosil and not sulfanilamide. The facts are (*1*) that Hörlein used and patented sulfanilamide in 1909 (2a) and that by the 1930s it was no longer re-patentable, and (*2*) that although Klarer and Mietzsch prepared what in 1932 proved to be a powerful antibacterial agent in mice, Domagk did not publish his clinical data until 1935. The suspicion will always linger that I. G. Farbenindustrie re-discovered and tested sulfanilamide first and spent the next few years in the early 1930s camouflaging ordinary sulfa into a new, complex, and above all, patentable compound—the red dye, Prontosil. Hörlein, who was connected with the story from beginning to end, never told any more than he wrote in 1935 (2b):

> Further work on the azo-compounds by our chemists Mietzsch and Klarer led to the discovery of bodies with an incomparably greater action on bacteria than that possessed by any of the azo-compounds mentioned. But even these new compounds had no effect on mice infected with bacteria. In the course of our investigations, however, Domagk observed a certain activity on the part of azo-compounds containing sulphonamide in the streptococcal sepsis of mice, thus furnishing an important starting point for the preparation of new experimental series.
>
> Azo-dyes with sulphonamide and substituted sulphonamide groups were first prepared by me in collaboration with Dressel and Kothe, twenty-five years ago. At that time we were engaged in elaborating dyes for textile purposes which, in the direct dyeing of wools, would possess a greater degree of fastness to washing and fulling than dyes free from sulphonamide, while possessing the same degree of fastness to light as the latter dyes; i.e., dyes which would enter into a more intimate combination with the protein-cells of the wool than the dyes free from sulphonamide.

The observation of Domagk on the action of one of these dyes on streptococci directed our subsequent work into a new channel. Numerous new azo-dye-containing sulphonamides were prepared, but the test object was no longer the wool fiber but the mouse infected with streptococci.

Artificial Kidney

This is a special case of interrelated "missed opportunities." Abel, Rowntree, and Turner in 1914 (3) published their experiments on vividiffusion in living animals but neither they nor anyone else seriously and successfully applied it to man until 1943 when Kolff did it in German-occupied Holland (4). You will say that no one could even try it in man until nontoxic anticoagulants and chemotherapeutic agents were available. But Abel and associates in 1913–14 used hirudin (that they themselves prepared from leeches), McLean published his discovery of heparin in 1916, and Best (5) noted that Schmidt had prepared a material similar to heparin in 1892 (6) and Doyon again in 1912 (7).

The point with respect to anticoagulants is that either no one saw a necessity for purifying heparin or hirudin to permit the artificial kidney to be used in man or, if clinicians saw a critical need, they lacked chemical expertise to do it themselves and had no chemical colleagues or pharmaceutical research laboratories to turn to. Charles Best, in retrospect, had no explanation of the failure to purify heparin for use in vividiffusion but did note that "after heparin became available many people stated that they had been thinking for many years of its use in cardiac and vascular surgery" (8).

The antibacterial agents needed could have been available in 1910 or 1917 had it not been for missed opportunities in this field (see above); and antibiotics could have been available in 1930 if Fleming had taken his observations a step further (from agar plates to experimentally infected mice) —another missed opportunity.

The Carotid Sinus and Reflex Control of the Circulation

Of all experiments in the physiology student laboratory, the one most certain to produce dramatic effects is the demonstration of the carotid sinus reflex. One can clamp both common arteries *below* their bifurcation and see an immediate rise in blood pressure (which does not occur if the branches are clamped *above* the bifurcation) or one can increase pressure in the extracranial carotid arteries and note immediate slowing of the heart and fall in blood pressure.

These observations date back at least to 1836 when Astley Cooper noted that occlusion of the common carotid arteries led to an increase in blood pressure; he attributed it to the effects of intracranial ischemia (9). At least five physiologists between 1838 and 1885 confirmed his observations and agreed with his explanation.

Now it is important to note that in 1893 Bayliss (10) showed that these cardiovascular changes could not be due to cerebral ischemia because occlusion of both common carotid arteries did not markedly change blood flow to the medulla oblongata; the vertebral arteries still provided adequate blood flow to this region. Leonard Hill also presented strong evidence against the cerebral ischemia explanation when, in 1896, he was able to ligate successively both common carotids and both vertebral arteries in dogs without causing any abnormal behavior in the animal on recovery from these operations (11); this was because blood still flowed through the fifth artery to the brain, the anterior spinal artery. Nevertheless, Porter and Pratt still reported in 1908 (12) that raising blood pressure in the carotid arteries caused slowing of the heart by affecting blood pressure in the medullary centers. And in the same year, Eyster and Hooker (13) artificially raised blood pressure in the carotid arteries to 200 mm Hg and recorded a marked bradycardia and hypotension (see figure 1a); this they attributed to "a direct effect of the increased blood pressure upon the cardioinhibitory centre" in the medulla. Note the strong resemblance to figure 1b taken from a paper by Hering, who in 1923 at last discovered the carotid sinus, its nerve, and the effect of stimulating the nerve endings electrically or mechanically (14).

It has been said: "We see what we look for and we look for only what we know." Eyster

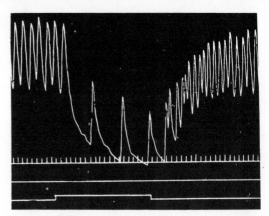

Fig. 1B. During the period indicated by the signal marker (bottom line), Hering stimulated the right carotid sinus nerve of a dog; the tracing shows an immediate fall in systemic arterial blood pressure and bradycardia.

and Hooker had all the information needed to find the carotid sinus in 1908. All they had to do was to look an inch higher in the neck of a living dog and see the bulging, pulsating origin of the internal carotids, literally enmeshed in nerve fibers. Anrep and Starling still wrote in 1925 "a mechanical rise in blood pressure in the brain inhibits the vasomotor centre and stimulates the cardioinhibitory centre" (15).

Nitrous Oxide, Ether, Local Anesthesia

Laughing gas parties were common in the early 1800s and Humphry Davy, who repeatedly inhaled nitrous oxide in his experiments of 1799, even suggested its use as a general anesthetic agent. But no one deliberately gave it to prevent pain until 1844—42 years of missed opportunities for how many physicians (and benefits to their patients).

Michael Faraday suggested in 1818 that ether be used to prevent surgical pain, and ether jags were a common form of social entertainment in the 1830s and 1840s; but no one gave it deliberately to prevent surgical pain until 1842.

Carl Koller, a young intern with his heart set on being an ophthalmologist, discovered in 1884 that cocaine was a superb local anesthetic for the eye. Yet since 1860, two years after the chemist Niemann had isolated cocaine from Peruvian coca leaves, it was well known that cocaine taken by mouth numbed the tongue. Koller's biographer, his daughter Hortense Koller Becker, wrote (16):

In 1862 Professor Schroff, in a paper read before

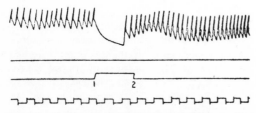

Fig. 1A. Between 1 and 2, Eyster and Hooker raised blood pressure to 200 mm Hg in the common carotid arteries of a dog while they recorded a decrease in blood pressure and heart rate from another artery.

the Viennese Medical Society, pointed out that cocaine numbed the tongue, narrowed the peripheral arteries, and widened the pupils by its action via the bloodstream or when applied locally. Nor was he the only one to have experimented upon the eye. These facts were commented upon by Mantegazza in 1859, De Marles in 1862, the Spaniard Moréno y Maiź in 1868, and by many others. In 1879 von Anrep at the Pharmacological Institute at Würzburg, wrote a comprehensive experimental paper in which he also described the locally numbing effects of cocaine and even the dilation of the pupil upon local application, and he suggested that this drug might some day become of medical importance. "Strangely enough," commented G. F. Schrady in an editorial in the Medical Record of November 8, 1884, "Anrep did not note that the conjunctiva was insensible, or if so did not appreciate the significance of this fact."

Hortense Becker notes that Koller had marked the following passage in his pharmacology text:

"Local effects: Injection under the skin as well as painting the mucous membrane, for example, the tongue—brings about the loss of feeling and pain. 15 minutes after painting it Anrep was incapable of distinguishing sugar, salt and sour at the treated spot. Even the needle pricks could no longer be felt there, whereas the other unpainted side reacted normally. The loss of sensibility lasted between 25 and 100 minutes.

"[The article concludes with] Therapeutic Uses: Up to now cocaine has not found any medical use. But on account of its powerfully stimulating effects on the psyche, respiration, and the heart, and also on account of its anesthetizing effect upon the mucous membrane, it might deserve experimental trial in quite a number of diseases. [Relative to the therapeutic use of the coca leaves:] There have been some experiments but no trustworthy ones over an extended period. They are, however, sold commercially and highly recommended for all possible needs."

Sigmund Freud had carried out what is still regarded as the classic pharmacological study of cocaine and the young Koller was closely associated with Freud in some of his work. Koller's daughter gives this account of why it was Koller, and not previous workers, who discovered that cocaine had great potential as a local anesthetic:

This is the chain of events which actually placed cocaine in my father's hand and focused his attention on it: Freud's interest in the drug, awakened primarily by the American literature on substituting it for morphine, by which method he hoped to help his suffering friend, Fleischl; the actual purchase of the scarce, expensive product [by Freud] and the request he made of my father to engage in experiments during the course of which my father was required to take it by mouth. These were the circumstances that prepared the way for his particular discovery, yet cocaine had been handled, taken by mouth, and its effect even upon the eye, observed for twenty-five years without its usefulness in surgery occurring to anyone. "Upon one occasion," my father said, "another colleague of mine, Dr. Engel, partook of some [cocaine] with me from the point of his penknife and remarked, 'How that numbs the tongue.' I said, 'Yes, that has been noticed by everyone that has eaten it.' And in the moment it flashed upon me that I was carrying in my pocket the local anesthetic for which I had searched some years earlier. I went straight to the laboratory, asked the assistant for a guinea pig for the experiment, made a solution of cocaine from the powder which I carried in my pocketbook, and instilled this into the eye of the animal." The young assistant in Stricker's laboratory, Dr. Gaertner, was the sole witness to my father's discovery ... he retold it in a 1919 newspaper of which he was medical editor:

"Now it was necessary to go one step further and to repeat the experiment upon a human being. We trickled the solution under the upraised lids of each other's eyes. Then we put a mirror before us, took a pin in hand, and tried to touch the cornea with its head. Almost simultaneously we could joyously assure ourselves, "I can't feel a thing." We could make a dent in the cornea without the slightest awareness of the touch, let alone any unpleasant sensation or reaction. With that the discovery of local anesthesia was completed. I rejoice that I was the first to congratulate Dr. Koller as a benefactor of mankind."

Koller's daughter continued:

My father was, of course, aware that local anesthesia had more general implications and was not by any means limited to operations on the eye. "I had started from the fact that the drug made the *lips* and *tongue* numb, but I limited myself to the eye, wishing to make a contribution to ophthalmology and also wishing to establish a claim to the much-coveted position of an assistant at one of the large eye clinics. I did, however, directly suggest to my friend, Jellinek [assistant to Schrötter in the laryngological clinic], that he make experiments on the nose, pharynx, and larynx. He reported the results at the same meeting of the *Gesellschaft der Ärzte* (October 17) at which I read my [second] paper."

It was Koller's intense desire to obtain this position in Vienna and his conviction that an important contribution to ophthalmology would

70

almost guarantee an offer that led him to solve the most serious problem in that specialty—how to operate painlessly and safely on the eye. General anesthesia was unsatisfactory because the patient often retched and vomited in the recovery period and because his conscious cooperation was frequently necessary during the operation. Ironically, because of strong anti-Semitism in Vienna, he never received the assistantship and, in 1888, he emigrated to America, where he became one of New York's most eminent ophthalmologists, showered with many honors.

Oral Diuretics

Oral diuretics as a class are one of the two most important new groups of drugs in the last 35 years—the other being chemotherapeutic and antibiotic drugs. Not many remember that sulfanilamide led to the discovery of chlorothiazide, the first of the oral diuretics.

In 1937, Hamilton Southworth at the Johns Hopkins Hospital noted that two of 50 patients treated with sulfanilamide began to breathe deeply. As a result, he studied 15 consecutive patients treated with sulfanilamide; the blood of each showed evidence of acidosis though none had *clinical* symptoms of acidosis (17). Pharmacologists at Hopkins then showed that a large single dose of sulfanilamide administered to dogs produced acidosis, and Strauss and Southworth demonstrated that in three normal human subjects, sulfanilamide led to acidosis, diuresis and increase in the renal excretion of sodium and potassium (18) (see figure 2).

Diuretics had long been an important part of treatment of congestive heart failure and edema but the only really effective diuretics in 1937 were mercurial diuretics and these required intravenous injection. Was sulfanilamide an effective oral diuretic that could at last replace intravenous injections of the organic mercurial compounds? And how did it produce diuresis?

In 1933, Roughton had isolated a new enzyme, carbonic anhydrase, from red blood cells and showed its property of greatly accelerating the reaction:

$$H_2O + CO_2 \rightleftharpoons H_2CO_3 \rightleftharpoons H^+ + H^-CO_3.$$

In 1940, Mann and Keilin found that some sulfonamides inhibit carbonic anhydrase; in 1941, Davenport and Wilhelmi found that carbonic anhydrase was present in the kidney, and, in 1945, Pitts and Alexander demonstrated the role

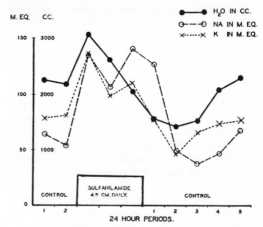

URINARY OUTPUT OF WATER, Na, AND K IN PATIENT L. H.

Fig. 2. After a control period of 2 days, Strauss and Southworth gave a subject 4.5 g sulfanilamide daily. Note diuresis and increased excretion of sodium (Na) and potassium (K).

of carbonic anhydrase in the exchange of hydrogen and sodium ions in the renal tubules and in the acidification of urine. Circumstantial evidence (though later shown not to be trusted) pointed to inhibition of carbonic anhydrase as the key to diuretic agents. Novello, Sprague, Beyer, and associates in the Renal Program at Merck, Sharp and Dohme synthesized a number of compounds in the sulfanilamide-carbonic anhydrase series and tested them for diuretic activity. They hit the jackpot with chlorothiazide (a compound resulting from ring closure of chlorodisulfamylaniline); it *is* a sulfonamide derivative, it *is* a carbonic anhydrase inhibitor, but its powerful diuretic action is *not* due to its ability to inhibit carbonic anhydrase (19).

Did the Hopkins group in 1937–1938 anticipate the train of events set into motion by Southworth's careful clinical observations? Dr. Robert Dripps asked this question of Southworth in 1972 and Southworth replied in part (20):

I have been back over the original papers and have tried to think back over those days. Working with Perrin Long at Johns Hopkins, I was in on the first excitement of sulfa drugs and was lucky enough one day to pick up the first case of acidosis associated with the use of sulfanilamide. [see (17)]. The subsequent work done with Margaret Strauss of the Biochemical Department was an attempt to work out why the acidosis developed and incidentally showed that large doses did increase the urine volume and the renal excretion of sodium and potassium [see (18)]. It also showed, interestingly enough, that some hemoconcentration was produced but Bob Loeb, who went over the paper with me at Presbyterian where I had moved at the end of '37, was suspicious of the figures on blood sodiums and would not let me publish them. No one knew then about carbonic acid anhydrase and we therefore couldn't explain the acidosis. By the time this paper came out, I was in the practice of medicine and was just winding up what I had done as a resident.

It is hard to remember just how much we did think of the diuretic possibilities of what we had found. I don't think it was very much and yet the paper went through the hands of Warfield Longcope and Robert F. Loeb so I was not the only one who failed to see the potential future significance. It is my vague recollection that we didn't take it too seriously because we were giving big doses (up to 6 to 8 gms) of a drug the toxic and allergic effects of which were just being described all around us, and which we only considered using in people who had quite serious infections. I don't, however, remember any of us considering that an analogue of the drug might be developed which would have this effect in smaller doses and with less toxicity. Also those were the days when diuresis was not considered as important as it was subsequently. We had Salyrgan and we thought it was quite good for the waterlogged cardiac.

Southworth missed the opportunity to develop or participate directly in the development of oral diuretics; "It was hard," he said in retrospect, "to realize that I was on the brink of something important [in 1937–38] and didn't really appreciate it." However, his astute clinical observations showed Beyer and his associates where to look. And that must be satisfying in itself.

OTHER MISSED OPPORTUNITIES

Karl Landsteiner won the Nobel Prize for discovering human blood groups and could have won it twice over for discovering the viral cause of poliomyelitis and his work on the Rh factor. But it was Ottenberg in 1911 and not Landsteiner in 1900 who first crossmatched blood to prevent human transfusion reactions.

Werner Forssmann catheterized his own heart but missed the opportunity to follow up and use his new tool for diagnostic purposes. He tried (21) but got crushed by the German geheimrat system. (See p. 114)

Marie Krogh devised a single breath test of diffusing capacity of the lungs but never used it for clinical diagnosis of disorders of the lungs or pulmonary capillary bed (22). However, she designed her test only to decide whether oxygen crossed the alveolar-to-capillary barrier by diffusion alone or in part by secretion. She had no need for it thereafter and in any case simple and rapid methods of gas analysis had to be invented before the test lent itself to use on large numbers of subjects and patients.

Waksman had a number of opportunities to discover streptomycin before 1944. The first was early in his scientific career; his main interest was then in soil (how it decomposed organic material added to it) and not in microbes, even though he did do studies on *Streptomyces griseus* between 1916 and 1919. Again, in 1932 he missed an opportunity when his pathologist friend, Beaudette, brought him a culture of tubercle bacilli apparently killed by a fungus growing on it; Waksman failed to study it. Then in the early 1940s his son Byron, now a prominent scientist in his own right but then a medical student, wrote to his father (23):

In reading the reprints you sent me, I was struck again with the urge to do some work in the direction of finding an effective *in vivo* antagonist to the tubercle bacillus. I was particularly impressed with the relative simplicity of the method you have used in isolating fungi-producing antibiotic substances, and I wondered if exactly the same method could not be used with equal ease to isolate a number of strains of fungi or actinomycetes which would act against *M. tuberculosis*. They could be tested after isolation against some more rapidly growing organism such as *M. phlei in vitro*, and finally against the tubercle bacillus itself *in vivo*. . . . . From the little reading I have done, it is my impression that no one as yet has published any work of this nature. There is no question that it has a great deal of practical value or would have if successfully concluded.

His father answered: "The time has not come yet. We are not quite prepared to undertake the problem." I wonder if this was a misunderstanding: the *son* was prepared to tackle the research while still a medical student; the *father* was not. In 1944, the father was prepared and isolated streptomycin (24).

Gross was the first to successfully ligate a patent ductus arteriosus in a child but when Taussig offered him the first crack at the now famous "blue-baby operation" he had no interest in it, and turned her down. Learning that she was thinking of moving to Boston, he advised her not to come where she would not be tolerated. "Stay where you are wanted," he said (25). She did, and so Gross left the field wide open for Alfred Blalock at Hopkins who eagerly collaborated with Taussig.

Hunt and Taveau in 1906 published a classic paper on the extraordinary physiologic activity of acetylcholine (26). In it they studied a number of other choline derivatives including succinylcholine. They completely missed its neuromuscular blocking effect because they worked on animals *curarized* at the onset of the experiment. As a result, succinylcholine never entered medical practice until 1949. Was this a missed opportunity for use of muscle relaxants in the practice of medicine and anesthesiology? Maybe not, for these reasons: (*1*) few surgeons or anesthetists in the early 1900s knew how to maintain artificial ventilation in man, (*2*) the deliberate paralysis of skeletal muscles, including the muscles of respiration, probably had to await the development of a new specialty of professional, medically trained anesthetists (in the 1940s), and (*3*) Meltzer and Auer in their experimental studies of insufflation respiration in dogs (27) routinely gave their animals an intravenous injection of curare sufficient to abolish any spontaneous or reflex movements. Though they stated that the dog's "life is as safe [with curare] as under regular artificial respiration," they never proposed its clinical use, nor did anyone else until 1942. I doubt that availability of a pure agent, such as succinylcholine, would have made surgeons any more comfortable about operating on a paralyzed patient.

Diphenylhydantoin (dilantin) was used for 20 years to decrease the excitability of cells in the motor cortex of epileptic patients before Leonard first used it to control ventricular tachycardia in man (28).

Local anesthetics were used experimentally for 48 years to reduce cardiac excitability in animals before James Southworth and associates finally used lidocaine to reverse ventricular fibrillation in man (29). Plenty of time for missed opportunities over these two decades, especially since it encompassed the important decades in which cardiac surgery began and matured.

Ganglionic blocking agents were known as early as 1915, when Burn and Dale clearly recognized that tetraethylammonium was a ganglionic "paralyzing" agent capable of blocking sympathetic nerve impulses to the heart and arterioles. But it was not until 1946 that Lyons and associates (30) used it to lower blood pressure in hypertensive patients by performing a "chemical sympathectomy." Were there missed opportunities for its use during this 31-year period? Probably "yes" in the 1930s and thereafter, but probably "no" before, because most physicians believed that patients with hypertension had initial renal disease and reduced renal blood flow. They believed that the resulting hypertension was compensatory or essential to maintain renal circulation and prolong the patient's life, even though it eventually caused cardiac hypertrophy and heart failure.

CONCLUDING REMARKS

Much has been said and written about lags between initial scientific discovery and final clinical application. In many instances, the lag was unavoidable because whole new branches of science had to come into being before the initial discovery could move forward (e.g., the invention of the microscope could not lead to antibiotics until it first led to the discovery of microbes, the germ theory of disease and the sciences of microbiology and pharmacology). Sometimes, however, an individual made observations crucial to an important next or even final step but didn't realize their significance. These "missed opportunities" cannot be labelled scientific discoveries "locked up" in a laboratory by an unconcerned scientist. They are an almost inevitable result of the background, training and environment of that scientist and his immediate goals and preoccupations that blind him to a new concept. It has been said that the eye often sees only that behind it and not what is in front of it. If it is any consolation to those who missed magnificent opportunities, remember that the world's greatest inventor, Thomas Edison, failed to see any useful application at all for his greatest scientific discovery, the "Edison effect," which later was the basis for the audion or vacuum tube that permitted the development of radio. And missed opportunities are not limited to science: Winston Churchill said, "Men occasionally stumble over the truth, but most of them pick themselves up and hurry off as if nothing had happened."

References

1. Heidelberger, M.: Personal communication to Robert Dripps, June 1, 1972.
2a. Hörlein, H.: German patent DRP 226239, May 18, 1909.
2b. Hörlein, H.: The chemotherapy of infectious diseases caused by protozoa and bacteria, Proc R Soc Med, 1935, *29*, 313–324.
3. Abel, J. J., Rowntree, L. G., and Turner, B. B.:

On the removal of diffusible substances from the circulating blood of living animals by dialysis, J Pharmacol Exp Ther, 1914, *5*, 275–316.

4. Kolff, W. J., and Berk, H. T. J.: Artificial kidney, dialyzer with great area, Geneesk Gids, 1943 *5*, 21.

5. Best, C. H.: Heparin and thrombosis, Harvey Lect, 1940-41, *36*, 66–90.

6. Schmidt, A.: Zur Blutlehre, Vogel, Leipzig, 1892.

7. Doyon, M.: Rapports du foie avec la coagulation du sang, J Physiol Pathol Gen, 1912, *14*, 229–240.

8. Best, C. H.: Personal communication to J. H. Comroe, November 23, 1972.

9. Cooper, A.: Some experiments and observations on tying the carotid and vertebral arteries, and the pneumo-gastric, phrenic, and sympathetic nerves, Guy's Hosp Rep, 1836, *1*, 457–475.

10. Bayliss, W. M.: On the physiology of the depressor nerve, J Physiol, 1893, *14*, 303–325.

11. Hill, L.: The Physiology and Pathology of the Cerebral Circulation, Churchill, London, 1896.

12. Porter, W. T., and Pratt, F. H.: The reactions of peripheral vasomotor areas, Am J Physiol, 1908, *21*, 16P; see also Porter, W. T.: On the percentile measurement of the vasomotor reflexes, Am J Physiol, 1914, *33*, 373–377, and Porter, W. T., and Pratt, J. H.: The state of the vasomotor centre in diphtheria intoxication, Am J Physiol, 1914, *33*, 431–440.

13. Eyster, L. A. E., and Hooker, D. R.: Direct and reflex response of the cardioinhibitory centre to increased blood pressure, Am J Physiol, 1908, *21*, 373–399.

14. Hering, H. E.: Der Karotisdruckversuch, Münch Med Wochenschr, 1923, *70*, 1287–1290.

15. Anrep, G. V., and Starling, E. H.: Central and reflex regulation of the circulation, Proc R Soc Lond [B], 1925, *97*, 463–487.

16. Becker, H. K.: Carl Koller and cocaine, The Psychoanalytic Quarterly, 1963, reprinted in *Cocaine Papers: Sigmund Freud*, ed. R. Byck, Stonehill, New York, 1974.

17. Southworth, H.: Acidosis associated with the administration of para-amino-benzene-sulfonamide (Prontylin), Proc Soc Exp Biol Med, 1937, *36*, 58–61.

18. Strauss, M. B., and Southworth, H.: Urinary changes due to sulfanilamide administration, Bull Johns Hopkins Hosp, 1938, *63*, 41–45.

19. Beyer, K. H., Baer, J. F., Russo, H. F., and Noll, R.: Electrolyte excretion as influenced by chlorothiazide, Science, 1958, *127*, 146–147.

20. Southworth, H.: Personal communication to Robert Dripps, 1972.

21. This volume, How to delay progress without even trying, pp. 114-119.

22. This volume, Harnessing carbon monoxide, pp. 27-30.

23. Waksman, S.: My Life with the Microbes, Simon and Schuster, New York, 1954.

24. Schatz, A., Bugie, E., and Waksman, S.: Streptomycin, a substance exhibiting antibiotic activity against Gram-positive and Gram-negative bacteria, Proc Soc Exp Biol Med, 1944, *55*, 66–69.

25. Harvey, A. M.: Adventures in Medical Research: A Century of Discovery at Johns Hopkins, Johns Hopkins University Press, Baltimore, 1976, pp. 236–237.

26. Hunt, R., and Taveau, R. de M.: On the physiological action of certain cholin derivatives and new methods for detecting cholin, Br Med J, 1906, *2*, 1788–1791.

27. Meltzer, S. J., and Auer, J.: Continuous respiration without respiratory movements, J Exp Med, 1909, *11*, 622–625.

28. Leonard, W. A.: The use of diphenylhydantoin (Dilantin) sodium in the treatment of ventricular tachycardia, Arch Int Med, 1958, *101*, 714–717.

29. Southworth, J. L., McKusick, V. A., Peirce, E. C., and Rawson, F. L.: Ventricular fibrillation precipitated by cardiac catheterization, JAMA, 1950, *143*, 717–720.

30. Lyons, R. H., Moe, G. K., Neligh, R. B., Hoobler, S. W., Campbell, K. N., Berry, R. L., and Rennick, B. R.: The effects of blockade of the autonomic ganglia in man with tetraethylammonium, Am J Med Sci, 1947, *213*, 315–323.

Publish and/or Perish

I've just finished an analysis of lags between scientific discovery and clinical application. In all, I've identified 17 different causes of lags. The one that has bothered the Administration and Congress the most in recent years—that university scientists "lock up" important discoveries in their laboratories—ranks numerically at the very bottom of the list, at least in the past 50 years.

It has not always been this way. I'm sure some early scientists decided not to publish at all in days when the reward for a real "breakthrough" was beheading or burning at the stake instead of today's Nobel prize. And even when burning went out of fashion, publication of some major discoveries was delayed until the authors could predict the reception awaiting them—acclaim or ridicule.

Three of the best-known instances of delay between completion of observations or experiments and their publication were those for the main works of Copernicus (31 years), Harvey (12 years), and Darwin (23 years).

Copernicus. His final work, *De Revolutionibus*, was published in 1543 (1). However, its essential concepts were included in his much earlier manuscript, *Commentariolus*, which may have been written as early as 1512. He kept revising it and adding fresh observations for almost 30 years and with each revision avoided the final step of full publication.

Historians give two possible reasons for his delay. The first is that he feared the opposition or displeasure of the Church or even persecution. If he feared this, it was not without some cause. Luther, on hearing of Copernicus's theory of a sun-centered universe, stated, ". . . this man subverts the whole field of astronomy. . . . I believe the Holy Scripture. After all, Joshua (10:13) commanded the sun to stand still and not the earth" (2). However, the Church took no positive action against the Copernican concept for more than 50 years—until Bruno had not only accepted most of the Copernican view but carried it a step further. In 1600, Bruno was burned at the stake for heresy; at the same time, Coperni-

cus's work was banned by the Church, a ban not lifted until 1822. And these drastic steps came before the Church realized the full impact of Copernicus's book; this came when Galileo developed his telescope in 1609 and soon provided visual proof that the earth was not the center of the universe as described in Genesis. This lag in the Church's appreciation of Copernicus's work meant that it was Galileo who risked defying the holy establishment, in 1616 and in 1633, in defense of a dead man's theory.

The second reason for Copernicus's delay—and the one given by most historians—was his fear of ridicule. Copernicus once said, "The contempt which I had to fear because of the novelty and apparent absurdity of my view nearly induced me to abandon utterly the work I had begun" (3). The concept that earth revolved once a day about its own axis without every loose object falling off was easy to ridicule in the 1500s and even centuries later.

In any case, Copernicus was subjected neither to persecution nor, during his life, to ridicule. This was because he delayed publication until he knew he had little time left on his spinning globe. In the winter of 1542-43, he suffered a paralytic stroke, with no hope of recovery. The first copy of his long-delayed book—an advance copy—was put in his hands on May 24, 1543 and several hours later, he died (4).

Harvey. Harvey discovered the circulation of the blood long before he published his small book, *De Motu Cordis,* in 1628. He presented his anatomic findings in a lecture in 1616 and had demonstrated them to students before that time. Why then did he delay for at least 12 years putting his observations and conclusions into print? Newman (5) points out Harvey's fear of possible charges of rash innovation or even of heresy. Harvey was apprehensive about writing a book and rightly so, for after its publication "he fell mightily in his practise and 'twas believed by the vulgar that he was crack-brained." Harvey himself said, "I not only fear injury to myself from the envy of the few, but I tremble lest I have mankind at large for my enemies" (5). William Cruikshank much later (1790) wrote: "When Harvey discovered the circulation, his opponents first attempted to prove that he was mistaken; but finding this ground untenable, they then asserted that it was known long before . . . when informed that the world at large were totally ignorant of the fact . . . except for Harvey, they once more shifted their ground, and said the discovery was of no use." (5a)

Darwin. Charles Darwin completed all of his observations needed for the *Origin of Species* in 1836, but did not publish his book until 1859. Why? Partly because he was innately cautious, partly because of chronic illness, partly because of other responsibilities, but also partly because of his fear that his concept would not be accepted and might even lead to persecution. In his notebooks for 1837-38 (6), Darwin wrote:

> Mention persecution of early astronomers. Then add chief good of individual scientific men is to push their science a few years in advance of their age. . . . Must remember that if they *believe* and do not openly avow their belief they do much to retard.

So early on, Darwin realized the potential importance of his observations to science, his obligation to publish them to avoid retarding scientific advance, *and* the consequences to his reputation if his ideas were not accepted. For 22 years, the consequences prevailed over the obligation. But the imperative to publish came in 1858 when Alfred Wallace independently discovered the principle of survival of the fittest and, knowing of Darwin's interest in the subject, sent a short paper to Darwin for his opinion. Darwin noted: "I never saw a more striking coincidence: if Wallace had my Ms. sketch written in 1842, he could not have made a better short abstract" (7, pp. 199-200). What might have become a historic struggle for priority was settled in a remarkable way. Darwin and Wallace sent a joint memoir to the Linnean Society on July 1, 1858 entitled, "On the tendency of species to form varieties; and on the perpetuation of varieties and species by natural means of selection" (8). Neither author was present at the meeting; there was no discussion and no sign of interest by the audience. In the annual Society report for that year, the President wrote: "The year . . . has not been marked by any of those striking discoveries which at once revolutionize, so to speak, the department of science on which they bear." Darwin, in his autobiography (7, p. 55), says the only published notice of the Darwin-Wallace joint production was by Professor Haughton of Dublin, who wrote that all that was new in them was false and what was true was old. (Note the similarity to the earlier criticism of Harvey's book!)

But Darwin now had to make a choice between not publishing at all and perishing *for certain,* or publishing and *possibly* perishing. He chose the latter. *Origin of Species* appeared in November 1859. It at once became a "best seller"; the first edition sold out on the day of publication and 16,000 copies were sold by 1876. From 1859 on, Evolution = Darwin, not Wallace, or Darwin and Wallace. But the two remained lifelong friends; Darwin secured a government pension for Wallace, and Wallace was one of Darwin's pallbearers.

Others who took years to publish were Long (7 years), Le Gallois (6 years), and Gley (17 years).

Long. Crawford Long was graduated from the University of Pennsylvania Medical School in 1839 and then established a country practice in Jefferson, Georgia. The counterparts of our present "glue sniffers" or "pot heads" were in that era the "laughing gas" inhalers. Some of these fun-loving lads asked Long to prepare some nitrous oxide for them to inhale at parties. According to Long: "I informed them that I had no apparatus for preparing or administering the gas, but that I had a medicine (sulphuric ether) which would produce equally exhilerating [*sic*] effects; that I had inhaled it myself, and considered it as safe as the nitrous oxide gas. I gave it to the gentleman who had previously inhaled it, then inhaled it myself and afterwards gave it to all persons present. . . . its inhalation soon became quite fashionable in this county. I noticed my friends, while etherized, received falls or blows, which I believe were sufficient to produce pain on a person not in a state of anesthesia and on questioning them, they uniformly assured me that they did not feel the least pain from these accidents" (9).

On March 30, 1842, he administered ether anesthesia while he removed an encysted tumor from the back of the neck of a patient who had repeatedly postponed the operation for fear of pain. When informed that the operation was over, the patient was incredulous until Long showed him the excised tumor.

Why did Long wait until 1849 to publish the results of his 1842 and later use of ether to produce surgical anesthesia? Long said: "I commenced a publication to the editor of the Medical Examiner. . . . I was interrupted when I had written but a few lines by a very laborious country practice from resuming my communication until the Medical Examiner for January 1847 was received which reached me in a few days after reading the December number [that number contained an abstract of Bigelow's paper in the *Boston Journal* describing Morton's use of ether] . . . I determined to wait a few months before publishing an account of my discovery and see whether any surgeon would present a claim to having used ether inhalation in surgical operations prior to the time it was used by me." Long further explained his reluctance in 1842 to publish his 1842 use of ether: "I was anxious, before making my publication, to try etherization in a sufficient number of cases to satisfy my mind that anaesthesia was produced by the ether and was not the effect of the imagination, or owing to any peculiar insusceptibility to pain in the persons experimented on. . . . There were physicians high in authority . . . who were advocates of mesmerism and recommended the induction of the mesmeric state as adequate to prevent pain in surgical operations. I was an unbeliever . . . and of the opinion that if the mesmeric state could be produced at all, it was . . . to be ascribed solely to the workings of the patient's imaginations. Entertaining this opinion, I was the more particular in my experiments in etherization."

The FDA would have been proud of Crawford Long but it was Morton, Wells, and Jackson who got credit for the first use of a general anesthetic agent. But otherwise, things went poorly for the latter three. They fought over priority and patent rights; Wells became insane and committed suicide at the age of 33, Jackson became insane, and Morton, impoverished and embittered, died of apoplexy at the age of 49. Long, who simply announced his earlier use of ether but never insisted on or fought for priority, had a happy and productive life until his natural death at the age of 63.

Le Gallois. This French scientist is remembered mainly for locating the medullary centers required for rhythmic breathing. But he was also one of the first to do research on fetal circulation and respiration and to note the resistance of the newborn and of cold-blooded animals to asphyxia, submersion, or opening the thorax. He did his research on the fetus and newborn in 1806, presented the results orally in 1808, and demonstrated his findings in 1809 but did not publish his *Le Principe de la Vie* until 1812, after a lag of 6 years (10). His simple explanation, "I have

been more careful in ascertaining the facts than eager to publish them!" assures him a place in my hall of fame.

Gley. We now come to what must be the most extraordinary lag between discovery and publication in the history of biomedical science (11).

In 1859, Langerhans, in his M.D. thesis, had described islands of cells scattered throughout the pancreas of the rabbit. In 1882, Languesse, a French histologist, named these the islets of Langerhans; because a year earlier Von Mering and Minkowski had removed the pancreas from dogs and noted that the dogs' urine was then loaded with sugar, Languesse proposed that islet cells secrete a substance that normally prevents glucose from appearing in urine.

If there were two types of secretory cells in the pancreas (exocrine, for digestion of fat in the intestine, and endocrine, to prevent loss of blood sugar in the urine), it should be possible to separate them. Gley attempted to do this, utilizing an old technic of Claude Bernard's, the injection of denatured gelatine backwards into the pancreatic duct to destroy the exocrine cells associated with these ducts. He then made an extract of what was left of the pancreas (the endocrine islet cells) and injected it into other dogs whose pancreas had been removed completely. The "clinical condition" of the injected dogs improved and the concentration of glucose in their urine decreased. Gley's report said in part:

> I have tried to find whether the sclerosed but nevertheless still functioning pancreas , prepared by the technic described, would yield the active material that it continued to produce. The extract, injected into dogs previously made diabetic by total removal of the pancreas, decreased considerably the quantity of sugar eliminated by these dogs. At the same time, it improved all of the symptoms of the diabetes. More complete experiments will permit me to determine for certain the mechanism of action of these extracts. [My translation]

But although his research and report were completed in 1905, the report was not published until 1922 (12)! In February 1905, Gley turned over his report, in a sealed envelope, to the Société de Biologie, not to be opened until Gley requested it. In December 1922, shortly after the first published reports of Banting and his associates on insulin (13), Gley, by now Professor of Physiology at the University of Paris, requested that the Société now open and publish his 1905 paper, "Sur la sécrétion interne du pancréas et son utilisation thérapeutique" (12).

Why this extraordinary sealing up of an important discovery for 17 years? On p. 1324 he says (my translation), "I have wished more than once to complete the research presented here but it required a great number of experimental animals at the time and, lacking the material means for lodging and maintaining these animals, I had to abandon the experiments each time. Now that Macleod has made known the results of his very interesting experiments [13], I no longer dream of resuming mine. And it is only just, for one who knows the difficulties and inherent disappointments in this type of research, to congratulate him on having conducted them so well." Despite his explanation, I have the feeling that Gley never really convinced himself of the accuracy of his experiments or of the importance of his results to medicine, or he would have gone through fire and water to have completed them in 1905.

These are six well-recorded delays in the transmission of scientific knowledge that must be attributed entirely to the scientist himself. What were the consequences of these delays? In the case of Le Gallois, the delay probably had a beneficial effect on biological science because Le Gallois stated for all to read (and emulate) his greater concern for accuracy than for priority; in retrospect, it did no harm because there was no important clinical need for his observations until 140 years later when hypothermia and infants with congenital heart defects entered the surgeon's domain.

In the case of Crawford Long, prompt publication might have saved lives and reduced suffering between 1842 and 1846, if an editor had accepted a manuscript submitted by a country doctor and if surgeons elsewhere had paid attention to it. However, the important lag was not between Long's use of ether and his publication but between Faraday's 1818 *suggestion* that ether might be an anesthetic agent and the 1840s application. I wonder if we shouldn't spend more time unearthing long-lost, untested suggestions and less in trying to discover who did what before whom!

In most cases, publication of unfinished work retards science, especially when not clearly labelled "Unfinished." But if Gley had published his experiments in 1905 as "Unfinished," with an invitation to others with better facilities to complete them, insulin might have been ready for diabetic patients 17 years earlier. Gley even had available a journal (the *Comptes Rendus de la Société de Biologie*) that often published the results of a single experiment.

As matters turned out, the delays by Copernicus and Harvey did not hold back science. Copernicus's 1543 publication required Galileo's telescope in the next century to provide convincing proof of his work and Harvey's *De Motu Cordis* had little impact until the 1660s and 1670s when experimental biology began to flourish with the beginnings of the Royal Society. Had Darwin delayed indefinitely in publishing, the theory of evolution would have been Wallace's, and Wallace, instead of Darwin, would have been on trial in the famous Scopes monkey case in Tennessee.

I believe that almost every scientist working today can get his work published, somewhere, once he decides to "write it up"; maybe it will be in the Bulletin of the Podunk County Medical Society rather than in a journal with international prestige or readership, or maybe it will be published only as an abstract. The main determinant of what is or is not published therefore seems to be the scientist, for it is he who decides to become or not become an author. Edison, for example, although he wrote about 1,300 patent applications, appears to have published only 10 papers, a total of 27 pages, between 1874 and 1900. Some well-known scientists have more than 800 published papers to their credit in their lifetime; others, equally well known, fewer than fifty. We have no way of learning how many experimental observations—right or wrong, momentous or trivial—have never been put into final manuscript form by hesitant, unconvinced, or indolent scientists, or by geniuses with far more ideas than time to complete work on them.

What to do with unpublished notes, observations, and ideas? Need these be "locked up" in a scientist's head or "little black book"? Many eventually find their way (either by hard or soft sell) into the work of colleagues, associates or research fellows. Some reach a much larger group of scientists, editors of journals permitting, in the form of unanswered questions and speculation. More later on the role of speculation in advancing science (see "Speculation on Speculation," pp. 99-105).

References

1. Copernicus, N.: De Revolutionibus Orbium Coelestium Libri Sex, ed. 1, Nuremberg, 1543.
2. Oberman, H. A.: in *The Nature of Scientific Dis-*

covery, O. Gingerich, ed., Smithsonian Institute, Washington, D. C., 1975, p. 139.

3. Schwartz, G., and Bishop, P. W.: Moments of Discovery, vol. 1, Basic Books, New York, 1958, p. 219.

4. Armitage, A.: Copernicus, The Founder of Modern Astronomy, Allen and Unwin, London, 1938, p. 60.

5. Newman, C. E.: The art of the De Motu Cordis, Br Med J, 1974, *1*, 616-21.

5a. Cruikshank, W.: Anatomy of the Absorbing Vessels of the Human Body, 2nd ed., London, Nicol, 1790.

6. Koestler, A.: The Act of Creation, Hutchinson, London, 1964, p. 136.

7. Charles Darwin's Autobiography, with His Notes and Letters Depicting the Growth of the *Origin of Species*, Sir Francis Darwin, ed., Schuman, New York, 1950.

8. Darwin, C., and Wallace, A. R.: On the tendency of species to form varieties; and on the perpetuation of varieties and species by natural means of selection, J Proc Linn Soc., 1858, pp. 45, 46-53, 53-62.

9. Long, C. W.: An account of the first use of sulphuric ether by inhalation as an anaesthetic in surgical operations, South Med Surg J, 1849, *5*, 705-713.

10. Le Gallois, J. J. C.: Expériences sur le Principe de la Vie, Chez D'Hautel, Paris, 1812.

11. Henderson, J. R.: Who discovered insulin?, Guys Hosp Gaz, 1971, *85*, 315-318.

12. Gley, E.: Action des extraits de pancréas sclérosé sur des Chiens diabétiques (par extirpation du pancréas), C R Soc Biol, 1922, *87*, 1322-1325.

13. Banting, F. G., Best, C. H., Collip, J. B., MacLeod, J. J. R., and Noble, E. C.: The effect of pancreatic extract (insulin) on normal rabbits, Am J Physiol, 1922, *62*, 162-176, 559-580.

Publisher's Dawdle: An Incurable Disease?

Like most people who complain about the weather, most scientists complain about long delays in publication, but few if any do anything about it. Roland and Kirkpatrick (1) divided into eight components the period between authors' hypotheses (conception of the idea) and date of publication of their manuscripts and determined the time required for each component. For papers dealing with laboratory or clinical investigation, the total time was about four years. The time for review and decision-making by the editors of journals was a little more than 1 1/2 months, for revision by authors about 3 months, and for the mechanics of publication (after final acceptance of a manuscript) about 5 1/2 months; the total time for "getting it published," once the manuscript was finished, was thus about 10 months.

It's the figure of 5 1/2 months, the mechanics of publishing, that puzzles me. Some editors take the position that since the process of research and writing a manuscript may take a year or two, why fuss about speeding up the mechanical process of publication by 4 to 5 months? But slow publication is an anachronism in the modern era of electronics and computers which have revolutionized not only the speed of making scientific measurements but also the process of printing and reproduction. A Sunday newspaper, one almost too heavy to lift, can be put together once a week. In some of its sections, it includes news that is only a few hours old and readers would scream if the "news" was any older. But a scientific journal, about 1/3 the weight, takes 5 1/2 months for the purely mechanical tasks of copy editing, typesetting, proofreading, printing, and binding!

It has not always been so. If we look way back through the Retrospectroscope into the seventeenth century, we see that the editor of the *Philosophical Transactions of the Royal Society*

stopped the press to publish Robert Hooke's experiments (2) proving that motion of the lungs and thorax was not essential to life as long as fresh air reached the alveoli; he accomplished alveolar ventilation without motion of the thorax or lungs by pricking many spots on the outer surface of the lungs with a sharp, pointed knife and then blowing a steady flow of air through the trachea, bronchioles, and alveoli, out to the surrounding air. The editor's explanation is reproduced in figure 1; in it, he notes that the experiment had been repeated as a demonstration before a public assembly, and that this obviously constituted satisfactory editorial review. The reception must have warranted instant publication and, since the industrial, electrical, and electronic revolutions and the U. S. Postal Service had not yet been invented, instant publication seems to have been a fairly simple matter.

In the nineteenth century, the Retrospectroscope shows that Roentgen's experiments on X-rays were published within weeks of the completed observations (3). No one knows when Roentgen completed the experiments reported in his December 28, 1895 paper but he presumably made his first observation on November 8, 1895. He then proceeded, to be sure that these were indeed previously unknown rays, to study the effect of various metals of different thicknesses on the passage of X-rays and to determine whether the rays could be refracted, reflected, condensed, or deflected by strong magnetic fields. These experiments, and his writing a ten-page paper, must have taken him until mid-December. Whether the *Sitzungsberichte* for December 1895 was actually published in late December or the first week in January 1896, we do not know. But, for certain, Roentgen had reprints (or preprints) before January 1, and, for certain, a complete English translation ap-

An Account
Of an Experiment made by M.Hook, of Preserving Animals alive by Blowing through their Lungs with Bellows.

This Noble Experiment came not to the Publisher's hands, till all the preceding Particulars were already sent to the Press, and almost all Printed off, (for which cause also it could not be mentioned among the Contents:) And it might have been reserved for the next opportunity, had not the considerableness thereof been a motive to hasten its Publication. It shall be here annexed in the Ingenious Author his own words, as he presented it to the Royal Society, Octob. 24. 1667. the Experiment it self having been both repeated (after a former successful trial of it, made by the same hand a good while agoe) and improved the week before, at their publick Assembly. The Relation it self followes;

Fig. 1. Prefatory comments to 1667 account by "M. Hook" (Robert Hooke) proving that life can be maintained without motion of the lungs.

peared in *Nature* in its January 23, 1896 issue, crossed the Atlantic, and was reprinted in *Science* in its February 14 issue. Incidentally, none of the three editors bothered to comment on the speed of publication in German, English, or American journals.

The world's record, however, was probably made in that same year by Thomas Cullen in Baltimore for his paper, "A rapid method of making permanent specimens from frozen sections by the use of formalin," which appeared in the *Johns Hopkins Hospital Bulletin* in 1895 (vol. 6, p. 67). According to Cullen, as reported by Harvey (4):

I tested the formalin method I had worked out on every sort of tissue and in every way I could think of. Then I went upstairs showing one of my sections to Dr. Welch and told him how I had hardened it and how long it had taken me. He looked at it and listened. Then he handed me a piece of tissue . . . "Take this and prepare it your way," he said. "If you make me a satisfactory specimen, I will be convinced." I took the tissue and made a specimen and brought it back. Popsy looked at it, looked at his watch and said, "Publish it." So I did. I wrote up the method and took my paper to Dr. Hurd, who was then editor of *The Johns Hopkins Hospital Bulletin*, the same night, but it was nearly too late. Dr. Hurd said he was sorry but the last copy for the next issue of the *Bulletin* had gone to the printer and mine would have to wait a month. I was going away on that comment, but he called me back and asked me how much space I would need to describe my hardening method. I said half a page, and he said "go ahead and

write it then." "It's written," I said, and gave it to him and it was in print in the *Bulletin* two days later.

At the beginning of this century, Dr. L. L. Hill of Birmingham, Alabama, performed the first successful operation on a heart in America; he sutured a stab wound in the heart of a 13-year-old boy. Dr. Hill operated on September 14, 1902 and kept his patient in the hospital until at least early October. His report related not only this experience but included a scholarly review of the world's literature on wounds of the heart and their management. He had previously reported on 17 such cases but brought his list up to 39 reports that had been published in at least four foreign language journals. This (while still attending to a busy practice) must have taken him into November. Yet his article was published in an American medical journal on November 29, 1902 (5).

In 1922, Schofield's discovery that hemorrhagic disease in cattle was caused by their munching on moldy sweet clover (and that plasma prothrombin was greatly decreased in these diseased animals*) was published so quickly that Schofield felt compelled to write an apology as his final paragraph (6):

This paper has been written very hurriedly as the editor was insistent that it appear in this issue.

*Later authors usually get credit for first noting the decreased plasma prothrombin, but Schofield states clearly on his page 77: "There is . . . a greatly diminished quantity of prothrombin [in the blood]."

I therefore ask the readers to be lenient in their criticism, not of the contents, but of the arrangement of the material presented.

A recent record in short gestation, on January 30, 1970, *Science* published its "Moon Issue" (7). It brought together in one issue 144 scientific articles dealing with the scientific aspects of the first scientific exploration of the surface of the moon. The total time from receipt of the authors' manuscripts to mailing the completed journal was 24 days! *Science* magazine was not shy in reporting its achievement in rapid publication of scientific reports; it presented in tabular form each step in the process and how long it took (table 1) (8).

This table is wonderfully informative: first, it shows each step in the process between receiving manuscripts and mailing them, professionally edited and printed in a journal, to 150,000 subscribers; and second, it shows how little time is really needed when someone makes up his or her mind to accord scientific articles the treatment regularly given by the daily press to murder, rape, war, and football games.

Once it demonstrated that it could be done, did *Science* continue to publish at this fast pace? Except for the staff of *Science* and individual contributors who keep logs, no one knows; I

TABLE 1

DATES OF START AND FINISH OF EACH STEP
IN THE PUBLICATION OF THE APOLLO 11
LUNAR SCIENCE CONFERENCE
ISSUE OF *SCIENCE*

Step	Dates
Receipt of manuscripts from authors	4–7 January
Reviewing of manuscripts	4–8 January
Authors' responses to reviews	5–8 January
Style editing and marking for printer	5–12 January
Redrafting and relettering illustrations	5–12 January
Authors' responses to style editing	5–23 January
Preparation of engravings	8–22 January
Typesetting	9–19 January
Proofreading of galley proofs	10–19 January
Pasteup of page dummies	13–20 January
Correction of galleys and makeup of pages	13–21 January
Proofreading of page proofs	17–24 January
Correction of pages	20–26 January
Proofreading of revised page proofs	21–27 January
Printing	23–28 January
Binding	28–30 January
Mailing	28–31 January

would guess that for some individual articles or letters it does publish quickly but that for most it does not.

Turning the Retrospectroscope into my own file cabinet, I learned that in late 1965, the Publications Committee of the American Heart Association asked me to be editor of *Circulation Research* for a 5-year term. I checked the time required for publication of accepted articles and found that it was about 6 months. I then asked the editor of *Proceedings of the National Academy of Sciences* for her publication schedule and learned that it was *6 weeks*. So my answer was easy: "If *Circulation Research* can match the publication schedule of PNAS, I'd like to take the job." The Publications Committee arranged a meeting for me with the publisher, printer, and engraver, at which I asked, "Can you put the printed journal in the mail 6 weeks after you get the last manuscript for it?" The answer came back immediately—"Sure." Taken by surprise, I asked, "Then why do you now take 6 months?" The answer was even more amazing—"No one ever asked us to do it in 6 weeks." "Will it cost more?" "No." So I signed an agreement with the American Heart Association; paragraph 12 stated:

It is understood that the Editor is vitally concerned with reducing the time between acceptance of a manuscript and its publication. The Association agrees to cooperate with the Editor to reduce this span and to pay for reasonable editorial staff required to meet the Editor's goal. It is further understood that if the Association is unable to meet the Editor's requirements on this point the Editor's term will conclude as of the December, 1967 issue upon notice given by him to the Publications Committee no later than January 1, 1967.

I never gave notice to the Committee because for the next 5 years, with minor exceptions, all articles accepted by the first of one month were in a bound journal in the mails on the 15th of the next month.†

Speedy publication has many advantages. Obviously, it speeds proper announcements of new advances of importance to physicians (and to their patients) and to other scientists; it speeds

† To keep everything honest, a "six-week" lag between accepting and publishing a manuscript in a monthly journal is six weeks only for those accepted near the monthly deadline; it's ten weeks for those that just missed the last deadline and so an average figure of eight weeks is about right. For a weekly publication, this range in lags would not apply.

publication of accurate accounts of other observations, less dramatic in themselves, but vitally important to the work of other scientists, possibly in unrelated fields; it could put an end to first announcement of "breakthroughs" in the "throw-away" medical journals, newspapers, and newsweeklies; and it might improve the quality of science by rechanneling scientific reports back into carefully edited journals and away from "quickie" journals that photograph and publish unreviewed, unrevised, unedited typewritten reports.

How are some heart and lung journals doing in 1976? Here are some figures for 6 journals during a 3-month period (table 2).

In their 1975 article, Roland and Kirkpatrick (1) divided the total time lapse between conception of the idea and final publication into eight components: planning time, research time, writing time, unexplained author delays, time for institutional editing, time for journal handling, revision time, and time for publication. I've never believed that one should hurry poorly conceived and badly done research through the planning and working stage and rush it off to an editor. I *do* believe that well-done work, accepted by critical reviewers, deserves as rapid publication as the funny papers. A lot of patients could die in a 5 1/2 month period between acceptance of the first paper on penicillin or sulfanilamide and its publication. Isn't it time that we catch up with the 1667 schedule of the Royal Society?

TABLE 2

TIME BETWEEN DATE OF ACCEPTANCE OF MANUSCRIPT AND DATE OF PUBLICATION OF JOURNAL

Journal	No. of Articles	Average Lag* (months)
Journal of Clinical Investigation (concise articles)	2	2.0
American Review of Respiratory Disease	47	3.2
Circulation Research	57	3.9
Respiration Physiology	33	3.9
Journal of Clinical Investigation (full articles)	84	4.2
Circulation	68	4.4
Chest	32	5.3

*These figures were calculated from the following data in each issue: Day #1 of the month printed on the journal's cover, and "date accepted," usually printed at the bottom of page 1 of each article in that issue. This calculation gives the *minimal* lag because (a) the official date of publication and mailing of a journal may be mid- or end-month and not day #1; (b) journals labelled October may actually be published later, even in the next month; and (c) no allowance is made for the weeks (?) that the journal is in the hands of the U. S. Postal "Service."

References
1. Roland, C. G., and Kirkpatrick, R. A.: Time lapse between hypothesis and publication in the medical sciences, N Engl J Med, 1975, *292,* 1273–1276.
2. Hooke, R.: An account of an experiment made by M. Hook[e], of preserving animals alive by blowing through their lungs with bellows, Philos Trans R Soc Lond, 1667, *2,* 539–540.
3. Röntgen, W. C.: Ueber eine neue Art von Strahlen, Sitzungsber Phys Med Gessel Würzburg, 1895, *134,* 132–141.
4. Harvey, A. M.: The second professor of gynecology and the department of art as applied to medicine, Johns Hopkins Med J, 1975, *137,* 224–234.
5. Hill, L. L.: A report of a case of successful suturing of the heart, and table of thirty-seven other cases of suturing by different operators with various terminations, and the conclusions drawn, Med Rec, 1902, *61,* 846–848.
6. Schofield, F. W.: A brief account of a disease in cattle simulating hemorrhagic septicaemia due to feeding sweet clover, Can Vet Rec, 1922, *3,* 74–78.
7. Science, 1970, *167,* 415–794.
8. *Ibid.,* p. 781.

. . . the soul of wit

Abraham Lincoln, on November 19, 1863, delivered his Gettysburg Address, one of the most elegant, famous, and widely quoted of modern speeches. Delivered on a Civil War battlefield, it was almost finished before the crowd became quiet. Few in the audience heard all or much of it. The Address contained only 272 words and, in print, was a single paragraph.

As a schoolboy, I (and I suppose all schoolchildren throughout America) memorized Lincoln's Address and recited it in the classroom. Never in my later scientific training, however, has anyone ever suggested that I memorize and recite a scientific article. I'm sure no candidate-article was as eloquent as Lincoln's Address, but some important discoveries or concepts were presented about as briefly. Here are a few; they include only complete accounts that stood alone and not abstracts that were enlarged upon later in a full article.

Benjamin Franklin, foremost scientist in the American Colonies, communicated in a one-page letter (one paragraph, 342 words, excluding his salutation) the details and conclusions of his famous kite and key experiment by which he demonstrated for the first time the "sameness" of lightning and "electric matter" stored in a Leyden jar (figure 1).

Korotkoff, in 1905, wrote a single paragraph describing how he modified Riva-Rocci's method to permit measurement of diastolic blood pressure and accurate recording of systolic pressure; his 1905 technic is essentially that used today. This paragraph is all that Korotkoff ever published on the subject (267 words in the English translation):

ON THE SUBJECT OF METHODS OF DETERMINING BLOOD PRESSURE

(From the clinic of Prof. S. P. Fedorov)

DR. N. S. KOROTKOFF:

On the basis of his observations, this reporter has arrived at the conclusion that a completely compressed artery in a normal condition does not produce any sound. Taking advantage of this situation the reporter proposes the sound method for determining the blood pressure in humans. The sleeve [cuff] of Riva-Rocci is placed on the middle 1/3 of the arm toward the shoulder. The pressure in the sleeve is raised quickly until it stops the circulation of the blood beyond the sleeve. Thereupon, permitting the mercury manometer to drop, a child's stethoscope is used to listen to the artery directly beyond the sleeve. At first no audible sound is heard at all. As the mercury manometer falls to a certain height the first short tones appear, the appearance of which indicates the passage of part of the pulse wave under the sleeve. Consequently, the manometer reading at which the first tones appear corresponds to the maximum pressure. With a further fall of the mercury in the manometer systolic pressure murmurs are heard which change again to a sound (secondary). Finally, all sounds disappear. The time at which the sounds disappear indicates a free passage of the pulse wave; in other words, at the moment the sounds disappear, the minimum blood pressure in the artery exceeds the pressure of the sleeve. Consequently, the reading of the manometer at this time corresponds to the minimum blood pressure. Experiments on animals gave positive results. The first sound-tones appear (10–12 mm.) sooner than the pulse, for the perception of which (r. art. radialis) the breakthrough of a greater part of the pulse wave is required.

Cooke and Barcroft, in 1913, recorded the first measurement of O_2 saturation of human arterial blood (four paragraphs, but only 180 words). Although Hürter had performed arterial puncture in Germany a year earlier, Barcroft took advantage of the then-current clinical technic for transfusion (inserting a cannula into the donor's artery and running arterial blood directly into the recipient's vein) to obtain blood without exposure to air or contamination with anesthetic gases. A year later, Hustin in Belgium hit upon citrate as a safe anticoagulant and in-

84

Oct. 19, 1752.

As frequent mention is made in the news papers from *Europe*, of the succefs of the *Philadelphia* experiment for drawing the electric fire from clouds by means of pointed rods of iron erected on high buildings, *&c.* it may be agreeable to inform the curious that the fame experiment has fucceeded in *Philadelphia*, though made in a different and more eafy manner, which is as follows :

Make a fmall crofs of two light ftrips of cedar, the arms fo long as to reach to the four corners of a large thin filk handkerchief when extended ; tie the corners of the handkerchief to the extremities of the crofs, fo you have the body of a kite ; which being properly accommodated with a tail, loop, and ftring, will rife in the air, like thofe made of paper ; but this being of filk is fitter to bear the wind and wet of a thunder guft without tearing. To the top of the upright ftick of the crofs is to be fixed a very fharp pointed wire, rifing a foot or more above the wood. To the end of the twine, next the hand, is to be ty'd a filk ribbon, and where the filk and twine join, a key may be faftened. This kite is to be raifed when a thunder guft appears to be coming on, and the perfon who holds the ftring muft ftand within a door, or window, or under fome cover, fo that the filk ribbon may not be wet ; and care muft be taken that the twine does not touch the frame of the door or window. As foon as any of the thunder clouds come over the kite, the pointed wire will draw the electric fire from them, and the kite, with all the twine, will be electrified, and the loofe filaments of the twine will ftand out every way, and be attracted by an approaching finger. And when the rain has wet the kite and twine, fo that it can conduct the electric fire freely, you will find it ftream out plentifully from the key on the approach of your knuckle. At this key the phial may be charged ; and from electric fire thus obtained, fpirits may be kindled, and all the other electric experiments be performed, which are ufually done by the help of a rubbed glafs globe or tube ; and thereby the famenefs of the electric matter with that of lightening completely demonftrated.

B. F.

Fig. 1. Letter from Benjamin Franklin to Peter Collinson describing his famous kite and key experiment. Many scientific communications in the 1700's were in the form of letters.

direct transfusions of venous blood replaced the artery-to-vein technic. Widespread use of arterial puncture for diagnostic purposes or physiologic investigation didn't surface until World War II.

Adolph Fick (1870) wrote only two paragraphs on the measurement of cardiac output; in the first, he outlined his principle, and in the second, gave a sample calculation based on reasonable data:

Herr Fick had a contribution on the measurement of the amount of blood ejected by the ventricle of the heart with each systole, a quantity the knowledge of which is certainly of great importance. Varying opinions have been expressed on this. While Thomas Young estimated the quantity at about 45 cc., most estimates in modern textbooks, supported by the views of Volkmann and Vierordt, run much higher, up to 180 cc. It is surprising that no one has arrived at the following procedure by which this important value is available by direct determination, at least in animals. One measures how much oxygen an animal absorbs from the air in a given time, and how much CO_2 it gives off. One takes during this time a sample of arterial and a sample of venous blood; in both samples oxygen content and CO_2 content are measured. The difference of oxygen content gives the amount of oxygen each cubic centimeter of blood takes up in its passage through the lungs; and as one knows how much total oxygen has been taken up in given time, one can calculate how many cubic centimeters of blood have passed through the lungs in this time, or if one divides by the number of heartbeats during this time, how many cubic centimeters of blood are ejected with each beat. The corresponding calculation with CO_2 quantities gives a determination of the same value, which provides a control for the other calculation.

Since for the demonstration of this method two gas pumps are needed, your reporter unfortunately is not in a position to communicate experimental data. He will only give, therefore, a calculation of blood flow in man according to this method, based on more or less arbitrary data. According to the experiments of Scheffer in Ludwig's laboratory, dog's arterial blood contains 0.146 cc. oxygen per cc. (measured at 0°C. and 1 atm. pressure); 1 cc. of venous blood contains 0.0905 cc. oxygen. Each cc. of blood therefore takes up 0.0555 cc. oxygen in its passage through the lungs. Let us assume the same in man. Assume, further that a man absorbs in 24 hours 833 grams of oxygen. This will occupy a space of 433,200 cc. at 0°C. and 1 atm. pressure. According to this, 5 cc. of oxygen would be absorbed by the lungs of a man each second. In order to effect this absorption,

5/0.0555 cc. of blood must perfuse the lungs per second, that is, 90 cc. Assuming, finally, 7 systoles in 6 seconds, each systole would then eject 77 cc. of blood.

Note Fick's statement that "It is surprising that no one has arrived at the following procedure by which this important value is available by direct determination," but he did no experiments because he had no "gas pumps" for measuring the O_2 or CO_2 content of blood. The first experimental determination based on his principle was reported 16 years later by Gréhant and Quinquaud (in a one-page paper) (C R Soc Biol *38:* 159-160, 1886).

William Dock in 1929 adapted the then-new cathode ray oscillograph to monitor and to record ECG (229 words); the CRO monitor is now routine in all operating rooms and intensive care units and, as such, is quite familiar to avid TV viewers.

Others who reported important discoveries in one page or less were the following:

Faraday (1818), who reported that inhalation of ether vapor produced effects similar to those of nitrous oxide.

O'Shaughnessy (1832), who discovered severe fluid and electrolyte disturbances in patients with cholera; within a year his work led to the first rational therapy of this scourge by Latta.

Pasteur (1882), who recounted his successful vaccination of sheep against anthrax; 100 per cent of those not vaccinated died, while 100 per cent of those vaccinated up to 8 months previously lived.

Hektoen (1907), who suggested that mixing blood of donor and recipient and examining the mixture for agglutinated red blood cells could eliminate transfusion reactions.

Carrel (1911), who described his technic of repeatedly passing tissue fragments cultured *in vitro* from an old to a fresh medium; this technic later became important in many fields, particularly in the culture of polio virus and preparation of polio vaccine.

Guthrie (1919), who demonstrated that blood vessels do not survive as such when transplanted from one animal to another but do provide a scaffolding or bridge for ingrowth of new tissue derived from the host.

Joliot and Curie (1934), who first announced the transmutation of one element to another (the alchemist's dream). They changed boron, magnesium, and aluminum into radionitrogen, radiosilicon, and radiophosphorus, respectively,

An Account
Of an Experiment made by M. Hook, of Preserving Animals alive by Blowing through their Lungs with Bellows.

I Did heretofore give this *Illustrious Society* an account of an Experiment I formerly tryed of keeping a Dog alive after his *Thorax* was all display'd by the cutting away of the *Ribbs* and *Diaphragme*; and after the *Pericardium* of the Heart also was taken off. But divers persons seeming to doubt of the certainty of the Experiment (by reason that some Tryals of this matter, made by some other hands, failed of success) I caus'd at the last Meeting the same Experiment to be shewn in the presence of this *Noble Company*, and that with the same success, as it had been made by me at first; the Dog being kept alive by the Reciprocal blowing up of his Lungs with *Bellowes*, and they suffered to subside, for the space of an hour or more, after his *Thorax* had been so display'd, and his *Aspera arteria* cut off just below the *Epiglottis*, and bound on upon the nose of the Bellows.

And because some Eminent Physitians had affirm'd, that the *Motion of the Lungs* was necessary to Life upon the account of promoting the Circulation of the Blood, and that it was conceiv'd, the Animal would immediately be suffocated as soon as the Lungs should cease to be moved, I did (the better to fortifie my own *Hypothesis* of this matter, and to be the better able to judge of several others) make the following additional Experiment; *viz.*

The Dog having been kept alive, (as I have now mentioned) for above an houre, in which time the Tryal had been often repeated, in suffering the Dog to fall into *Convulsive* motions by ceasing to blow the Bellows, and permitting the Lungs to subside and lye still, and of suddenly reviving him again by renewing the blast, and consequently the motion of the Lungs: This, I say, having been done, and the Judicious Spectators fully satisfied of the reality of the former Experiment; I caused another pair of Bellowes to be immediately joyn'd to the first, by a contrivance, I had prepar'd, and pricking all the outer-coat of the Lungs with the slender point of a very sharp pen-knife, this second pair of Bellows was mov'd very quick, whereby the first pair was alwayes kept full and alwayes blowing into the Lungs; by which means the Lungs also were alwayes kept very full, and without any motion; there being a continual blast of Air forc'd into the Lungs by the first pair of Bellows, supplying it as fast, as it could find its way quite through the Coat of the Lungs by the small holes pricked in it, as was said before. This being continued for a pretty while, the Dog, as I exspected, lay still, as before, his eyes being all the time very quick, and his Heart beating very regularly: But, upon ceasing this blast, and suffering the Lungs to fall and lye still, the Dogg would immediately fall into Dying convulsive fits; but be as soon reviv'd again by the renewing the fulness of his Lungs with the constant blast of fresh Air.

Towards the latter end of this Experiment a piece of the Lungs was cut quite off; where 'twas observable, that the Blood did freely circulate, and pass thorow the Lungs, not only when the Lungs were kept thus constantly extended, but also when they were suffer'd to subside and lye still. Which seem to be Arguments, that as the *bare* Motion of the Lungs *without fresh Air* contributes nothing to the life of the Animal, he being found to survive as well, when they were not mov'd, as when they were; so it was not the subsiding or moveless-ness of the Lungs, that was the immediate cause of Death, or the stopping the Circulation of the Blood through the Lungs, but the *want* of a sufficient *supply of fresh Air.*

I shall shortly further try, whether the suffering the Blood to circulate through a vessel, so as it may be openly exposed to the fresh Air, will not suffice for the life of an Animal; and make some other Experiments, which, I hope, will throughly discover the *Genuine use of Respiration*; and afterwards consider of what benefit this may be to Mankinde.

Fig. 2. Robert Hooke's account of experiments proving that pulmonary blood, flowing through lungs distended with air, could maintain life even in the absence of rhythmic inflation and deflation of the lungs. (*Hook,* in the title, is printer's error.)

and won a third Nobel Prize for the Curie family.

Alvarez and Cornog (1939), who first produced tritium in the Berkeley cyclotron.

Pattle (1955), who observed stable pulmonary edema foam and speculated that the surface tension of lung bubbles is zero.

Lehmann (1946), who noted that pathogenic tubercle bacilli have an increased uptake of O_2 in the presence of salicylates and first used para-amino salicylic acid as a bacteriostatic agent against tubercle bacilli.

Somewhat more verbose were the following:

Hooke (1667), who required a page-and-a-half to present proof that rhythmic movements of the lung were not necessary for life if the lungs were inflated by a stream of air (figure 2). Hooke missed the one-page-or-less category because he also included in his article a bit about artificial ventilation, a technic for continuous positive airway pressure (though scarcely applicable clinically because he pricked the outer layer of the lungs with the "slender point of a very sharp penknife" to maintain a continuous flow of air *through* the alveoli), proof that pulmonary blood flow without ventilation could not maintain life and a suggestion that extracorporeal oxygenation of blood was feasible (really *aeration,* since there was no oxygen in 1667).

Henry (1803), who required two pages to present his law relating partial pressure of a gas in a liquid to the quantity dissolved in it.

Von Behring and Kitasato (1890), who needed one-and-a-half pages to tell the medical world of immunization against diphtheria and tetanus; they were awarded the Nobel Prize in 1901 for this work.

Curie, Curie, and Bémont (1898), who used two-and-a-half pages to announce the discovery of radium in pitchblende (another Nobel Prize-winning discovery).

Hering (1924), who took two pages to describe the carotid sinus reflex.

Bayliss and Muller (1928), who needed two pages to describe and illustrate their rotary, roller pump, later known by a variety of names, such as the DeBakey pump (three pages).

Urey, Brickwedde, and Murphy (1932), who used one-and-a-half journal pages to announce the preparation of deuterium.

Stanley (1935), who needed one-and-a-half pages to announce the isolation from infected tobacco plants of a crystalline protein with the properties of tobacco-mosaic virus.

Enders, Weller, and Robbins (1949), who ex-pended one-and-three-quarter pages to present the cultivation of polio virus in human embryonic tissue, which led to the Nobel Prize for them and polio vaccine for all.

Clements (1957), who took one-and-a-half pages to quantify the surface-tension lowering properties of pulmonary surfactant ("anti-atelectasis factor").

Some wrote very long articles that are known today largely for a single paragraph. Henry Head's 70-page paper "On the regulation of respiration" (1889) is remembered mainly for one paragraph on page 13, in which he parenthetically described "Head's paradoxical reflex." And Christian Bohr's 33-page paper (1891) is remembered by most for his equation for respiratory dead space, stated in a few lines on page 248.

It's pretty hard nowadays to join this very select club of those who have written (and had published) a very short, important paper. You can try but I doubt that you'll succeed. Editorial boards resist accepting either long papers or very short papers (unless the latter are carefully segregated in a special section, suggesting that they are grade B and not grade A contributions). I suspect that today some of those mentioned earlier in this article would have received letters from the editor such as these:

Dear Dr. Korotkoff:

Thank you for permitting us to read your interesting manuscript. We regret that we cannot publish it in its present form. You may wish to resubmit it after you have (1) compared data obtained by your method with that obtained by the Riva-Rocci method in a large number of subjects of different ages and different arm circumferences, (2) verified the accuracy of your method against direct measurements of systolic and diastolic arterial blood pressure in animals, and (3) done statistical analysis of the data.

Sincerely,
The Editors

Dear Professor Fick:

Thank you for sending us your interesting suggestion for measuring cardiac output. We regret that we do not publish ideas unsupported by data and are returning your paper forthwith.

Sincerely,
The Editors

88

Dear Dr. Hooke:

We have read your communication entitled "Preserving animals alive by blowing through their lungs with bellows." We note that you have been sending us a number of short communications, none of which has been suitable for publication. We suggest that you consider combining all of these into one longer, more substantial manuscript that might contain enough new information to make it worthy of acceptance.

Respectfully,
The Editors

References

Alvarez, L. W., and Cornog, R.: Helium and hydrogen of mass 3, Phys Rev, 1939, 56, 613.

Bayliss, L. E., and Müller, E. A.: A simple high-speed rotary pump, J Sci Instr, 1928, 5, 278-279.

von Behring, E. A., and Kitasato, S.: Ueber das Zustandekommen der Diphtherie-Immunität und der Tetanus-Immunität bei Thieren, Dtsch Med Wochenschr, 1890, 16, 1113–1114.

Bohr, C.: Ueber die lungenathmung, Skand Arch Physiol, 1891, 2, 236–268.

Carrel, A.: Rejuvenation of cultures of tissues, JAMA, 1911, 57, 1611.

Clements, J. A.: Surface tension of lung extracts, Proc Soc Exp Biol Med, 1957, 95, 170–172.

Cooke, A., and Barcroft, J.: Direct determination of the percentage saturation of arterial blood with oxygen in a normal person, J Physiol, 1913, 47, xxxv.

Curie, P., Curie, M., and Bémont, G.: Sur une nouvelle substance fortement radio-active, contenue dans la pechblende, C R Acad Sci, 1898, 127, 1215–1217.

Dock, W.: The use of the cathode ray oscilloscope for electrocardiography, Proc Soc Exp Biol Med, 1929, 24, 566.

Enders, J. F., Weller, T. H., and Robbins, F. C.: Cultivation of the Lansing strain of poliomyelitis virus in cultures of various human embryonic tissues, Science, 1949, 109, 85–87.

Faraday, M.: Effects of inhaling the vapour of sulphuric ether, J Sci Arts, 1818, 4, 158-159.

Fick, A.: Uber die Messung des Blutquantums in der Herzventrikeln, S B Phys-Med Ges Würzburg, July 9, 1870, xvi. English translation from "Circulation of the Blood: Men and Ideas," ed. Fishman, A. P., and Richards, D. W., New York, Oxford University Press, 1964, pp. 96-97.

Franklin, B.: New Experiments and Observations on Electricity Made at Philadelphia in America, ed. 3, part I, D. Henry and R. Cave, London, 1760, pp. 106–108.

Guthrie, C. C.: End-results of arterial restitution with devitalized tissue, JAMA, 1919, 73, 186–187.

Head, H.: On the regulation of respiration, J Physiol, 1889, 10, 1–70.

Hektoen, L.: Isoagglutination of human corpuscles, JAMA, 1907, 48, 1739–1740.

Henry, W.: Experiments on the quantity of gases absorbed by water, at different temperatures, and under different pressures, Proc R Soc Lond, 1803, 1, 103–104.

Hering, H. E.: Die Änderung der Herzschlagzahl durch Änderung des arteriellen Blutdruckes erfolgt auf reflektorischem Wege, Pflügers Arch, 1924, 206, 721–723.

Hooke, R.: An account of an experiment made by M. Hook[e], of preserving animals alive by blowing through their lungs with bellows, Philos Trans R Soc Lond, 1667, 2, 539–540.

Joliot, F., and Curie, I.: Artificial production of a new kind of radio-element, Nature, 1934, 133, 201–202.

Korotkoff, N. S.: K voprosu metodakh uzsledovaniya krovanovo devleniya, Voen Med Akad Izvestiia, 1905, 11, 365. Translated by A. S. Badger, Cardiovasc Res Cent Bull, 1967, vol. 5, pp. 57–74.

Lehmann, J.: Determination of pathogenicity of tubercle bacilli by their intermediate metabolism, Lancet, 1946, 1, 14–15. Para-aminosalicylic acid in the treatment of tuberculosis, Ibid., 15–16.

O'Shaughnessy, W. B.: Experiments on the blood in cholera, Lancet, 1831–1832, 1, 490.

Pasteur, L.: Sur des expériences de vaccination charbonneuse, Bull Séances Soc Agr France, 1882, 42, 74–75.

Pattle, R. E.: Properties, function, and origin of the alveolar lining layer, Nature, 1955, 175, 1125–1126.

Stanley, W. M.: Isolation of a crystalline protein possessing the properties of tobacco-mosaic virus, Science, 1935, 81, 644–645.

Urey, H. C., Brickwedde, F. G., and Murphy, G. M.: A hydrogen isotope of mass 2, Phys Rev, 1932, 39, 164–165.

"Tell It Like It Was"

When I first used this instrument (1), I wrote that I did not intend to use the Retrospectroscope to uncover who did what before whom, but rather to analyze how and why important discoveries (and sometimes rediscoveries) came about. I can tell you unequivocally that it's a hard job—largely because of the rigid format and style of the modern scientific article. Scientists presumably spend a lifetime in science because of the joy of discovery, but this joy rarely comes through to the reader of their scientific articles. Worse, for those seriously interested in learning more about the process of scientific discovery, the scientist, once he changes into the role of author, rarely "tells it like it was"; he conforms to the IMRAD style—Introduction (concise and impersonal), Methods, Results And Discussion—and leaves out, "Why did I do it? Was my initial idea right or wrong? How did I get on the right track?"

Schilling, in an article published in 1958 (2) laid it on the line in his subtitle: "Science as Lived by Its Practitioners Bears but Little Resemblance to Science as Described in Print." He then went on to say:

...the findings of science are usually presented to students and the public as straightforward, logical developments, rather than in such a way as to reveal how they actually evolved—haltingly, circuitously, with many false starts, and often even illogically. While there are, of course, very good reasons for this, the fact is that, in the absence of further explanation, it leaves the uninitiated with a thoroughly misleading idea of the processes of science.

Six years later, Medawar also took scientists to task for *doing* their research one way, and *telling* it another way (3). In his "Is the Scientific Article Fraudulent? Yes; It Misrepresents Scientific Thought" he writes:

...I do not, of course, mean "Does the scientific paper misrepresent facts?" and I do not mean that the interpretations you find in a scientific paper are wrong or deliberately mistaken. I mean the scientific paper may be a fraud because it misrepresents the processes of thought that accompanied

or gave rise to the work that is described in the paper.

That is the question, and I will say right away that my answer to it is "yes." The scientific paper in its orthodox form does embody a totally mistaken conception, even a travesty, of the nature of scientific thought....

Once in a while, a scientist does tell us, in his initial report, how he came upon his discovery. Roentgen did (see "The Inside Story" [4]). So did Sidney Ringer (forever famous for Ringer's solution), whose discovery of the essential role of calcium and potassium in normal cardiac contraction and rhythm was all-important to much of today's basic and clinical research on the heart.

Calcium and Cardiac Contraction

How did Ringer make his celebrated discovery? Here are his words in the 1883 *Journal of Physiology* (5):

After the publication of a paper in the *Journal of Physiology*, Vol. III, No. 5, entitled "Concerning the influence exerted by each of the Constituents of the Blood on the Contraction of the Ventricle," I discovered that the saline solution which I had used had not been prepared with distilled water, but with pipe water supplied by the New River Water Company. As this water contains minute traces of various inorganic substances, I at once tested the action of saline solution made with distilled water and I found that I did not get the effects described in the paper referred to. It is obvious therefore that the effects I had obtained are due to some of the inorganic constituents of the pipe water.

Water supplied by the New River Water Company contains 278.6 parts of solids per million.

They consist of:

Calcium	38.3	per million.
Magnesium	4.5	"
Sodium	23.3	"
Potassium	7.1	"
Combined Carbonic Acid	78.2	"
Sulphuric Acid	55.8	"
Chlorine	15	"
Silicates	7.1	"
Free Carbonic Acid	54.2	"

90

[The actual total of the solids listed is 283.5 parts per million.]

This water is faintly alkaline to test-paper from bicarbonate of lime. Saline made with this water I found at first rounds the top of the trace of each contraction and later greatly prolongs diastolic dilatation, and that these effects are completely obviated by about 1 c.c. of 1% solution of potassium chloride solution to the 100 c.c. of circulating saline. So that with this addition the saline thus made forms an excellent artificial circulating fluid for the heart, as in some experiments I found the ventricle fed by this mixture would continue beating well for more than four hours, indeed at the end of that time the contractions were almost as good as at the commencement of the experiment, when the ventricle was fed with blood mixture. . . .

The heart's contractility cannot be sustained by saline solution nor by saline containing potassium chloride, nor with saline solution containing bicarbonate of soda, nor by saline solution containing bicarbonate of soda and potassium chloride; but after contractility has ceased, the addition of a lime salt will restore good contractility. The addition too of a calcium salt to any of the above solutions will sustain contractility. I conclude therefore that a lime salt is necessary for the maintenance of muscular contractility. . . .

If these two salts are not present in the correct proportions then the trace becomes abnormal. If too little potassium is present, the contractions become broader etc. and there results fusion of the beats. If too much potassium is present, or too little lime salts, then the contraction of the ventricle is imperfect, and by increasing the quantity of potassium salt the beat becomes weaker and weaker till it stops.

Ringer's account gives me the picture of a man puzzled by the results of his earlier experiments, unwilling to accept them, and checking every possible error in technic. He found the error and at once identified the important role of calcium ions in cardiac function. A conventional paper by Ringer would have given us *calcium* but not the important lesson to all future scientists: check the composition and purity of all reagents.

Protamine-Heparin Antagonism

Chargaff and Olson told it "like it was" when they discovered a new action of protamine in 1937 (6):

. . . the animal organism seems able to dispose of it [heparin] in a comparatively short time. Whether this is brought about by rapid combination of the heparin with the proteins of the tissues or of blood, by its excretion, or by its destruction,

it is not yet established. We have attempted to protract the short lived activity of heparin by combination with a protamine, *viz.* salmine. This was done in view of the promising results obtained with the combination of insulin and protamine: In the case of heparin the effect was unexpected: the anticoagulant action of heparin *in vivo* was entirely stopped by protamine. The significance of these findings and some possible practical applications will be discussed later in this paper. . . .

Their hypothesis, although quite reasonable, was wrong; their result, although totally unexpected, turned out to be of considerable clinical importance. Because editors forever remind us that paper, printing, binding, and mailing are all very expensive, it's important to note that Chargaff and Olson took only 56 words—well worth it—to tell scientists that the *un*expected may sometimes be worth more than the expected result.

The Discovery of Heparin

A lot of scientists have told us, several decades later, how it really happened at the time of their initial discovery.

One of these was Jay McLean, who discovered heparin in 1916 but didn't "tell it like it was" until 1957. Indeed, in 1916 he scarcely told anything at all; neither the title of his article, "The Thromboplastic Action of Cephalin," nor his conclusions mention his discovery of heparin or of a new anticoagulant (7). He began his article as follows:

In 1912 Howell reported the results of a study of the thromboplastic action of the tissues in which he showed that the active substance is a phosphatid having the general properties of cephalin. . . . At the suggestion of Dr. Howell I have undertaken a re-examination of this subject to determine if possible whether the thromboplastic effect may be attributed to an impurity, or is a property of the cephalin itself, and also to determine in how far a similar property is exhibited by other related phosphatids.

The remainder of the article's eight pages dealt with factors that *hasten* blood coagulation (thromboplastic factors) rather than retard it, except for these two sentences in which McLean mentions a new anticoagulant:

The heparphosphatid on the other hand when purified by many precipitations in alcohol at 60° has no thromboplastic action and in fact shows a marked power to inhibit the coagulation. The anticoagulating action of this phosphatid is being studied and will be reported upon later.

Even his conclusions say nothing about his momentous discovery of a powerful naturally-occurring *anti*coagulant. His conclusions were:

1. Cephalin when prepared as pure as possible exhibits marked thromboplastic activity, as indicated by its effect in increasing the thrombic action of fresh serum.

2. Cephalin exhibiting this reaction has been prepared from the liver, heart and brain.

3. The other phosphatids that have been described, lecithin, cuorin, heparphosphatid and sphingomyelin have no thromboplastic action.

4. Evidence is presented to show that this property of cephalin is not due to adherent impurities, but is a characteristic property of the cephalin itself.

In 1957, shortly before his death, McLean recounted the actual story (8). His father and uncle were graduated from the University of California Medical School (1867 and 1876 respectively) and his uncle was a professor of surgery and dean there. Jay McLean wanted to be an academic surgeon. His cousin, Herbert McLean Evans, then on the Anatomy staff at Johns Hopkins Medical School, convinced Jay that, to achieve his goal, he should come to Hopkins to be a physiologically-trained surgeon rather than go elsewhere and be an anatomically-based surgeon! Going to the state medical school near his home meant far less expense than going to a private school in Baltimore and the McLean family finances were at an all-time low. The 1906 earthquake and fire in San Francisco levelled both the family's house and the stepfather's place of employment. To finance his third year of premedical education (required by Hopkins), he dropped out of college for 15 months to work first as a "mucker," then as chuck-tender, apprentice miner, and finally as millhand who actually pressed the ore into gold bricks. With these earnings, he finished college but was broke again. So he drilled oil wells for 15 months and made enough money to get him through the first year of medical school at Berkeley, waiting for acceptance by Hopkins for the next year. At this point he received a letter from Hopkins turning him down. McLean's reaction was to buy a railroad ticket and go off to Baltimore where he promptly introduced himself to the dean. The next day, Hopkins had an unexpected vacancy and accepted McLean for the next year's class.

An interesting sidelight to this story is that McLean worked his way East on the advice of his cousin, then an Associate Professor at Hopkins. McLean met his cousin for the first time, in 1915, the day before McLean boarded the train to Baltimore; his cousin had just arrived in San Francisco to become Professor of Anatomy at the University of California! Evans went West where he became the world's greatest experimental endocrinologist; McLean went East to discover heparin!

McLean had a year to wait in Baltimore and decided to spend it doing research. Here are parts of his account (8).

I promptly paid the fees for a year as a medical student, taking no medical school courses. I immediately called on Dr. Howell and told him of my desire to prepare for an academic career in surgery and that I wished to devote one whole year to physiological research now. I felt that I could never do it after graduation for that would interfere with the house officer progress on a surgical staff. I told him then that I wanted a problem I could reasonably hope to finish and publish in one academic year entirely by myself. I wanted to determine if I could solve a problem by myself. I told him my savings would just last one year, and after that I would have to work a year before returning to school.

He gave me the problem of determining the value of the thromboplastic substance of the body. He thought this to be kephalin (cephalin), obtained from brain but, of course, knew the thromboplastic material from brain to be a mixture—a crude extract, though a powerful thromboplastic agent. . . .

My problem was to determine what portion of this crude extract was the active accelerator of the clotting process and to that end, to prepare cephalin as pure as possible and determine if it had thromboplastic action. I was also to test the other components of the crude ether-alcohol extract. . . .

It was this determination to become a physiology-based surgeon rather than an anatomy-based surgeon that led to the discovery of heparin. . . . I suggested to Dr. Howell that it might be profitable to extract the lipoids (phosphatides) from many different organs. . . . In my reading of the German chemical literature on phosphatides, I found articles by Erlandsen and Baskoff in which they described extracts of heart and liver secured by a process similar to that for obtaining cephalin from brain. Therefore, these products might be heart and liver cephalin, but were named cuorin (from the heart) and heparphosphatide (from the liver); hence the name heparin. I suggested this research problem as a logical supplement to the problem Dr. Howell had given me. He had not known about cuorin or heparphosphatide. . . . I had saved batches of cuorin and heparphosphatide and from time to time tested these in serum plasma to determine whether or not the cephalin from the heart and liver deteriorated and lost its thromboplastic power as did that from the brain. If I had not saved them, I would probably not have found heparin....

The various batches were tested down to the point of no thromboplastic activity, but two of those first prepared appeared not only to have lost their thromboplastic action, but actually to retard slightly the coagulation of the serum-plasma mixture. I had in mind, of course, no thought of an anticoagulant, but the experimental fact was before me; and I retested again and again until I was satisfied that an extract of liver (more than heart) possessed a strong anticoagulant action after its contained cephalin had lost its thromboplastic action.

I went one morning to the door of Dr. Howell's office, and standing there (he was seated at his desk) said, "Dr. Howell, I have discovered antithrombin." He smiled and said, "Antithrombin is a protein and you are working with phosphatides. Are you sure that salt is not contaminating your substance?"

I told him I was not sure of that, but it was a powerful anticoagulant. He was most skeptical. So I had the Diener, John Schweinhant, bleed a cat. Into a small beaker full of its blood, I stirred all of a proven batch of heparphosphatides, and I placed this on Dr. Howell's laboratory table and asked him to tell me when it clotted. It never did clot.

He still did not believe that I had discovered a natural anticoagulant, but it was at this point that he became associated in my research problem, namely the study of the effects of my anticoagulating substance (heparphosphatide), which gave greater yield and higher coagulating potential than cuorin *in vivo* in dogs. When I demonstrated new batches to him *in vitro*, and he became satisfied that it did actually inhibit the coagulation of the serum-plasma test mixture as well as whole blood *in vitro*, we planned the first *in vivo* experiment with a dog and administered the heparin intravenously.

[This was as far as Dr. McLean progressed in his history of the discovery of heparin before he developed his fatal illness and died November 14, 1957.—Ed.]

One learns more about the process of scientific discovery from the 1957 account than from the 1916 article. One learns how important it was for science that the Professor (Howell) gave an inexperienced student a free hand to make mistakes or discoveries. One learns how important it was that the student explored his unexpected and contradictory observations instead of ignoring them. And how important it was that he convinced his doubting professor that, with heparin added, the blood "never did clot"!

Citrate as an Anticoagulant

It's pretty hard, in 1976, to realize that between 1900 and 1915 the accepted method for giving a blood transfusion was to anastomose, by a long and delicate surgical procedure, the artery of a donor to the vein of the patient. There were no indirect transfusions because there was no way to keep blood liquid outside of the body except by defibrinating it (by whipping it with broomstraws) and defibrinated blood often caused serious reactions. In 1914, a young Belgian physician, Dr. Hustin, found that when sodium citrate was added to blood, blood stayed liquid long enough to permit indirect transfusion.

Why did Hustin use citrate? Here are excerpts from his conventional 1914 paper (9) (my translation from his French):

Blood transfusion, the introduction of blood from one individual into the circulation of another, is a very old therapeutic technic which has been revived in the last few years by the efforts of the American surgeon, Crile....

For two centuries, physicians have tried to join vessels of a donor directly to those of the recipient. But the failures of this method were numerous because the tubes used to join the vessels provoked clotting of the blood and obstruction of the tube. In the past several years experiments with suturing vessels have demonstrated the importance of the endothelial lining and the role played by tissue juices in blood coagulation. . . . New technics of vascular suture give good results but they present numerous problems: they require a longer and very delicate operation; an imperfection in one step may often lead to total failure of the procedure; there is no certain way of measuring the amount of blood transfused at any given time, except for the overall condition of the donor and recipient . . . the need to bring the vessels of the donor and recipient into direct contact increases the donor's chance of being infected by the recipient; because of the complexity of the technic, one must obtain from one donor the entire quantity of blood needed and transfuse it all at once . . . in spite of precautions, clots can form at the site of the anastomosis and either stop blood flow there or be dislodged into the circulation....

[Hustin then discussed two ways of delaying blood coagulation. One was to decrease the concentration of electrolytes in blood by adding isotonic sodium chloride, Ringer's, or glucose solution; possibly these acted to dilute the calcium concentration of the blood. The other was to add "dispersing substances," particularly sodium citrate. His table (see below) showed that blood plus isotonic glucose plus citrate kept blood from clotting for as long as 45 to 67 minutes (line 8) compared with dilution only with salt solution (line 7) or with glucose solution (line 11). He then proceeded to transfuse citrated blood from dog to dog, rabbit to rabbit, man to dog, and finally man to man.]

The technic of the transfusion that I have described requires two steps. One allows a certain amount of venous blood to flow into an equal amount of isotonic glucose-citrate solution, by means of one or several venipunctures (about 150 ml of blood with each puncture from an average-sized vein). This liquid is then poured into ordinary serum apparatus; it is then injected into a vein after transcutaneous puncture. . . .

He summarized his findings as follows:

1. The technic of transfusion that we have used requires no complicated surgical operation but only several venipunctures.

2. It permits precise measurement of the quantity of blood transfused, a matter of great importance to the safety of the donor.

3. It eliminates transferring an infection from the patient to the donor.

4. One can transfuse as often as necessary; several donors can be used at the same time.

5. Between the time of collection and infusion, one can submit the blood to certain manipulations (removal of carbon monoxide and replacement with oxygen; different types of irradiation).

6. In many of the cases in which transfusion is indicated, the heart of the patient needs to be strengthened and glucose is known to be a nutrient of the first order for cardiac muscle fibers.

7. The delay in blood coagulation is long enough to permit a slow transfusion and so prevent overburdening the right heart.

In 1960, Hustin wrote another article on blood transfusion (10), telling what had motivated his 1914 work and why he was successful. Here are his words (my translation from the French):

Pekelharing and Sabattini's physiological studies in 1902 were, for a long time, ignored by clinicians; at least not a single clinician had thought of using the anticoagulant properties of sodium citrate for blood transfusion. I was not even aware of its anticoagulant properties when, in 1913, I undertook my first attempts of blood transfusion in the Laboratory of Physiology at the University of Brussels. At that time, I knew only of Gengou's work—that sodium citrate had dispersing properties and rendered stable a suspension of mastic.

It was not by looking for a new method of transfusion that I conceived of the technique of transfusing citrated blood. If this had been my intention, it is probable that I would have followed the usual tracks and that I would have succeeded, at best, in improving on some procedure or some apparatus already known. My goal was quite different, as you will see.

It happened that one day, at the hospital, I found myself standing by a man dying from inhalation of illuminating gas. I told myself that one could save his life if only one could withdraw part of his blood, remove the carbon monoxide blocking its hemoglobin, and then reinject the withdrawn blood once it had been purified and properly oxygenated. But to achieve this plan of treatment, first it was necessary, after withdrawing blood from the patient, to maintain the blood in a fluid state during the time required to extract the toxic gas. It was at this moment that I realized the possibility of stabilizing the blood by means of sodium citrate, since this salt had demonstrated its property of maintaining mastic in suspension.

I then undertook "in vitro" attempts; first I had to make sure that sodium citrate acted on blood as it did on mastic; i.e., that sodium citrate

COMPOSITION OF THE MIXTURE

	Coagulation Time	
	Beginning (Minutes)	End (Minutes)
1. Blood + saline solution + 50 centigr. % citrate	12	15
2. '' + '' + 40 ''	5	13
3. '' + '' + 30 ''	5	15
4. '' + '' + 20 ''	5	15
5. '' + '' + 10 ''	4	22
6. '' + '' + 5 ''	—	9
7. '' + saline solution ———————————	4	8
8. '' + glucose solution + 50 centigr. % citrate	45	67
9. '' + '' + 30 ''	25	32
10. '' + '' + 10 ''	9	15
11. '' + glucose solution ———————————	—	12

prevented it from becoming a gel; then I had to determine the amount of citrate needed for delaying blood coagulation for at least half an hour. . . . For reasons that would be too long to report here, I also added glucose so I came to use a glucose-citrate mixture as my anticoagulant solution.

If, at that time, I had pursued my initial goal—that of saving patients intoxicated by carbon monoxide—I would have looked for some means of extracting the carbon monoxide contained in the blood. But I did not because I realized that my researches had led me, unintentionally, to an entirely new method of transfusion: the glucose-citrated transfusion. In order to reach this new objective, I had only to demonstrate that reinjection of blood, made uncoagulable by sodium citrate, could be performed without danger for the patient.

I then injected a dog with some citrated blood that had been withdrawn from another dog; thereafter I injected a dog with blood sampled from a human being; finally, on March 27, 1914, I performed at St. John Hospital in Brussels, the first transfusion of glucose-citrated blood, from one man to another man.

One might wonder why transfusion with citrated blood was not discovered shortly after the discovery of anticoagulant properties of sodium citrate in 1896. One might further wonder since, at the beginning of the century, the dangers of transfusion had been overcome and the interest of the medical world in transfusion had been revived by the techniques that imaginative surgeons had devised to anastomose blood vessels. . . . Without any doubt, particular circumstances in certain men's life have often played a role in their inventions or discoveries. The first circumstance was that, while acting as a surgeon at the hospital in 1910, I had undertaken experimental work on animals in the Physiological Laboratory of the University of Brussels. As part of this, I often had to withdraw from dogs a certain amount of blood which I had maintained in a fluid state by shaking it with glass beads, so that I could then perfuse it through the vessels of isolated organs. The concept of making blood incoagulable was then familiar to me. To treat carbon monoxide poisoning, I had to change only one thing: to replace the mechanical action of the glass beads by the chemical action of sodium citrate. The second circumstance was that my hospital activities had initiated me to the current problems associated with blood transfusion. So I was led to leave a problem of limited interest—the treatment of carbon monoxide intoxication—for a problem of much wider interest, that of blood transfusion.

The idea of citrated transfusion was then born quite naturally from a mind formed by two different disciplines, a physiological and a clinical one, the hospital environment raising the question to solve, the laboratory providing the elements for the answer.

Microvascular Surgery

One of the great cardiovascular advances was microvascular surgery, introduced by Jacobson and Suarez in a modest, conventional 2-page paper in 1960 (11). Here are some excerpts from it:

> Results of arterial surgery have been uniformly poor in vessels below 4 mm. in diameter. The reason, it seems to us, is purely technical. A 1 mm. error in suture placement results in thrombosis in a 2 mm. anastomosis but has little significance when one works on large vessels.
>
> Techniques have been developed for performance of vascular anastomosis under the dissecting microscope. Far greater accuracy in suture placement is obtained. . . . Bits of adventitia not visible to the naked eye can be removed. The surgeon can tie knots so that intimal edges almost exactly coapt.
>
> One hundred per cent patency rates have been found in the carotid arteries of 20 dogs and 6 rabbits observed up to 4 months. The vessels averaged 3.2 and 1.4 mm. respectively. . . .
>
> It is our belief that the techniques presented will extend vascular surgery to many previously inaccessible areas.

Clear and concise, but it doesn't tell *why*, after otologists had been operating with the aid of magnifying lenses and microscopes for almost 40 years, no vascular surgeon picked up the ball until 1960. I wrote to Jacobson in 1972 and he told me how it really happened (Jacobson, J. H.: Personal communication, Aug. 7, 1972):

> In 1959 I completed a seven-year residency at New York's Presbyterian Hospital and stayed on there for a short while as an attending surgeon. In 1960 I was appointed the Director of Surgical Research at the University of Vermont and was able to transfer a sizable USPHS grant entitled "Factors in the Development of Collateral Circulation." It was this money that allowed us to do the initial work in microsurgery.
>
> Just before leaving Presbyterian Hospital, I wandered into one of the Ear, Nose, and Throat operating rooms and was allowed to look through the Zeiss microscope they were using. I'm sorry to say that there was no sudden recognition of its potential value in vascular surgery.
>
> Some months later, on my arrival in Vermont, one of the pharmacologists asked for help in completely denervating the canine carotid artery. The only way to really accomplish this with certainty was to divide a segment of the vessel and re-anastomose the divided ends. In attempting to do this, it was immediately evident that the problem was

not in the ability of the hand to do but rather the eye to see. Early experimentation was carried out using ocular loupes and large magnifying glasses placed over the operative field. These proved unsatisfactory for one reason or another and finally I remembered looking through the ENT microscope.

A Zeiss microscope was borrowed from the operating room and used in the performance of a small vessel anastomosis. The experience was very much like looking at the moon for the first time through a powerful telescope; a wealth of previously unappreciated detail was seen for the first time and minor surgical errors became glaringly apparent. I should add at this point that before going to medical school I had worked in the area of cell physiology under Dr. L. V. Heilbrunn, and had also spent several summers at Woods Hole. I interject this because, in thinking back, it becomes obvious to me that I probably would not have attempted to interpose a microscope between my eyes and the surgical field had the use of dissecting microscopes not been second nature to me by that time.

One final question: Why did the Vermont pharmacologists want to study a denervated carotid artery? Here are a few lines from their 1962 paper (12):

Our present experiments ... were designed to determine whether the altered sensitivity of the reserpine-treated and denervated tissues to noradrenaline, tyramine and nicotine was correlated with changes in the noradrenaline content of the artery.... Denervation of the artery was performed by two different methods: first, by arterial stripping; secondly, by removal and reversal of an arterial segment with subsequent anastomosis using the method described by Jacobson and Suarez (1960).

Now we know why microvascular surgery began in 1960. A surgeon, fascinated by research because of stimulating experiences at Woods Hole Biological Laboratories and with an inspiring general physiologist, Lewis Heilbrunn, was asked by two pharmacologists to lend his technical skill to help solve a basic problem on the sensitivity of denervated arteries. Conventional surgical technics then available to him were obviously inadequate but instead of his saying, "Sorry, it's impossible," he came up with microvascular surgery, which in turn led to many other new surgical methods for opening closed ducts or tubes, including re-opening a ligated vas deferens. We still don't know why a Jacobson didn't come along in 1930, 1940, or 1950. Maybe there wasn't anyone with the same combination of sur-

gical and research training, inquisitiveness, patience, and willingness to help a couple of basic scientists working on an esoteric problem.

Penicillin

In 1940, Chain and associates (13) published their first report on the chemotherapeutic action of penicillin in experimentally infected mice. The report essentially said that it was about time to study naturally occurring chemotherapeutic substances and the group started with a study of penicillin. Here are excerpts from this historic article, which was written in a fairly conventional format:

In recent years interest in chemotherapeutic effects has been almost exclusively focused on the sulphonamides and their derivatives. There are, however, other possibilities, notably those connected with naturally occurring substances. It has been known for a long time that a number of bacteria and moulds inhibit the growth of pathogenic micro-organisms. Little, however, has been done to purify or to determine the properties of any of these substances. The antibacterial substances produced by *Pseudomonas pyocyanea* have been investigated in some detail, but without the isolation of any purified product of therapeutic value.

Recently, Dubos and collaborators (1939, 1940) have published interesting studies on the acquired bacterial antagonism of a soil bacterium which have led to the isolation from its culture medium of bactericidal substances active against a number of gram positive micro-organisms. Pneumococcal infections in mice were successfully treated with one of these substances, which, however, proved to be highly toxic to mice (Hotchkiss and Dubos 1940) and dogs (McLeod et al. 1940).

Following the work on lysozyme in this laboratory it occurred to two of us (E. C. and H. W. F.) that it would be profitable to conduct a systematic investigation of the chemical and biological properties of the antibacterial substances produced by bacteria and moulds. This investigation was begun with a study of a substance with promising antibacterial properties, produced by a mould and described by Fleming (1929). The present preliminary report is the result of a cooperative investigation on the chemical, pharmacological and chemotherapeutic properties of this substance.

Fleming noted that a mould produced a substance which inhibited the growth, in particular, of staphylococci, streptococci, gonococci, meningococci and *Corynebacterium diphtheriae*, but not of *Bacillus coli, Haemophilus influenzae, Salmonella typhi, P. pyocyanea, Bacillus proteus* or *Vibrio cholerae*. He suggested its use as an inhibitor in the isolation of certain types of bacteria, especially *H. influenzae*. He also noted that the injection into animals of broth containing the substance, which he called "penicillin," was no more toxic than plain broth, and he suggested that the substance might be a useful antiseptic for application to infected wounds. The mould is believed to be closely related to *Penicillium notatum*. Clutterbuck, Lovell and Raistrick (1932) grew the mould in a medium containing inorganic salts only and isolated a pigment—chrysogenin—which had no antibacterial action. Their culture media contained penicillin but this was not isolated. Reid (1935) reported work on the inhibitory substance produced by Fleming's mould. He did not isolate it but noted some of its properties.

During the last year methods have been devised here for obtaining a considerable yield of penicillin, and for rapid assay of its inhibitory power. From the culture medium a brown powder has been obtained which is freely soluble in water. It and its solution are stable for a considerable time and though it is not a pure substance, its anti-bacterial activity is very great. Full details will, it is hoped, be published later.

[The authors then presented their work on the pharmacology and toxicity of penicillin in normal animals, the effects on bacteria *in vitro* and the therapeutic effect of penicillin in mice experimentally infected with streptococci, staphylococci, and *Clostridium septique*.]

Summarising the data given in the table we see that in the final streptococcus experiment (no. 2) whereas 25/25 controls died, 24/25 treated animals survived. With *Staphylococcus aureus* the final experiment (no. 2) shows 24/24 deaths of the controls and 21/24 survivals among the treated. Lastly, with *Cl. septique* when the larger doses of penicillin were given (bottom line) the figures are 25/25 control deaths and 24/25 treatment survivals.

[The investigators then presented their conclusions.]

The results are clear cut, and show that penicillin is active *in vivo* against at least three of the organisms inhibited *in vitro*. It would seem a reasonable hope that all organisms inhibited in high dilution *in vitro* will be found to be dealt with *in vivo*. Penicillin does not appear to be related to any chemotherapeutic substance at present in use and is particularly remarkable for its activity against the anaerobic organisms associated with gas gangrene.

In 1971, Chain (who had become a Nobel Laureate in 1945) wrote an article entitled "Thirty Years of Penicillin Therapy" (14), in which he "told it like it was":

In 1935, a few months after his appointment to the Chair of Pathology at Oxford, I was invited by Professor H. W. Florey, as he then was, to join his staff at the Sir William Dunn School of Pathology....

When Florey and I in our first meetings discussed the future possible research programme of the biochemical section in his Department which I was to organize, Florey drew my attention to a very striking lytic phenomenon in which he, himself, had been interested for some years (Goldsworthy & Florey 1930). In 1924, Alexander Fleming (Fleming 1924), a bacteriologist working at St. Mary's Hospital, London had made the observation that tears, nasal secretion and egg-white contained a substance which was capable of dissolving thick suspensions of a saprophytic bacterium which Fleming had isolated from the air. The bacterium was termed by Fleming *Micrococcus lysodeicticus*. The active lytic substance had obvious enzymic properties, but the substrate on which it acted in the bacterial cell was not known, and Florey suggested to me that it would be interesting to attempt to isolate and characterize this substrate, if indeed lysozyme was an enzyme. The reason why Florey was interested in lysozyme was not so much its antibacterial power which was of a very limited range, but the fact that, in addition to the sources I have just mentioned, it also occurred in duodenal secretions, and Florey thought at that time that it might play a role in the mechanisms of natural immunity and, in particular, could be involved in the pathogenesis of duodenal ulcers.

The study of the biochemical mode of action of a powerful bacteriolytic agent, as lysozyme obviously was, was a problem exactly representative of the kind which has always attracted my particular interest. I therefore took up Florey's suggestion with enthusiasm and started the work in 1936 with a Ph.D. student, L. A. Epstein, an American Rhodes scholar. We were able to show that lysozyme was an enzyme of polysaccharidase nature acting on a polysaccharide which we could isolate from dried bacterial cells of *M. lysodeicticus*.

[Chain then recounts his literature survey of bacteriolytic agents which led him to observations on inhibition of growth of one bacterial species by another (without actual lysis), to the phenomenon of microbial antagonism, and to Fleming's work on *Penicillium notatum*.]

I should like to point out that the possibility that penicillin could have practical use in clinical medicine did not enter our minds when we started our work on penicillin. A substance of the degree of instability which penicillin seemed to possess according to the published facts does not hold out much promise for practical application. If my working hypothesis had been correct and penicillin had been a protein, its practical use as a chemotherapeutic agent would have been out of the question because of anaphylactic phenomena which inevitably would have followed its repeated use. From the scientific point of view, however, the problem of purifying penicillin and isolating the substrate on which I thought it acted was of interest and hence well worth pursuing.

I started to work on penicillin in 1938, long before the outbreak of the war. The frequently repeated statement that the work was started as a contribution to the war effort, to find a chemotherapeutic agent suitable for the treatment of infected war wounds, has no basis. The only reason which motivated me to start the work on penicillin was scientific interest. I very much doubt, in fact, whether I would have been allowed to study this problem at that time in one of the so-called "mission oriented" practically minded industrial laboratories. The research on penicillin, which was started as a problem of purely scientific interest but had consequences of very great practical importance, is a good example of how difficult it is to demarcate sharp limits between pure and applied research.

One wonders why some of the substance of these last two paragraphs was not included in the 1940 report instead of the less informative "following the work on lysozyme in this laboratory it occurred to two of us that it would be profitable to conduct a systematic investigation of the chemical and biological properties of the antibacterial substances produced by bacteria and moulds." Perhaps the original manuscript "told it like it was" and the editor of the journal cut it out.

CONCLUDING REMARKS

We all are "frauds" at one time or another. In 1945, Robert Dripps and I tried whenever possible in our laboratory course in pharmacology to demonstrate the action of drugs in unanesthetized man instead of in anesthetized cats or dogs or pithed frogs. That year, we decided to demonstrate in man the highly specific neuromuscular block produced by tubocurarine. We realized that the safest way was to produce a local block, i.e., to give tubocurarine intra-arterially, preferably into the brachial artery, while the corresponding arm veins were occluded. We asked for a volunteer and gave him a very small dose of d-tubocurarine intra-arterially. To our astonishment, huge wheals and flares soon covered much of his forearm. We immediately thought that our subject was sensitive to curare preparations. Another student volunteered and we repeated the experiment and got the same result. Now we decided to skin test the third volunteer; intracutaneous injection produced a wheal and flare similar to that following histamine. At this point, a student said, "How about skin-testing all of us?" We did—and all 13 soon had characteristic histamine-like wheals. That's how we discovered that tubocurarine liberated histamine from the skin of man.

But that's not how we wrote our report (15)! We wrote a typical IMRAD article that gave no indication of why or how we did the study. I'm sure we never considered any other format in 1945; we simply conformed to the pattern.

There's little doubt that most scientists advocate impersonal, cold, unrevealing scientific writing, devoid of human interest or even of speculation. Lord Brain, in a reply to Medawar's use of the word "fraud" (3), said, "...it does not seem to me to follow that the structure of the scientific paper, the object of which is to communicate something to the reader, should necessarily correspond to the logical process by which the discovery was made" (16). Lord Brain is correct if all that scientists want to know are the methods, data, and conclusions. Medawar is correct if it's important to science to learn how discoveries have come about. Maybe we can have both. Let scientists use their IMRAD manuscripts to tell how they would have done their experiments if they had proceeded with impeccable logic from the first experiment to the last; this will be comforting to their ego. But let them send with the manuscript a sealed envelope that contains an account that "tells it like it was"— the envelope to be opened upon the author's death or award of the Nobel prize, when the ego no longer needs comforting.

References

1. Comroe, J. H., Jr.: Retrospectroscope: Pulmonary diffusing capacity for carbon monoxide, Am Rev Respir Dis, 1975, *111*, 225–228.

2. Schilling, H. K.: A human enterprise. Science as lived by its practitioners bears but little resemblance to science as described in print, Science, 1958, *127*, 1324–1327.

3. Medawar, P. B.: Is the scientific paper fraudulent? Yes; it misrepresents scientific thought, Sat Rev, Aug 1, 1964, pp. 42–43.

4. This volume, The inside story, pp. 7-11.

5. Ringer, S.: A further contribution regarding the influence of the different constituents of the blood on the contraction of the heart, J Physiol

(Lond), 1883, *4*, 29–42.

6. Chargaff, E., and Olson, K. B.: Studies on the chemistry of blood coagulation, J Biol Chem, 1937, *122*, 153–167.

7. McLean, J.: The thromboplastic action of cephalin, Am J Physiol, 1916, *41*, 250–257.

8. McLean, J.: The discovery of heparin, Circulation, 1959, *19*, 75–78.

9. Hustin, A.: Principe d'une nouvelle methode de transfusion muqueuse, J Med Bruxelles, 1914, *12*, 436–439. (For "muqueuse" read "sanguine.")

10. Hustin, A.: Renouveau de la transfusion sanguine au début du XX siècle, Acta Chir Belg, 1960, *8*, 762–780.

11. Jacobson, J. H., and Suarez, E. L.: Microsurgery in anastomoses of small vessels, Surg Forum, 1960, *11*, 243–245.

12. Macmillan, W. H., Smith, D. J., and Jacobson, J. H.: Response of normal, denervated, and reserpine-treated arteries to sympathomimetic amines and nicotine in dogs, Br J Pharmacol Chemother, 1962, *18*, 39–48.

13. Chain, E., Florey, H. W., Gardner, A. D., Heatley, N. G., Jennings, M. A., Orr-Ewing, J., and Sanders, A. G.: Penicillin as a chemotherapeutic agent, Lancet, 1940, *2*, 226–228.

14. Chain, E.: Thirty years of penicillin therapy, Proc R Soc Lond [Biol], 1971, *179*, 293–319.

15. Comroe, J. H., Jr., and Dripps, R. D.: The histamine-like action of curare and tubocurarine injected intracutaneously and intra-arterially in man, Anesthesiology, 1946, *7*, 260–262.

16. Brain, W. R.: Structure of the scientific paper, Br Med J, 1965, *2*, 868–869.

Speculation on Speculation

A legitimate public concern is how to speed up scientific discovery and its application to clinical medicine and surgery. Several years ago, I listed 18 steps between the initial idea and full clinical application and noted that delay *could* occur at any one of these (1). However, I ruled out one of these as a factor of importance—a scientist's indifference toward publishing his work for others to read. It is true that historically there have indeed been some notable delays between an initial discovery and its publication, especially in past centuries, when public disclosure of what we would now call a remarkable discovery was likely to endanger the life of the scientist; scientists then had an understandable reluctance to become authors. And in European scientific circles in the nineteenth and early twentieth centuries, we must confess that there was a curious phenomenon called "the sealed letter" (2). But in modern times, scientists seem to report their discoveries with either prudent or immodest promptness; the weight of *Index Medicus*, about 5 pounds per month, which prints only title, authors, and journal reference for each article, with not even a minuscule summary, is proof enough of authors' urge to publish for all to read, confirm, extend, apply, or deny.

However, if we're honest, we can't rule out all 18 steps. There *are* steps where speeding up might well be accomplished. One of these I've labelled "Publisher's Dawdle" (3). Another is getting newly published information to the next man along the line. One problem here may be not what's *in* the published article, but what's *not* in it. In the myriads of articles that appear yearly in our journals, what is usually *not* included is speculation—an author's ideas or suggestions reached by contemplation, reasoning, conjecture, or surmise but not yet supported by sufficient hard data to merit separate publication. I speculate that we might speed the advance of medical science by inviting all authors to in-clude some speculation, labelled clearly as such in their scientific articles, to follow Introduction, Methods, Results and Discussion—and to precede and not to be confused with the author's well-fortified Conclusions. *Pediatrics* now does this by asking authors to include a paragraph headed "Speculation and Relevance, or Implications," but most journals frown on such a practice.

What does and does not qualify as reasonable, legitimate speculation?

(*a*) It should not be science fiction of the Tom Swift or Star Trek type (predictions of what the next century might bring). This would exclude Benjamin Franklin's 1749 speculation on his electrical cooker (in his April 29 letter to Peter Collinson):

> It is proposed to put an end to them [electrical experiments] for this season, somewhat humorously, in a party of pleasure on the banks of Skuylkil. Spirits, at the same time, are to be fired by a spark sent from side to side through the river, without any other conductor than the water; an experiment which we some time since performed, to the amazement of many.

> A turkey is to be killed for our dinner by the electrical shock, and roasted by the electrical jack, before a fire kindled by the electrified bottle: when the healths of all the famous electricians in England, Holland, France, and Germany are to be drank in electrified bumpers, under the discharge of guns from the electrical battery (4).

On the other hand, Eadweard Muybridge's speculation might be acceptable since, in 1872, he had indeed invented motion pictures, and Edison a little later had put together a reasonably good phonograph. In 1898 Muybridge wrote, in the preface to his book *Animals in Motion*:

> The combination of such an instrument [motion pictures] with the phonograph has not, at the time of writing, been satisfactorily accomplished; there

can, however, be little doubt that in the—perhaps not far distant—future, instruments will be constructed that will not only reproduce visible actions simultaneously with audible words, but an entire opera, with the gestures, facial expressions and songs of the performers, with all the accompanying music, will be recorded . . . for the instruction or entertainment of an audience long after the original participants shall have passed away (5).

His speculation became reality in 1927 with the production of "The Jazz Singer"; whether Muybridge's speculation ignited the spark of invention and development required for "talkies" is not known.

(b) The speculation can and should include fields completely outside the author's interest or competence, such as the 1896 suggestion that newly discovered X-rays be used to check passengers' luggage for concealed bombs, or a later suggestion that microvascular surgical technics might be used to reconstruct successfully a ligated vas deferens (when the owner had new plans that required an open duct), or the suggestion that an oral diuretic, designed for relieving patients with congestive heart failure of their excess fluid collections, might lower blood pressure in patients with essential hypertension.

(c) The speculation must not be an obvious next step in the author's continuing investigation if he has already bolstered his speculation by pilot experiments.

Adhering to this qualified definition, let's look into the Retrospectroscope and see what we can learn. We *cannot* learn how many investigators included speculation (useful or impractical) in their manuscripts because we can look only at what escaped the editor's scissors or blue pencil; however, we can look at some speculation that has been published and estimate its impact on the advance of medicine.

SPECULATION WITH NO IMPACT

Extracorporeal Oxygenation

Hooke in 1667 wrote:

> I shall shortly further try, whether the suffering the Blood to circulate through a vessel, so as it may be openly exposed to the fresh Air, will not suffice for the life of an Animal; and make some other Experiments, which, I hope, will thoroughly discover the Genuine use of Respiration; and afterwards consider of what benefit this may be to Mankinde (6).

This, the first speculation on extracorporeal oxy-genation of blood, predictably had no impact on medicine. Oxygen, microbiology, anticoagulants, blood groups, anesthesia, and modern surgery still had to be discovered. Extracorporeal oxygenation *did* become useful for organ perfusion in physiologic laboratories in the nineteenth century, but it is unlikely that this can be attributed to Hooke.

The Stewart Clamp

In 1910, G. N. Stewart, a physiologist well known for his indicator-dilution principle, needed a device to occlude an artery only partially (for operations on its wall), permitting blood flow to continue through the remainder of the vessel. He described his clamp in the *Journal of the American Medical Association;* because he was not a surgeon, presumably he published it in a clinical journal only to call it to the attention of surgeons. He speculated freely for them:

> Such clamps might be employed to arrest hemorrhage from a wound in a large vessel which could not be clamped completely without detriment, and during the suturing of the wound; possibly in the treatment of sacculated aneurism in some situations; in performing lateral anastomosis of bloodvessels in cases where it is undesirable to completely occlude one or both of the vessels for the time required in the operation; in performing lateral implantation of one vessel on to another which must not be totally occluded; in inserting a cannula laterally into a vessel without stopping the circulation when there is no convenient branch of the vessel which might be used, or where it is disadvantageous to occlude such a branch; in narrowing experimentally the lumen of a vessel without temporarily occluding it, especially when a diminution of the lumen by a definite amount is desired, etc. (7)

As far as I know, the first use of Stewart's clamp, 36 years later, was in 1946 when it became the Potts' clamp and was used to permit aorta-pulmonary artery anastomosis to relieve cyanosis in blue babies. Because Potts was unusually generous in giving credit to the work of Blalock and Taussig that preceded his operation, but never mentioned Stewart's clamp, I can only surmise that Potts never saw Stewart's article even though it was written in English and published in the *JAMA.*

Freeze Drying

In 1909, Shackell, trying to measure accurately the glycogen content in liver and muscle of steers, ran into the problem of rapid postmortem hydrolysis of glycogen; to stop this hydrolysis, he devised a method of rapid freezing followed by vacuum desiccation. He realized that freeze-drying had wide applications to the preservation of sera, of other components of blood, of viruses (e.g., of rabies), and of food. He wrote:

> Experiments so far indicate that all materials, especially those unstable substances associated with immunity work, can be desiccated as outlined and can be indefinitely preserved.
>
> It is generally recognized that no chemical changes take place in perfectly dry substances. The products of this method are for all purposes entirely moisture-free. Deterioration in them is therefore absolutely precluded, providing the ordinary precautions of stoppered containers are taken to prevent contact with atmospheric moisture. If necessary, substances after drying can be hermetically sealed *in vacuo*.
>
> The special value of the method in medicine lies undoubtedly in the field of serum-therapy. One of the great practical problems has been the prevention of auto-degeneration in serums and toxins. It has been found possible, however, by the use of this method to obviate autolysis of such typically unstable substances as the complement of guinea-pig serum and the virus of hydrophobia.
>
> Though but a few of the most important results of the method have been mentioned in the present paper, the writer and his colleagues appreciate the probability of its widely extended application to many current problems, several of which are being attacked at the present time (8).

Shackell wrote only one other paper on freeze-drying, dealing largely with preserving rabies virus. In these two papers, he tossed out enough ideas to excite basic and applied scientists, in universities and industry, for years to come. But (except for Gersh's use of it to prepare histologic sections in 1932) no one used the new method until 1935, and it had little application until World War II, when it became important in the large scale production of preserved dried plasma and penicillin. Finally industry applied it in the food business and among other things it led to the production of a best seller—instant freeze-dried coffee.

Why did Shackell's experiments and speculation go unnoticed for almost 25 years? Elser and co-workers (9) in 1935 wrote:

> Shackell fully appreciated the value of his discovery, particularly in the field of immunology, but apart from publishing a paper in association with Harris dealing almost entirely with the preservation of the virus of rabies, he apparently failed to continue this line of investigation and for some unaccountable reason his work did not receive the attention from immunologists which in our opinion it deserved. Possibly, the appearance of the original communication in the American Journal of Physiology not commonly consulted by bacteriologists and the fact that subsequent papers stressed the value of the method in connection with the conservation of rabies virus may be in part responsible for the lack of progress made in this field during the time that has intervened.

SPECULATION WITH IMPACT

On the other hand, some speculation seems to have been picked up reasonably quickly by others, whose work then led to specific medical advances.

Flame Photometry

Barnes in 1945 speculated on a wide variety of uses of this new technic: for continuous analysis of salts in water, for determination of sodium and potassium in soil samples, and in the analysis of biologic materials (10). Of the latter, he said:

> Some of the most interesting uses to which these instruments have already been put concern the analysis of biological materials. In the hands of several clinical research workers, the flame photometer has been used successfully to analyze such materials as whole blood, blood serum, urine, body fluids, and tissue residues. These analyses, which are usually both difficult and time-consuming as a result of the very nature of the samples and the small size of the average samples which are available, may readily be performed. For the determination of sodium in blood serum, a sample of as little as 0.1 ml. can be satisfactorily analyzed after diluting by a factor of 1 to 100. The potassium content of serum could conceivably be determined on a 0.1-ml. sample after diluting to 2.5 ml. but a 0.5-ml. sample is much to be preferred. This fact, plus the speed with which the analyses may be completed, makes possible certain studies which have hitherto been impossible.
>
> Thus, in the clinical laboratory, the flame photometer has proved itself to be a most valuable instrument in connection with research on metabolic studies, the rapid diagnosis, and the treatment of certain diseases.

Obviously, pilot studies had already been done but this paragraph (published in *Industrial and Engineering Chemistry*, a nonmedical journal) stimulated widespread use of the new instrument. By 1947, Hald had reported careful studies of Na^+ and K^+ in biologic materials and an important new tool was available for basic and clinical research and clinical diagnosis and care.

Blood Oxygen Tension

Davies and Brink were primarily interested in measuring the O_2 consumption of nerves and sympathetic ganglia. To do this, they constructed an O_2 electrode that worked well in saline solutions. They dabbled a bit in measuring blood Po_2 and ran into a few practical problems that they believed could be solved. Their main interests lay elsewhere but Brink did, in 1950 (11), offer this suggestion to others:

The electrode was used for several experiments, but the agar plug finally became ineffective. The principal reason is that agar does not adhere firmly to a glass surface. Further development of electrode coatings is desirable. Other tests indicate that a collodion membrane is effective but can be used only where mechanical damage to the electrode tip is not likely to occur.

The measurement of dissolved O_2 in whole blood seems of sufficient importance to warrant more development of these methods for this purpose. The platinum electrode has the distinct advantage over the dropping Hg type that it can be inserted in the flowing blood of the experimental animal. In fact, by means of a motor-driven syringe it would be possible to draw blood from a human subject at a uniform rate and measure the dissolved O_2 therein. The flow rate could be as low as 3 cu mm/min, as in the flow respirometers used in this laboratory. *It is apparent that the component parts exist for successful development of an electrical instrument for measurement of dissolved O_2 in whole blood in situ. All that is required is an intensive program of development of the electrode for this specific purpose. Those interested in using the measurements must decide whether such a development is justified.* (Italics added)

Leland Clark did have a specific need for such an electrode; he ingeniously solved the problem 3 years later (12). The Clark electrode was soon widely used in basic and clinical research and clinical care.

Humoral Transmission of the Nerve Impulse

G. L. Brown attributes the beginnings of this novel concept to the speculations of T. R. Elliott in 1904. Elliott, after demonstrating that adrenalin secreted by the adrenal medulla does not directly stimulate either sympathetic ganglia or nerves, but does excite *peripheral* tissue (e.g., smooth muscle) innervated by sympathetic nerves, speculated (13):

Therefore it cannot be that adrenalin excites any structure derived from, and dependent for its persistence on, the peripheral neurone. But since adrenalin does not evoke any reaction from muscle that has at no time of its life been innervated by the sympathetic, the point at which the stimulus of the chemical excitant is received, and transformed into what may cause the change of tension of the muscle fibre, is perhaps a mechanism developed out of the muscle cell in response to its union with the synapsing sympathetic fibre, the function of which is to receive and transform the nervous impulse. *Adrenalin might then be the chemical stimulant liberated on each occasion when the impulse arrives at the periphery.* (Italics added)

Further advance waited for 10 years but then came in successive studies by Dale, Loewi, Feldberg, Brown, Gaddum, and Cannon, and opened whole new fields in physiology and pharmacology.

In 1948 Ahlquist speculated that Elliott's receptors were of two types, alpha and beta adrenoreceptors (13a); his predictions led to a search for agonists and antagonists (blockers) of beta receptors and to finding new drugs for treating arrhythmias and hypertension. Laragh (13b) noted that Ahlquist's pharmacological manuscript was turned down by the *Journal of Pharmacology and Experimental Therapeutics* (too much speculation?) and was published in the *American Journal of Physiology*.

Transfusion Reactions

Landsteiner in 1900 discovered that immunologically there were three different types of human blood (14). In that paper, he did not speculate that transfusion of blood of one type from a donor to a recipient whose blood was a different type might cause hemolysis or agglutination of red blood cells; transfusions continued without previous matching of blood, and so did transfusion reactions. But in 1907, Hektoen published a brief article in the *JAMA* (15) that contained no data but did contain the following speculation:

By means of a refined technic Crile recently transfused blood from normal to diseased human beings, and with apparent success. The occurrence of isoagglutinins in human blood suggests that under special conditions homologous transfusion might prove dangerous by leading to erythrocytic agglutination within the vessels of the subject transfused. It has not been possible to conduct animal experiments on this point because of failure to demonstrate isoagglutinins in the serum of suitable animals. *It may be pointed out, however, that the possible danger here indicated can be avoided by the selection of a donor whose corpuscles are not agglutinated by the serum of the recipient and whose serum does not agglutinate the corpuscles of the latter* [italics added]; that is to say, donor and recipient should belong to the same group and preferably to Group I or II. The actual isoagglutinative relation of the donor and the recipient are readily determinable in a short time in the manner already outlined.

By 1911, Ottenberg introduced direct cross-matching of blood from donor and recipient, and transfusion reactions for the most part came to an end. When Hustin in 1914 made indirect transfusion possible by adding a new anticoagulant, citrate, to blood, blood transfusions at last became a safe and practical therapeutic measure.

The Cardiac Pacemaker

In 1951, Callaghan and Bigelow, like others before them, tried to pace an animal's heart with an electrode in contact with the natural pacemaker, the sino-atrial node; in their experiments, they tried to achieve this contact by passing an electrode down the superior vena cava. However, they noted that "from the practical aspect . . . intimate contact with the sino-auricular node is not essential for good control since distances up to three quarters of an inch from the nodal area were adequate." They speculated that the time had come to apply this to the human heart beset by serious iatrogenic arrhythmias that occurred during intracardiac procedures (16).

Within a year, Zoll tried first an intraesophageal electrode and then subcutaneous needles (placed on opposite sides of the thorax) in man and successfully paced the human heart. And eventually others used transvenous pacing of the human heart much as Callaghan and Bigelow had suggested from their work on animals.

Nitrous Oxide and Ether Anesthesia

Humphry Davy in 1800 speculated that "As nitrous oxide in its extensive operation appears capable of destroying physical pain, it may probably be used with advantage during surgical operations in which no great effusion of blood takes place" (17). Davy's former pupil, Michael Faraday, wrote in 1818,

> In trying the effects of the ethereal vapour on persons who are peculiarly affected by nitrous oxide, the similarity of sensation produced was very unexpectedly found to have taken place. One person who always feels a depression of spirits on inhaling the gas, had sensation of a similar kind produced by inhaling the [ether] vapour (18).

Physicians did not immediately act on these suggestions. Whether they failed to read them or were fearful of using these gases or vapors (despite the incalculable benefits of a general anesthetic agent), we cannot say. But someone noted them, because "laughing gas" parties became pretty common thereafter. One adventurous group asked Dr. Crawford Long in 1842 to prepare some nitrous oxide for an evening's lark; he replied that he didn't have the apparatus for making the gas but he did have some ether and that would do the trick just as well. As a result of these parties and the obvious analgesia that ether or nitrous oxide conferred on those injured after falling, Long deliberately used ether for surgical anesthesia in 1842, and Colton and Wells used nitrous oxide in 1844.

THOUGHTS ON SPECULATION

I haven't done a systematic analysis of how many authors, in what periods of time and in what cultures, have speculated (beyond the facts on which they based conclusions or recommendations) and whether their speculation was right or wrong. Nor have I tried to determine numerically how many investigators were strongly influenced by earlier speculation of others and how long it took them to be so influenced. Accurate data on this are hard to obtain because the rigid, stereotyped format of today's scientific paper favors an author who would like to avoid acknowledging the source of his ideas or hypothesis.

However, of a random sampling of 50 articles* in which authors *did* speculate, only 4 proved later to be wrong. These were Sir Almroth Wright in 1894 on oral administration of citrate or calcium to influence blood coagulation in man (he suggested that citric acid, given orally, would diminish blood coagulability by bonding lime salts in blood); Howell and Holt, who in 1917 assigned no clinical importance to heparin except as a cause of hemophilia; and Hering (1923) and Koch and Mies (1929), who thought that ineffective carotid sinus function was an important cause of hypertension in man. The other 46 tossed out good ideas later shown to be worthy of investigation by others.

If this analysis of randomly selected articles suggests that speculation has greater potential for

---

* All of these were "key articles" crucial to clinical advances in cardiovascular medicine or surgery (19).

good than for harm, why do scientific articles contain little or no speculation?

(1) First is the ancient dictum that "a scientist must never go beyond his facts."

(2) Even though speculation is put into a separate section and boldly labelled, it may still come through to some readers as "conclusions."

(3) Space in journals is expensive and when a reviewer of a manuscript says "cut it in half," the first thing to go is speculation.

(4) A serious problem, especially for young investigators, is that speculation gives away to others an author's best ideas for future research which he is entitled to follow up, at least within a reasonable period of time. Speculation by scientists working in industrial scientific laboratories of course gives competitors leads to highly profitable products.

(5) A closely related problem is that speculation can be an unethical device for an author to claim later on that an important discovery was really his work though he put in no actual experimental time or effort to establish the validity of his idea.

(6) Finally, there's the rationalization that it's not worth the effort because "you can lead a horse to water but you can't make him drink."

I believe that the time has now come when we should give speculation a fair trial and evaluate its impact on scientific advance. It could provide worthwhile research projects for those who cannot distinguish between the more and the less important or for those who lack originality but are technically superb at completing important research projects proposed by others (and I think many horses will drink water from another well when they realize theirs is dry). It might put to an experimental test some ideas that otherwise die when a brilliant scientist dies. And if we could bring together into one journal well-edited speculation from many fields of science, we might speed entry of a whole new set of ideas and concepts into biomedical research and greatly extend the scope of a scientist's reading.

Finally, if we believe in the power of private enterprise, here's a way of letting individual scientists decide for themselves which of many promising leads to explore instead of being "directed" by non-scientists who are convinced that *someone* must act.

Addendum

I'd like to see speculation become a respected

and valuable component of each scientific article in each journal, but it seems easier to start a new journal than to change an existing one! Just about 20 years ago a new journal, *Perspectives in Biology and Medicine,* appeared, "designed to communicate heuristic ideas," and invited readers to submit new hypotheses and concepts. Although its articles have always been interesting to read, relatively few have dealt specifically with "generalizations, working hypotheses, leisurely interpretation and speculation that the reader might carry to the laboratory and to the bedside," and I don't think it has fulfilled its promise.

Recently another journal, *Medical Hypotheses,* has appeared on the scene (20). Let David F. Horrobin, its editor, tell why he added one more to the 3,000 biomedical journals now in existence:

The physical and chemical sciences long ago recognized that observations are not superior to hypotheses in generating scientific progress nor are hypotheses superior to observations. Both are necessary. While the ideal research worker may be one who is equally able to generate hypotheses and to test them experimentally, these sciences also recognized that such paragons are very rare indeed. Most scientists are much better at either one or the other activity. In physico-chemical fields this is fully accepted and the contributions of both theoretical and experimental scientists are recognized.

In contrast in the biomedical sciences there seems to me much ignorance of the way in which scientific advance actually occurs. . . . [Biologists] have failed to recognize adequately that observation is always more effective when disciplined and channelled by hypothesis. . . . Most scientists now active in the biomedical field are competent observers whose ability to generate ideas is either naturally absent or has been stultified by the prevailing philosophy. As a result they spend their time in making more and more detailed observations of the same sorts of phenomena. In contrast a few have far more ideas than they could possibly investigate but their potential contribution is largely nullified because they are allowed to publish only in those areas where they have done experimental or clinical work. If only these differences of ability and emphasis could be accepted and recognized then the people with ideas (who may often be inept experimenters) could generate a steady flow of new concepts which might rejuvenate the work of those whose primary skill is in observation.

Medical Hypotheses won't accomplish my goal of sprinkling reasonable, legitimate speculation in each article in each journal; it won't reach many individual subscribers ($60/6 issues) or carry many hypotheses to them (about eight articles every two months)—but it's a brave start. If it doesn't let history, philosophy, sociology, and politics of science crowd out hypotheses, journal #3,001 should be a valuable addition to the present 3,000.

References

1. Comroe, J. H., Jr.: What's locked up? (editorial), Am Rev Respir Dis, 1974, *110*, 111-114.
2. This volume, Publish and/or perish, pp. 74-78.
3. This volume, Publisher's dawdle: An incurable disease?, pp. 79-82.
4. Franklin, B.: New Experiments and Observations on Electricity Made at Philadelphia in America, ed. 3, part I, D. Henry and R. Cave, London, 1760.
5. Muybridge, E.: Animals in Motion, 1898, reprinted by Dover Publications, New York, 1957.
6. Hooke, R.: An account of an experiment made by M. Hook[e], of preserving animals alive by blowing through their lungs with bellows, Philos Trans R Soc Lond, 1667, *2*, 539-540.
7. Stewart, G. N.: A clamp for isolating a portion of the lumen of a blood-vessel without stopping the circulation through the vessel, JAMA, 1910, *55*, 647-649.
8. Shackell, L. F.: An improved method of desiccation with some applications to biological problems, Am J Physiol, 1909, *24*, 325-340.
9. Elser, W. J., Thomas, R. A., and Steffen, G. I.: The desiccation of sera and other biological products (including microorganisms) in the frozen state with the preservation of the original qualities of products so treated, J Immunol, 1935, *28*, 433-473.
10. Barnes, R. B., Richardson, D., Berry, J. W., and Hood, R. L.: Flame photometry: A rapid analytic procedure, Indust Eng Chem Anal Ed, 1945, *17*, 605-611.
11. Brink, F., Jr.: Methods in Medical Research, vol. 2, Year Book Medical Publishers, Chicago, 1950, pp. 175-177.
12. Clark, L. C., Jr., Wolf, R., Granger, D., and Taylor, Z.: Continuous recording of blood oxygen tensions by polarography, J Appl Physiol, 1953, *6*, 189-193.
13. Elliott, T. R.: On the action of adrenalin, J Physiol, 1904, *31*, xx-xxi.
13a. Ahlquist, R. P.: A study of the adrenotropic receptors, Am J Physiol, 1948, *153*, 586-600.
13b. Laragh, J.: Honors for two great leaps forward, Cardiovasc Med, 1976, *1*, 277-278.
14. Landsteiner, K.: Zur Kenntnis der antifermentativen, lytischen und agglutinierender Wirkungen des Blutserums und der Lymphe, Centralbl Bakteriol Parasit Infekt, 1900, *27*, 357-362.
15. Hektoen, L.: Isoagglutination of human corpuscles, JAMA, 1907, *48*, 1739-1740.
16. Callaghan, J. C., and Bigelow, W. G.: An electrical artificial pacemaker for standstill of the heart, Ann Surg, 1951, *134*, 8-17.
17. Davy, H.: Researches, Chemical and Philosophical; Chiefly Concerning Nitrous Oxide, or Dephlogisticated Nitrous Air, J. Johnson, London, 1800.
18. Faraday, M.: Effects of inhaling the vapour of sulphuric ether, Q J Sci Arts, 1818, *4*, 158-159.
19. Comroe, J. H., Jr., and Dripps, R. D.: Scientific basis for the support of biomedical science, Science, 1976, *192*, 105-111.
20. *Medical Hypotheses*, D. F. Horrobin, ed., Clinical Research Institute, 110 Pine Ave. West, Montreal, H2W 1R7, Canada.

Lags

Congress, in the interest of promoting the health of the public, has shown considerable concern about (1) *too-rapid* introduction of laboratory discoveries into clinical practice and (2) *too-slow* introduction. Obviously what we need is a *just-right* interval between scientific discovery and clinical application. The introduction of insulin in the 1920s came pretty close to *just-right*, although some clinicians resisted this new-fangled material for more than a decade. Thalidomide obviously was used much too quickly and too widely, though few if any could have predicted the tragic events that followed its use and not even the most cautious pharmacologists thought of screening tests for fetal damage in a variety of animal species. X-rays were used almost instantly throughout the world after their discovery in 1895; however, when reports of tissue damage began to flow in, they also proved to have been applied clinically too quickly and too widely. Was the 1955 introduction of Salk polio vaccine *too-rapid* or *just-right?* Even Congress debated whether that vaccine had been introduced prematurely and devoted 27 pages of a congressional report to the matter.

On the other hand, some lags between discovery and application, such as that in the use of intermittent positive pressure ventilation during clinical intrathoracic operations (1), have been very long indeed. Here are a few more examples of long lags.

Measurement of residual volume of the lungs. The greatest scientific event of the eighteenth century was the discovery of oxygen and the Chemical Revolution that it generated. Interest in the therapeutic use of oxygen, and other gases that might be respirable, ran high and led Thomas Beddoes to raise funds to build the Pneumatic Institution near Bristol in England. It opened in 1798, one of the earliest medical centers combining facilities for both medical care and research. Beddoes invited Humphry Davy, then 20 years old, to join the staff as Director of the Laboratory. Davy's first achievement there was to purify nitrous oxide and to test its effects,

first on cats, rabbits, and goldfinches, and then on himself and his friends, among whom were Joseph Priestley and Samuel Taylor Coleridge. In 1800, he recorded the results of his studies, including the observation that "as nitrous oxide . . . appears capable of destroying physical pain, it may probably be used with advantage during surgical operations"—a suggestion not tested clinically until 44 years later.

Among other gases prepared by Davy was hydrogen. Davy built his own spirometer, filled it part way with a measured volume of hydrogen, and breathed it back and forth "for rather less than half a minute, making in this time seven quick respirations." He then expired fully into the spirometer and measured the amount and concentration of hydrogen in it. He reasoned that if no hydrogen had been absorbed by blood flowing through the lungs, the hydrogen that was no longer in the spirometer must be in his lungs. Now, knowing the amount of hydrogen in his lungs and assuming that the concentration of hydrogen was the same in the spirometer and in his lungs, he calculated (figure 1) his residual lung volume to be 37.5 cu in or 614 ml—a somewhat low value, but, as Davy wrote, "my chest is narrow, measuring in circumference but 29 inches and my neck rather long and slender (2)."

Hutchinson did his monumental study on vital capacity and its subdivisions in 1846 but reported no measurements of residual volume or total capacity. Sixty years after Davy's work, Gréhant used a hydrogen method to measure functional residual capacity (FRC) (3,4). This was followed by another long, relatively quiet period until 1923, when Van Slyke and Binger used a hydrogen-rebreathing test to measure FRC (5). They reported no measurements on patients; clinical measurements of FRC finally began at McGill in 1930 (130 years after Davy's report) when Christie developed his oxygen method.

Estimation of changes in intrapleural pressure during breathing. Today, evaluation of the mechanical properties of the lungs is an integral

I refpired at 59° 102 cubic inches of hydrogene apparently pure, for rather lefs than half a minute, making in this time feven quick refpirations.

After the complete expiration, when the common temperature was reftored, the gas occupied a fpace equal to 103 cubic inches nearly. Thefe analifed were found to confift

Carbonic acid ..	4,0
Oxygene	3,7
Nitrogene	17,3
Hydrogene	78,0
	103,0

Now as in this experiment, the gas was increafed in bulk only a cubic inch ; fuppofing that after the compleat expiration the gas in the lungs, bronchia and fauces was of nearly fimilar compofition with that in the airholder, and that no hydrogene had been abforbed by the blood, it would follow that 24 cubic inches of hydrogene remained in the internal organs of refpiration, and confequently, by the rule of proportion, about 7,8 of the mixed refidual gas of the common air. And then the whole quantity of refidual gas of the lungs, fuppofing the temperature 59°, would have been 31,8 cubic inches ; but as its temperature was nearly that of the internal parts of the body, 98°, it muft have filled a greater fpace; calculating from the experiments of Guyton and Vernois,* about 37,51 cubic inches.

Fig. 1. Davy's method for measuring residual gas in his lungs (2).

part of testing for pulmonary function. To assess these, one must know the forces acting on the lung, and this requires measuring or estimating intrapleural pressure. Carl Ludwig (1847) was the first to report measurements of intrapleural pressure in living animals (6). He introduced a water-filled tube capped with a rubber balloon between the parietal and visceral pleurae and connected the tube to a mercury manometer.

This system provided data in animals on the forces acting on the surface of the lung but could hardly be applied to healthy man or used routinely in a pulmonary function laboratory. The question whether it was possible to find a safe way to measure pressure outside the lungs but inside the thoracic cage was answered in 1878 by Luciani (7). Acting on a suggestion by Ceradini, he simply put a tube in the intrathoracic esophagus and measured pressure changes in the flabby-walled esophagus; the tube had numerous holes near the lower end (sometimes covered with a small rubber balloon) and was connected to a Marey capsule that recorded pressure changes more faithfully than the sluggish, less sensitive mercury manometer. Luciani's esophageal sound (figure 2) seemed to work well and provide reasonable data. And certainly everyone would agree that swallowing a balloon-catheter was a lot safer for the patient than putting a needle in his thorax. But the method was never applied to man until 1949!

Why not? Possibly it was lack of interest on the part of physiologists. There were indeed giants in respiratory physiology at the turn of the century but not many with an interest in the mechanics of breathing. Those who *were* interested in forces, pressures, and flow of air at that time failed to take advantage of the improved manometers for measuring blood pressure (see below) and, possibly on that account, managed to "do in" the use of the esophageal balloon. Heynsius (1882) criticized esophageal pressures because these were considerably lower than intrapleural pressure and were inconsistent; he attributed these problems to the thickness of the esophageal wall and irregular contractions of smooth muscle provoked by the catheter-balloon acting as a foreign irritant (8). Meltzer (1892) agreed with him and this concurrence put an end to the esophageal balloon for several decades (9).

Wirz, who did important work on pressure-volume and pressure-flow relationships in 1923, measured intrapleural pressure directly. In his paper, he reviewed other methods, including Luciani's; apparently without doing any studies using an esophageal balloon, he dismissed the method with the statement that it had "only

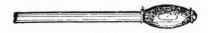

Fig. 2. Luciani's esophageal sound used by him to estimate intrapleural pressure in animals (7).

small historical importance. Based on incorrect premises, it never contributed anything to perfect the methods or broaden the view of the problem (10)." And, in so saying, he banished it for another 26 years.

In the meantime, those who wanted to learn about the mechanical properties of healthy, human, living lungs had no choice but to puncture the pleural cavity cautiously. This caution was well expressed by Aron, the first to measure intrapleural pressure in healthy man (1896); in 1900 he wrote, "It is perhaps debatable whether an experiment of this kind on a living, healthy human being is justified. However, trusting the reliability of today's asepsis and antisepsis, I decided to risk it. . . . I was not brave enough to repeat it too often (11)." Ronald Christie did it again in 1934 (12), but Mead (13) wrote that between 1896 and 1961 probably fewer than ten persons served as normal subjects for direct measurement of intrapleural pressure.

In 1949, Hermanus Johannes Buytendijk completed his thesis for the Ph.D. degree at the University of Groningen; it was entitled "Esophageal Pressure and Lung Elasticity." He used an esophageal balloon and a thin copper membrane manometer. His thesis, written in Dutch, took a while to be noticed by many English-speaking physiologists. In 1952, when Dornhorst and Leathart wrote a paper on measuring esophageal pressure (with a free polythene tube without a balloon), in which they concluded that "the pressure in the esophagus is readily measured and is a satisfactory index of general intrathoracic pressure" (14), Buytendijk's thesis had not yet come to their attention. When his Ph.D. thesis was translated into English, it provided convincing evidence that the method was indeed reliable in man and opened the way for routine examination of pulmonary compliance.

There are two morals to this saga of the esophageal balloon. One is that when a scientist achieves the status of being an "authority," he then has an additional responsibility—of *not holding back* the advance of science by pronouncements that discourage certain lines of investigation. The other is that "non-authorities" have the responsibility of not accepting authoritative pronouncements without question.

Strain gauge. Today pulmonary physiologists use strain gauges routinely to measure transairway or transpulmonary pressure, and cardiovascular physiologists use them daily to measure intravascular and intracardiac pressures. But there was a long, tortuous path between the first use of the mercury U-tube manometer by Poiseuille in 1828 and the first use of the strain gauge manometer by Lambert and Wood in 1947. Because the inertia of the mercury and friction between it and the glass prevented the mercury manometer from recording true pressures in a dynamic system, a 119-year search went on for an accurate, precise, sensitive, yet rugged and dependable manometer. This period saw the rise and decline of Marey and Chauveau's rubber membrane manometer, Fick's spring manometers, Hürthle's steel spring manometer, a series of optical manometers designed by Frank, Wiggers, Hamilton, Kubicek, and Green, and the electrical capacitance manometers of Lilly, Warburg, and Hansen.

Yet for the last 71 years of this search, the principle of the strain gauge was known; it had been published by Herbert Tomlinson in 1876 in the *Proceedings of the Royal Society of London* (15). The object of his research was "to determine the relation between increased resistance to the passage of an electric current and stretching force," and he concluded that "the temporary increase per cent of resistance of a wire when stretched in the same direction as the flow of the current is exactly proportional to the stretching force." He did not speculate on the possible usefulness of this precise relationship and apparently his study was not applied in industry or medicine until Simmonds patented the bonded strain gauge in 1942 and licensed it to the Baldwin Locomotive Works (16). Shortly thereafter, suitable wires became available commercially, and soon found many applications.

Lambert and Wood were the first to report on the use of a strain gauge to measure blood pressure (17). In 1945, they were attempting to develop direct methods for continuous recording of arterial blood pressure in subjects exposed to positive acceleration in the Mayo Clinic's human centrifuge. A few years earlier, Louis Statham, a physicist at the Curtiss-Wright Airplane Company of Buffalo, N.Y., had developed the "unbonded strain gauge." Statham patented the device and started his own Statham Laboratories in Los Angeles in 1943. He made one for Lambert and Wood in 1946 that they adapted to measure fluid pressure. Over a period of years, they requested and obtained from Statham transducers with improved dynamic response characteristics capable of measuring faithfully a wide variety of blood and air pressures.

Why did it take 71 years from discovery of the principle of the "strain wires" to its application for measuring blood pressure? In part, this was due to lack of suitable amplifiers, galvanometers, and recorders. Braun devised the cathode ray tube in 1897; Einthoven constructed a sensitive string galvanometer in 1903; Gasser, Erlanger, Forbes, and Thacher built electron tube amplifiers, a cathode ray oscilloscope, and a rapid photographic recorder between 1920 and 1922, but these were not ideal for high frequency recording. Lambert and Wood sidestepped these problems in 1947 by using a rugged, sensitive Heiland galvanometer commonly employed at that time by geophysicists; it required no amplifier. Shortly thereafter Bardeen, Brattain, and Shockley developed the transistor and industry provided a wide variety of amplifiers and recorders suitable for physiologic measurement.

Sometimes I think that Congress and the Administration believe that failure to recognize a significant achievement is a characteristic limited to scientists. Yet the talent of Vincent van Gogh, today acclaimed as one of the world's great painters, went unrecognized in his lifetime; Herman Melville, now believed by many to be America's greatest novelist, was practically unknown for 30 years after his death, and his greatest work, *Moby Dick*, was a critical failure and a financial disaster during his life; and Franz Schubert died before there was any recognition of his musical genius. And to these three could be added hundreds of now-famous authors, painters, composers, and even statesmen whose achievements were not acclaimed for many decades. Could it be that lack of clairvoyance is a widespread human failing and not a special characteristic of biomedical scientists?

References

1. This volume, Inflation — 1904 model, pp. 110-113.
2. Davy, H.: Researches, Chemical and Philosophical, Chiefly Concerning Nitrous Oxide or Dephlogisticated Nitrous Air and its Respiration, Johnson, London, 1800.
3. Gréhant, N.: Recherches sur la mesure du volume des poumons de l'homme, C R Acad Sci, 1860, *51*, 21-23.
4. Gréhant, N.: Perfectionnement du procédé de mesure du volume des poumons par l'hydrogène, C R Soc Biol Mem, 1887, *39*, 242-244.
5. Van Slyke, D. D., and Binger, C. A. L.: The determination of lung volume without forced breathing, J Exp Med, 1923, *37*, 457-470.
6. Ludwig, C.: Beitrage zur Kenntnis des Einfluss der Respirations bewegungen auf den Blutlauf im Aortensysteme, Arch Anat Physiol Wiss Med, 1847, 242-302.
7. Luciani, L.: Delle oscillazioni della pressione intratoracica e intraddominale, Arch Sci Med, 1878, *2*, 177-224.
8. Heynsius, A.: Ueber die Grösse des negativen Drucks im Thorax beim ruhingen Athmen, Arch Ges Physiol, 1882, *29*, 265-311.
9. Meltzer, S. J.: On the respiratory changes of the intrathoracic pressure, measured in the mediastinum posterior, J Physiol, 1892, *13*, 218-238.
10. Wirz, K.: Das Verhalten des Druckes im Pleuraraum bei der Atmung und die Ursachen seiner Veranderlichkeit, Arch Ges Physiol, 1923, *199*, 1-56.
11. Aron, E.: Der intrapleurale Druck beim lebenden gesunden Menschen, Arch Pathol Anat Physiol, 1900, *160*, 226-234.
12. Christie, R. V.: The elastic properties of the emphysematous lung and their clinical significance, J Clin Invest, 1934, *13*, 295-321.
13. Mead, J.: Mechanical properties of lungs, Physiol Rev, 1961, *41*, 281-330.
14. Dornhorst, A. C., and Leathart, G. L.: A method of assessing the mechanical properties of lungs and air-passages, Lancet, 1952, *2*, 109-111.
15. Tomlinson, H.: On the increase in resistance to the passage of an electric current produced on wires by stretching, Proc R Soc Lond, 1876, *25*, 451-453.
16. Simmonds, E. E.: U. S. Patent No. 2,292,549, 1942.
17. Lambert, E. H., and Wood, E. H.: The use of a resistance wire, strain gauge manometer to measure intraarterial pressure, Proc Soc Exp Biol Med, 1947, *64*, 186-190.

Inflation—1904 Model

When general anesthesia was discovered in 1846,[*] the practice of surgery exploded in many directions. Previously limited to procedures that the surgeon could complete swiftly with lightning slashing and stitching and that the patient could tolerate with the help of morphine, alcohol, or "biting the bullet," surgeons could now perform a variety of operations that required longer periods of dissection, probing, excision, and careful repair.

But this did not include intrathoracic operations. For a variety of reasons (1), cardiac surgery didn't "take off" until almost 100 years after Morton first demonstrated the use of ether, and pulmonary surgery was still pretty dangerous business until the mid-1930s. The first successful lobectomy in man was performed by Ferdinand Sauerbruch in 1908 and the first successful one-stage pneumonectomy by Evarts Graham in 1933 (2); before 1933 an entire lung had been removed from 2 patients, but in each, the surgeon simply ligated the root of the lung and allowed the tissue to slough out!

What held back pulmonary surgery? The main problem seems to have been pneumothorax and inability of the surgeons to cope with it. In 1904, Sauerbruch, the great German surgeon, finally hit upon a way to prevent it (3). His reasoning was simple: The lungs normally function in a box, the thoracic cage, where pressure is subatmospheric (negative); this overcomes the elastic recoil of the lungs and keeps them expanded, even at end-expiration. Therefore, to avoid

pneumothorax, all one need do is put the *patient* (except for his head) in a box and keep the *box* at subatmospheric pressure; then when the thorax is opened surgically, atmospheric pressure acting on the patient's nose and mouth outside the chamber will keep the lungs expanded, since the lungs are within the negative pressure chamber.

Sauerbruch first worked with animals and a cuirass-type chamber that enclosed only the dog's thorax; the chamber had 2 sleeve-type openings that permitted him to work with both hands inside it. He then built a larger chamber that enclosed all of the dog (except for its head) and all of the surgeon; the surgeon could now sit in relative comfort and leisurely open the thorax and operate on the lung. Pressure within the chamber was kept at 10 mm Hg less than room pressure and this pressure difference prevented the dreaded pneumothorax.

Sauerbruch was now ready to operate on human lungs. For this, he built a special negative-pressure room that could accommodate the patient, the surgeon, and the surgeon's assistants (figure 1). It even had an antechamber fitted as an air lock so that assistants could enter or leave the main chamber without altering its negative pressure (figure 2). Sauerbruch's chamber excited the interest of surgeons throughout Europe and thoracic surgeons in Berlin, Cologne, Vienna, St. Petersburg, and other medical centers soon installed this new device. It probably reached the ultimate in size in Willy Meyer's "Universal Negative Pressure Chamber" set up in the Rockefeller Institute in New York City in 1909 (4). One thousand cubic feet in volume, it could contain 17 persons in all: the patient, the surgeon, the surgeon's assistants, visitors, an engineer to maintain the air pressure, and 2 anesthetists; the latter, along with the patient's head, were in a *positive* pressure chamber within the negative pressure room!

Yet, despite the ingenuity and inventiveness

---

[*] For practical purposes, 1846 marked the beginning of anesthesia for surgical operations. However, Joseph Priestley is known to have prepared nitrous oxide in 1776 and Davy suggested its use in surgical operations in 1800; Faraday commented on the anesthetic properties of ether in 1818 and Crawford Long used ether anesthesia in 1842 when he excised a patient's tumor (Long did not report his discovery until 1849).

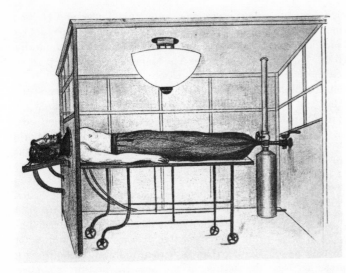

Fig. 1. A Sauerbruch constant negative (subatmospheric) pressure chamber.

of those who conceived these elaborate devices that captured the imagination of the surgical world, no one thought of *ventilation. Inflation* of the lungs, *yes,* but *ventilation,* the process by which fresh air enters alveoli and alveolar air leaves, *no.* The only goal was to keep the lungs inflated *continuously,* and, at all costs, to prevent even temporary deflation. True, the patient could move his thorax and continue to make respiratory movements. However, the lung in the *open* hemithorax remained motionless (unless air was sucked from it into the other lung during inspiration) and respiratory movements of the lung in the *closed* hemithorax must have been inadequate for the exchange of O_2 and CO_2, considering the handicaps imposed by a mobile mediastinum, deep anesthesia, and further depression of breathing caused by reflexes from fully inflated lungs.

Since every schoolboy or schoolgirl now learns how to maintain ventilation in an apneic person by repeated cycles of blowing into the patient's mouth and then allowing expired air to escape, the negative pressure devices spawned by Sauerbruch in the early 1900s are hard to explain. And they are practically inexplicable when we add that, in 1543, Andreas Vesalius rhythmically ventilated the lungs of a pig (5); in 1667, Robert Hooke did the same for a dog whose thoracic cage had been completely removed (6); and throughout the nineteenth century physiologists used bellows and pumps to

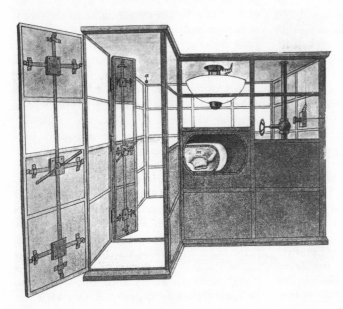

Fig. 2. Another constant negative pressure chamber with an air lock antechamber to allow personnel to enter and leave the main chamber during an operation.

provide rhythmic artificial ventilation for animals employed in laboratory experiments.

If there was little or no communication between physiologists and surgeons in Sauerbruch's time, there should have been more between surgeons and surgeons. In 1899, Rudolph Matas, professor of surgery at Tulane and an eminent thoracic surgeon, wrote in the Annals of Surgery:

> The procedure that promises the most benefit in preventing pulmonary collapse in operations on the chest is the artificial inflation of the lung and the rhythmical maintenance of artificial respiration by a tube in the glottis directly connected with a bellows. Like other discoveries, it is not only elementary in its simplicity, but the fundamental ideas involved in this important suggestion have been lying idle before the eyes of the profession for years. It is curious that surgeons should have failed to apply for so long a time the suggestions of the physiological laboratory, where the bellows and tracheal tubes have been in constant use from the days of Magendie (1783-1855) to the present, in practising artificial respiration on animals (7).

In 1893, Fell of Buffalo described an apparatus he devised to maintain artificial respiration in patients with opium poisoning; it was identical to that used in physiological laboratories except that it provided the option of using either a tracheal cannula inserted through a tracheotomy or a mask (8). O'Dwyer soon eliminated the danger of tracheotomy and the inefficiency of a mask by using an endotracheal tube (devised in 1880 by Macewen [9]). O'Dwyer commented simply, "In the performance of artificial respiration by any means, it is important to remember that all we have to do is to get air into the lungs, and give it sufficient time and room to escape, the power generated and stored up in overcoming the resistance to inspiration being amply sufficient to carry on expiration" (9a). The external end of O'Dwyer's endotracheal tube had 2 branches: one branch conducted fresh air to the lungs from a foot-operated bellows while the operator's thumb closed the other branch; expiration occurred when he removed his thumb. Matas recommended use of the Fell-O'Dwyer apparatus and it was used at least once in 1899 by his associate, Parham, with "brilliant" success, but it never caught on. Quénu and Longuet used an airtight helmet and positive pressure in 1896 (10), and in 1904, Brauer revived the Quénu-type helmet and positive pressure. But both of these techniques used *continuous* positive pressure; only Tuffier and Hallion (11), working in François-Franck's physiology laboratory, ventilated the lungs rhythmically, but no one except Matas seems to have paid attention to their report.

Today no one uses large negative-pressure chambers for intrathoracic operations. When and why did modern endotracheal rhythmic positive pressure ventilation come about? World War I probably had something to do with the elimination of these cumbersome chambers (except in Germany, where they were still used in the 1930s, so great was the prestige of Sauerbruch), because they were hard to set up near the front lines where they were most needed. The introduction of the Meltzer-Auer technique, far simpler than any other, was also responsible for the decline of the negative pressure chamber, although, curiously enough, it also ignored the matter of gas exchange (12). This new technique needed no boxes, chambers or special rooms; all it required was an endotracheal tube and a source of compressed air. When the tube filled just enough of the trachea and when the pressure bottle delivered slightly more air to the trachea than initially could flow out between the tube and the tracheal wall, a positive pressure developed in the distal airways and alveoli that kept them continuously inflated when the surgeon opened the thorax. Although Meltzer and Auer's opening sentence was, "The object of the function of respiration is to supply the animal with oxygen and to remove carbon dioxide," they never measured blood O_2 or CO_2 and, because their dogs recovered, simply took it for granted that "under these conditions the supply of oxygen and removal of carbon dioxide take place apparently in physiological fashion."

Rhythmic inflation of the lungs gradually replaced continuous distention. Crafoord (13) credits his former chief, K. H. Giertz, with demonstrating in 1914–1916 that (1) there was no essential difference in pulmonary ventilation accomplished by negative versus positive pressure and (2) rhythmic insufflation during inspiration followed by free outflow during expiration was clearly superior to all other methods of managing ventilation and preventing pneumothorax during operations on the lungs. Other factors were the introduction of direct-vision laryngoscopy by Chevalier Jackson, which made it far easier for non-experts to insert an endotracheal tube (14); the invention of the first closed-circuit anesthesia apparatus by Dennis Jackson (15), who designed it to recycle expensive anesthetic gases and so reduce the cost of anesthesia to the poor; the introduction of a simple to-and-fro closed-circuit rebreathing system by Ralph Waters (16); the change-over from clinical anesthesia to academic anesthesiology with a strong research component; the introduction of rapid or even continuous methods for measuring O_2 and CO_2 in blood and air; and the demonstration by Dripps (17) and by Beecher and Murphy (18) of harmful effects of CO_2 accumulation during anesthesia, even when hypoxia was prevented by supplying high concentrations of O_2 to the patient.

What lessons can we learn by using the Retrospectroscope to look at this curious era of the negative pressure chamber? Several: (1) Scientists and clinicians usually advance progress but sometimes retard it. (2) An impressive piece of hardware, backed by a highly prestigious designer, can hold back progress for decades. (3) It was difficult for surgeons to understand (a) that a transpulmonary pressure difference of 770 minus 760 mm Hg inflated the lungs the same amount as one of 760 minus 750 and (b) that, because diffusion over long distances is a very slow process, adequate gas exchange requires alveolar ventilation. (4) A trip—in either direction—across the street that separated basic science (physics or physiology in this case) from clinical departments could have accelerated the advent of successful pulmonary surgery by at least 50 years. (5) Finally, what are we, with our infinite wisdom and magnificient technical advances, doing today that will appear primitive, curious, or even stupid 50 years from now?

References

1. Comroe, J. H., Jr., and Dripps, R. D.: Ben Franklin and open heart surgery, Circ Res, 1974, 35, 661-669.
2. Graham, E. A., and Singer, J. J.: Successful removal of an entire lung for carcinoma of the bronchus, JAMA, 1933, 101, 1371-1374.
3. Sauerbruch, F.: Zur Pathologie des offenen Pneumothorax und die Grundlagen meines Verfahrens zu seiner Ausschaltung. Mitteilung Grenzebeit Med Chir, 1904, 13, 399-482.
4. Meyer, H. W.: The history of the development of the negative differential pressure chamber for thoracic surgery, J Thorac Surg, 1955, 30, 114-126.
5. Vesalius, A.: Pulmonis motuum, De Humani Corporis Fabrica Libri Septem, Oporinus, Basel, 1543, p. 658. [Follows p. 661 owing to incorrect numbering by printer.]
6. Hooke, R.: An account of an experiment made by M. Hook(e), of preserving animals alive by blowing through their lungs with bellows, Philos Trans R Soc Lond, 1667, 2, 539-540.
7. Matas, R. On the management of acute traumatic pneumothorax, Ann Surg, 1899, 29, 409-434.
8. Fell, G. E.: Fell Method—forced respiration—report of cases resulting in the saving of twenty-eight human lives. History and a plea for its general use in hospital and naval practice, Proc Section of General Medicine, Pan American Medical Congress, Washington, D. C., Sept. 7, 1893, p. 309.
9. Macewen, W.: Clinical observations on the introduction of tracheal tubes by the mouth instead of performing tracheotomy or laryngotomy, Br Med J, 1880, 2, 122-124, 163-165.
9a. O'Dwyer, J.: An improved method of performing artificial forcible respiration (with exhibition of instruments), Arch Ped, 1892, 9, 30-34.
10. Quénu, E., and Longuet, F.: Note sur quelques recherches expérimentales concernant la chirurgie thoracique, C R Soc Biol (Paris), 1896, 48, 1007-1008.
11. Tuffier, T., and Hallion, L. Opérations intrathoraciques avec respiration artificielle par insufflation, C R Soc Biol (Paris), 1896, 48, 951-953.
12. Meltzer, S. J., and Auer, J.: Continuous respiration without respiratory movements, J Exp Med, 1909, 11, 622-625.
13. Crafoord, C.: Some aspects of the development of intrathoracic surgery, Surg Gynecol Obstet, 1949, 89, 629-637.
14. Jackson, C.: The technique of insertion of intratracheal insufflation tubes, Surg Gynecol Obstet, 1913, 17, 507-509.
15. Jackson, D. E.: A new method for the production of general analgesia and anaesthesia with a description of the apparatus used, J Lab Clin Med, 1915, 1, 1-12.
16. Waters, R.: Clinical scope and utility of carbon dioxid filtration in inhalation anesthesia, Curr Res Anesth Analges, 1924, 3, 20-22, and 26.
17. Dripps, R. D.: The immediate decrease in blood pressure seen at the conclusion of cyclopropane anesthesia: "Cyclopropane Shock," Anesthesiology, 1947, 8, 15-35.
18. Beecher, H. K., and Murphy, A. J.: Acidosis during thoracic surgery, J Thorac Surg, 1950, 19, 50-70.

How To Delay Progress Without Even Trying

It's difficult to identify the "who, when, and where" of advances in medicine and surgery because it's a rare advance indeed (such as the use of digitalis by William Withering) that can be clearly related to the astuteness of one person at one time and place. It's a bit easier to identify the "who, when, and where" of some *delays* in progress along a frontier in medical science. To become a "who" who *held up* the advance of science, one must meet certain criteria. These include: (*1*) The scientist or clinician must be a highly respected "eminent authority" or "geheimrat" in some field; (*2*) he must have strong convictions; (*3*) he must not hesitate to utter these forcibly in his writing, lecturing, or both; (*4*) he must in *this* instance be *wrong,* although he surely doesn't recognize his error; and (*5*) no one dares to challenge him. Let me give you a few examples of some "whos" who have met these criteria.

Thoracic Surgery

I've already stated my belief that pulmonary surgery was held back for almost 90 years by the failure of surgeons and anesthetists to use simple, well-known, and effective ways of rhythmically ventilating lungs in an open thorax (1). I estimate that 20 to 25 of these 90 years of delay can be attributed to the convictions of an influential authoritarian surgical "geheimrat," Ferdinand Sauerbruch, who, beginning in 1904, performed his operations in an elaborate negative-pressure chamber and ignored the advice (even plea) of Rudolph Matas to use a simple device that inflated and deflated lungs rhythmically instead of producing constant inflation.

This was the same Professor Sauerbruch who later, in 1929-30, had as an intern a young surgeon named Werner Forssmann, who had just published a paper on right heart catheterization in man (for which he was to receive a Nobel Prize 27 years later). Let Forssmann (2) tell of his experiences with Sauerbruch:

> Every time I attempted to talk to the Old Man [about the work on right heart catheterization] I got the feeling that independent think-

ing was regarded as a dangerous threat. This applied not only to scientific questions but also to problems with patients. An extraordinary inflexibility of thought reigned over the department, a rigid dogma based upon the teachings of Sauerbruch. Any divergent opinions were considered heresy. . . . I often wondered why Sauerbruch's surgical department, in itself so excellent, produced so many dull and uninspired doctors. Later I found the answer in a biography of Peter the Great by the eighteenth-century Russian historian M. M. Sherbatov. "How could men remain virile and steadfast when in their youth they had trembled before the rod of their superiors and been praised only for servility?"

And later when Forssmann ventured to express to Sauerbruch the hope that he might qualify for a lectureship, Sauerbruch responded, "You might lecture in a circus about your little tricks, but never in a respectable German university." And when Forssmann protested quietly, Sauerbruch screamed, "Get out! Leave my department immediately." He did, and returned to Eberswalde where he had done his 1929 cardiac catheterization.

Treatment of Essential Hypertension

It is difficult to realize today, when supermarkets sell stethoscopes and manometers for measuring blood pressure and there is a vigorous national mission to reduce high blood pressure by use of antihypertensive drugs, that one hundred years ago physicians thought of high blood pressure only as part of Bright's (kidney) disease. It was not until 1905 that physicians could actually *measure* blood pressure and even in the 1930s were fearful of lowering a patient's high blood pressure because of the belief that it was compensatory and therefore required to force adequate amounts of blood through the kidneys and probably other vital organs. It was not until the 1950s and 1960s that epidemiologic studies, particularly those at Framingham, Massachusetts, supported by the National Heart Institute, convinced physicians that untreated essential hypertension, even though moderate or mild, shortened life and that high blood pressure demanded vigorous, continuing treatment.

What held back treatment of essential hypertension? One obvious "what" was that there was no noninvasive, clinical method for measuring systolic and diastolic blood pressure until 1905. That meant that until then it was impossible to learn anything about the effect of very high, high, or moderately high blood pressure on the life span of man. But even when it was apparent that malignant hypertension was a serious, life-threatening disease, physicians doubted the wisdom of lowering high blood pressure. Why? Largely, according to Irvine Page, because of Ludwig Traube, who in 1856 formulated the concept that patients with hypertension *needed* high blood pressure for survival—that it was *essential* to overcome high resistance in narrowed renal arterioles and so maintain excretion of urine (3). He believed it important for the patient's survival that his left ventricle should hypertrophy and maintain a high arterial pressure. Cohnheim, the great German pathologist, promoted Traube's concept.

It was a courageous team (Dr. Rowntree and Dr. Adson and their patient, "a 33 year old, 185 pound man with a blood pressure of 230/130") that showed in 1925 that surgical sympathectomy lowered the patient's blood pressure and he, *mirabile dictu,* instead of dying, actually improved.* A year later, Reid found that lowering blood pressure in hypertensive patients did not impair renal function, and in 1934 Page legitimized deliberate lowering of blood pressure in patients with malignant hypertension when, using the then-new technic of urea clearance, he found well-maintained renal function despite a lower blood pressure. And so 78 years after Traube's dictum was published, the *treatment* of hypertension became *essential,* rather than the *disease.*

Poliomyelitis

In May 1909, Landsteiner and Popper (4) obtained portions of the spinal cord of two patients who had died of poliomyelitis, and injected some of this tissue into the peritoneal cavities of monkeys. One developed paralysis of its lower limbs and died on the sixth day after inoculation; both monkeys, at autopsy, had

---

*I go against established surgical custom by applying the adjective "courageous" to the *patient* as well as to his physicians; see pp. 131-135.

spinal cord lesions similar to those of patients with poliomyelitis.

Until that time, the cause of the disease was unknown. There had been an epidemic of poliomyelitis along the Atlantic seaboard in 1907 and Simon Flexner, director of the new Rockefeller Institute for Medical Research, began intensive research on the cause of the disease and of its epidemic nature. In 1907 he had attempted to transfer the disease by introducing cerebrospinal fluid from patients into the spinal canal and peritoneal cavity of lower animals; he failed. However, in 1909 he succeeded and reported, "The chart shows unmistakably that by employing the *intracranial* method of inoculation, it is possible to carry the virus of epidemic poliomyelitis successfully through a series of *monkeys.* It is highly probable that the transmission may be carried on indefinitely. . . . the outlook for securing a fuller understanding of this disease will be immeasurably improved" (italics added) (5). Indeed, not long thereafter (1911), Flexner issued a press release announcing that his staff had already discovered how to prevent the disease and a cure was just around the corner (6). Yet a safe and effective vaccine did not come for 40 years. Why?

Some workers in the field (6) believe that Flexner, one of the most respected and powerful scientists in America, held back scientific advance in poliomyelitis by insisting that (1) for experimental work, the human disease could be transferred only to monkeys, (2) poliovirus could grow only in nerve tissue, especially in the brain, and (3) the portal of entry of poliovirus was invariably the nasopharynx and that the virus traveled in or along nasopharyngeal nerves to reach the brain. Insistence on point (1) severely limited research on poliomyelitis to well-endowed institutions because monkeys were expensive and there was no National Institutes of Health to pay for them; insistence on point (2) made it difficult to grow poliovirus in quantities needed to produce vaccines; insistence on point (3) precluded work on an oral vaccine of either killed or attenuated poliovirus. As pointed out by Professor Gard in presenting the Nobel Prize for 1954 (7), "Of all tissues, nerve tissue is the most specialized, the most exacting and consequently the most difficult to cultivate. As there seemed to be no alternative to the use of human brain tissue, the general resignation is easily understood."

In the late 1930s and throughout the 1940s,

dogma began to crumble. Armstrong showed that polio could be produced experimentally in the cotton rat; Trask, Vignec, and Paul found poliovirus in the stools of polio patients; Burnet and Jackson showed that the virus entered the body of cynomolgus monkeys after *oral* administration; Sabin, and Howe and Bodian, established the gastrointestinal tract as a portal of entry; and Horstmann found poliovirus in circulating *blood* after giving the virus *orally* to monkeys. Finally, Enders, Weller, and Robbins showed in 1949 that poliovirus could indeed be grown in non-neural tissue; in the same year Bodian, Morgan, and Howe learned that only three (and not fourteen) basic immunologic types of poliovirus were needed for immunization. A safe and effective polio vaccine was *then* right around the corner—even an oral vaccine.

Penicillin

On first thought, it seems unfair, in the case of penicillin, even to consider that one or more scientists held back the advance of medical science, since Fleming published his laboratory discovery in 1929 and Chain, Florey, and associates described the remarkable chemotherapeutic effects of penicillin in experimentally infected mice in 1940 and in therapeutic trials in patients a year later. In 1945, all three won the Nobel Prize in Physiology or Medicine. Yet Fleming, in his 1929 paper (8), was curiously unenthusiastic about his work. He did say that penicillin "appears to have some advantages over the well-known chemical *antiseptics* . . . a more powerful inhibitory agent than is carbolic acid and it can be applied to an infected *surface* undiluted, as it is non-irritant and non-toxic" (italics added) and "penicillin is certainly useful to the bacteriologist for its power of inhibiting unwanted microbes in bacterial cultures." And it is baffling that although he found that "penicillin is non-toxic to animals in enormous doses . . . it does not interfere with leucocyte function to a greater degree than does ordinary broth," he never infected a mouse with penicillin-sensitive microorganisms to determine whether his nontoxic penicillin, administered systemically, could save the life of the mouse—an experiment easy to do and one that would have required no more than a few hours of his time.

Why? Ernst Chain, co-winner of this Nobel Prize, in 1971 commented in retrospect on Fleming's 1929 work (9):

I have mentioned that Fleming had injected 0.5 ml of the penicillin-containing culture fluid into mice without any toxic effects. His culture fluid must have contained at least 1-2 units of penicillin per millilitre. It has always amazed me that Fleming did not carry out exactly the same experiment on mice infected with streptococci. No chemical knowledge was required for such an experiment. Had he done this, he would certainly have got *some* chemotherapeutic effect though, maybe, not so striking as the one which we obtained with the more purified preparation. It would have been impressive enough, however, to stimulate chemists into action to get the active principle in a purified form, which actually was not a very difficult operation, and in this they would undoubtedly have succeeded with the result that humanity would have had penicillin at its disposal ten years earlier than it did. The reason why Fleming did not even attempt to carry out this simple experiment, is, in my opinion, that the whole atmosphere in the Institute where he worked, the Inoculation Department of St. Mary's Hospital, was not conducive to this approach; it was, in fact, positively unsympathetic to experiments of this kind. The Director and Head of the Inoculation Department was Sir Almroth Wright, who believed that antibacterial therapy could only be based on immunological techniques, and any attempt to use chemicals was doomed to failure, as all the available experience had shown that they would be more harmful to the host than to the invading bacteria. "Stimulate the phagocytes" was his motto and dogma (he was the model for the doctor [Sir Colenso Ridgeon] in George Bernard Shaw's play *The Doctor's Dilemma*), and he would not readily admit any other view. Fleming was his pupil and junior collaborator, and became himself a strong advocate of immunotherapy and was openly sceptical about the potentialities of chemotherapy. . . . it was, after all, six years before the discovery of prontosil and the sulphonamides. [However, it was some years *after* Ehrlich's synthesis of "606" (Salvarsan or arsphenamine), effective against spirochetes without killing their human host, and *after* the successful use of "Bayer 205" (suramin), which killed trypanosomes, again leaving the host alive—*my note*.]

Despite Leonard Colebrook's defense of Almroth Wright (10), Wright does emerge as "the villain of the piece" (to use Hare's expression [11]). Sir Almroth Wright was an eminent and outspoken experimental pathologist at St. Mary's Hospital who passionately believed that bacterial infections could be conquered only by stimulating the body's natural defense mechanisms and that chemotherapy potent enough to be toxic to bacteria in the host must also be toxic to the host. Wright *almost* used citrate as an anticoagulant for indirect blood transfusions in 1894 but didn't. He was *almost* the first to vaccinate man against typhoid fever, but he was second. His laboratory was *almost* the first to discover the first chemotherapeutic agent against bacteria (6 to 7 years before sulfanilamide) but he wasn't interested in penicillin. Although knighted Sir Almroth Wright, some preferred to call him "Sir Almost Right." In fairness to Wright, Ernst Chain was sure that Wright did not *prevent* Fleming from carrying out chemotherapeutic experiments at St. Mary's. As Chain put it (9):

> However, despite the generally unsympathetic attitude to the possibilities of antibacterial chemotherapy which prevailed in the twenties at the Inoculation Department of St. Mary's Hospital, no one in that Department, and least of all Almroth Wright, would have prevented Fleming from carrying out the simple experiment of injecting the crude penicillin-containing culture medium into a mouse infected with a penicillin-sensitive bacterium if he had wanted to. He did not perform it because he did not think that it was worthwhile trying. I mention this aspect of the history of the penicillin discovery as a good example of how preconceived ideas in science can stifle imagination and impede progress; there exist many others of the same type. It is always dangerous when any generally accepted theories or any kind of central dogmas are taken too seriously.

Sir Henry Dale, in his obituary on Fleming, said (12):

> Neither the time when the discovery was made, nor, perhaps, the scientific atmosphere of the laboratory in which he worked, was propitious to such further enterprise as its development would have needed. Repeated failure had caused opinion then to harden, almost into a settled conviction, against the possibility of a successful chemotherapy of the common bacterial infections. Sir Almroth Wright himself had no belief in such a possibility.

Discovery of Oxygen

It's hard to believe that before 1776, there was neither an American Declaration of Independence nor oxygen. Mayow almost discovered oxygen in 1674. He demonstrated that only *part* of air was necessary for life and that part was re-

moved both by respiration and by fire (combustion). This part he called "nitro-aerial spirits." He enclosed an animal and a lighted lamp in a vessel (fortunately, over water that absorbed CO_2) so arranged that air could not enter. The lamp died first (because, as Mayow pointed out, it exhausted the particles immediately around the flame); the mouse died a little later (later, because its breathing brought in particles from a distance). He stated that gills of fish function as lungs and fish survive in water only because it contains nitro-aerial spirits. (He observed that fish cannot live in boiled water since boiling removes the vital substance.) However, he did not realize that the vital substance was a gas that could be isolated.

No one followed up on Mayow's work. Instead, along came Georg Ernst Stahl, physician to the King of Prussia from 1716 to 1734, and his "upside-down" phlogiston theory of combustion. It's hard to explain this "almost-right" theory in a paragraph but it's something like this: All combustible materials contain something that, on heating, is transformed into fire; this "something," since it becomes fire, he named "phlogiston." Combustible materials consisted of a calx or ash combined with phlogiston (which escaped during burning, leaving the ash behind). Fire died out in closed spaces because when air became saturated with phlogiston, no more could leave the combustible material. There was a serious problem with the phlogiston theory: metals when heated gained weight; they then lost weight when converted by charcoal back to metal. Stahl explained away this matter of weight *gain* (when phlogiston was supposed to *leave*) by attributing negative weight to phlogiston (giving it a tendency to float upward).

The discovery of oxygen came 100 years after Mayow's observations. On August 1, 1774, Joseph Priestley, using a 12-inch "burning glass" facing the summer sun, heated mercuric oxide and so released a gas. The chemical equation, as we know it, was:

$$2 \text{ Hg} + \text{O}_2 \text{ (air)} \xrightarrow{+ \text{ heat}} 2 \text{ HgO}$$

$$2 \text{ HgO} \xrightarrow{+ \text{ intense heat}} 2 \text{ Hg} + \text{O}_2$$

This he reported to the Royal Society in March 1775. On March 8, 1775, he exposed a mouse to gas he had released from mercuric oxide and found the gas "was much better than common air." Priestley was the first man to breathe O_2, the first to note the beauty and vivacity of a flame in O_2, the first to suggest the use of O_2 and flame to melt platinum and to suggest the use of O_2 in exploding gun powder.

But he didn't really know that he discovered oxygen; he insisted to his death that he discovered "dephlogisticated air." Scheele, who independently discovered oxygen (probably in 1773, although he did not publish until 1777), was also an ardent phlogistonist and also completely entangled in Stahl's theory. And so the discovery of the real significance of oxygen was delayed until 1776 when Lavoisier, completely free of previous dogma, realized its chemical nature and its role in combustion, named it oxygen, initiated the "Chemical Revolution" and ended the phlogiston era.

I'm fascinated by Priestley's own comments on his discovery of "dephlogisticated air." He said (13):

> When the decisive facts did at length obtrude themselves upon my notice, it was very slowly, and with great hesitation, that I yielded to the evidence of my senses. And yet, when I reconsider the matter, and compare my last discoveries relating to the constitution of the atmosphere with the first, I see the closest and the easiest connexion in the world between them, so as to wonder that I should not have been led immediately from the one to the other. That this was not the case, I attribute to the force of prejudice, which, unknown to ourselves, biasses not only our *judgments*, properly so called, but even the perceptions of our senses: for we may take a maxim so strongly for granted, that the plainest evidence of sense will not intirely [sic] change, and often hardly modify our persuasions; and the more ingenious a man is, the more effectually he is entangled in his errors; his ingenuity only helping him to deceive himself, by evading the force of truth.

Here is Priestley, himself hopelessly entangled in an incorrect theory—the phlogiston concept—warning others to stick to the evidence and not give in to their prejudices! Claude Bernard, 100 years later, wrote, "It is the things we *do* know that are the great hindrance to our learning the things that we do *not*."

Cardiac Surgery

Aristotle (ca. 350 B.C.) wrote, "The heart alone of all viscera cannot withstand injury." I suspect that Aristotle's views prevailed until the nineteenth century, because even after the discovery of ether and nitrous oxide and the attack by surgeons on many organs, none touched the heart. As late as 1883, Billroth, Europe's greatest surgeon, still respected Aristotle when he stated: "A surgeon who tries to suture the heart deserves to lose the esteem of his colleagues" (14). No one challenged Billroth until 1897 when Ludwig Rehn sutured a knife wound in a man's heart and the patient survived. A few years later, a surgeon in Alabama again challenged Billroth and sewed up a stab wound in the heart of a 13-year-old boy; the surgeon's name was Dr. Luther L. Hill, who, having studied abroad under Lord Lister, quite naturally named his son Lister Hill (later the U.S. Senate's staunchest supporter of the National Institutes of Health, including the National Heart Institute).

Mackenzie, England's great cardiologist, gets the credit for holding back surgical repair of damaged heart valves because of his strong conviction that one need not worry about the state of the valves as long as the heart muscle is healthy. In 1902 Brunton suggested slitting open fused mitral valve leaflets, and in 1925 Souttar, in London, actually performed an operation on the mitral valve. But after Souttar successfully dilated the stenotic valve by pushing his finger through the orifice, he never did a second operation. Why? Souttar wrote, "It was an article of faith with physicians that the valves were of no importance and that the only thing that mattered was the condition of the heart muscle. In that atmosphere I was unable to obtain another case in spite of this one complete success." Such was Mackenzie's influence in the field of cardiology! John McMichael recalls (15):

> I was present at a discussion meeting of the American Heart Association in 1948 on the rival mitral valvotomies of Harken and Bailey. Dr. Sam Levine recounted how he had written to James Mackenzie to tell him about Elliot Cutler's first effort to open up a stenosed mitral valve in 1923: he read from a letter from Mackenzie: "Dear Sam, What a foolish thing to try to do. Have you forgotten that the myocardium is all-important?"

Measurement of Cardiac Output in Man

Arthur Grollman, the great authority on measurement of cardiac output, held back for a decade the use of indicator dilution technics and the direct Fick method because of supreme confidence in his own acetylene method. In his book *The Cardiac Output of Man in Health and Disease*, Grollman stated unequivocally

(16): "Because of its obvious superiority, this gas has displaced other foreign gases for determining the cardiac output. . . . The only criticism that can be levelled against acetylene as a gas for determining cardiac output is its taste. . . . on repeated use, this initial distaste . . . gives way to one of pleasure."

He then demolished the dye dilution technic by pronouncing: "Its underlying assumptions are so complex as to render the results quite questionable. . . . The required arterial punctures and the injection of a foreign substance into the blood stream would in themselves render the injection method undesirable and it is unlikely, therefore, that it will find any wide application to cardiac output studies." When cardiologists began to catheterize the right heart of man, they soon got around to measuring cardiac output by both the direct Fick method and the acetylene method; the latter, found to give values far too low, went to its grave.

CONCLUDING REMARKS

In my opening paragraph, I gave my formula for "How to delay progress without even trying." Fortunately, all five components must be in the recipe or it won't work. It's going to be very hard to eliminate the first four components from our biomedical research family. The hope for the future lies in eliminating the last of the five.

References

1. This volume, Inflation — 1904 model, pp. 110-113.
2. Forssmann, W.: Experiments on Myself. Memoirs of a Surgeon in Germany, Droste, Dusseldorf, 1972 (English edition, St. Martin's Press, New York, 1974).
3. Traube, L.: Ueber den Zusammenhang von Herz und Nierenkrankheiten, Hirschwald, Berlin, 1856.
4. Landsteiner, K., and Popper, E.: Uebertragung der Poliomyelitis acuta auf Affen, Z Immunitätsforsch Exp Ther, 1909, 2, 377-390.
5. Flexner, S., and Lewis, P. A.: The transmission of acute poliomyelitis to monkeys, JAMA, 1909, 53, 1639.
6. Paul, J. R.: A History of Poliomyelitis, Yale University Press, New Haven, 1971.
7. Gard, S.: Presentation speech for 1954 Nobel Award. Nobel Lectures, Physiology or Medicine, 1942-1962, Elsevier, Amsterdam, 1964, pp. 443-447.
8. Fleming, A.: On the antibacterial action of cultures of a penicillium, with special reference to their use in the isolation of B. influenzae, Br J Exp Pathol, 1929, 10, 226-236.
9. Chain, E.: Thirty years of penicillin therapy, Proc R Soc Lond [Biol], 1971, 179, 293-319.
10. Colebrook, L.: Almroth Wright, Provocative Doctor and Thinker, Heinemann, London, 1954.
11. Hare, R.: The Birth of Penicillin and the Disarming of Microbes, Allen and Unwin, London, 1970.
12. Dale, H. H.: in Obituary. Sir Alexander Fleming, Br Med J, 1955, 1, 732-735.
13. Priestley, J.: Experiments and Observations on Different Kinds of Air, vol. II, Johnson, London, 1775.
14. Billroth, T.: Quoted in Jeger, E.: Die Chirurgie der Blutgefässe und des Herzens, Hirschwald, Berlin, 1913, p. 295.
15. McMichael, J.: A Transition in Cardiology: The Mackenzie-Lewis Era, Royal College of Physicians, London, 1976.
16. Grollman, A.: The Cardiac Output of Man in Health and Disease, Charles C Thomas, Springfield, 1932.

The Clouded Crystal Ball

In "How to delay progress . . ." (1), I suggested one pretty dependable way for a scientist to hold back progress — to be highly respected, authoritative, articulate, internationally famous, and, in his *current* views, hypothesis, prediction, or suggestion, *to be wrong*. I gave a few classic "for instances" of scientists who achieved this combination and the consequences of their "achievement." I'm sure I shocked some readers by suggesting that even the best of scientists or clinicians can, once in a while, be wrong. Everyone knows that statesmen, presidents, kings, generals, admirals, economists, critics of music, art, literature, and theater, sociologists, judges (even of the Supreme Court), FBI, and CIA occasionally make mistakes whose consequences range from modest to catastrophic. But over the past few years, public opinion polls have consistently placed research scientists way at the top of the list of professions rated on their integrity and the public's respect, trust, and esteem for them.

I surely don't want to reduce the public's confidence in scientists to a lower level, such as that accorded to Supreme Court Justices or Congressmen or Presidents, but it *is* important to scientists, to the public, and to their Congressmen to learn whether even eminent scientists may occasionally be wrong—not deliberately or maliciously—but in their estimate or conviction of where the "big pay-off" will be in science.

In the good old days, it didn't affect other scientists (and their work) very much if one scientist tried to be clairvoyant but wasn't, because each scientist was free to ignore or follow up the prediction or advice of another. Times have changed, and with change has come greater probability that predictions on where to put the public's money will do good or harm or both. When Congress set up Institute after Institute in the NIH (presumably with advice from scientists), it changed priorities for research for any scientist who needed NIH support for his work. When, again with advice from scientists, Congress greatly increased the budgets of one or two

Institutes and decreased the research buying power of other Institutes, it again re-ordered national priorities. Whenever Congress earmarked any part of its appropriation for a specific project, it again re-ordered priorities. When one of the Institutes assigned more of its money for contract-supported or commission-directed or panel-recommended research, it again re-ordered the pattern of biomedical research.

For good, for bad, for both? No one knows. For a several-billion-dollar organization operated by scientist-administrators, with the advice of working scientists, and for the over-all advance of science, it is remarkable that the NIH does little or no continuing research on the effectiveness of new ways of setting priorities in achieving its goals. The data on clairvoyance in science are all in their files—from the day of the first NIH research contract and the first commissioned-mandated research program to today. How much money was awarded to each? for what? on what time schedule? on or against whose advice? How many have or have not made it to the finish line? What exciting new ideas, concepts, diagnostic technics, and cures have come from these new ways of supporting research? How many have made it to Stockholm and the Nobel Prize? Is the huge cancer research program on schedule?

Until someone objectively analyzes recent performances in the art of clairvoyance, it seems worthwhile to look into the Retrospectroscope and see whether eminent scientists have ever been wrong in their predictions of what's going to be terribly important or utterly worthless.

SOME PREDICTIONS IN BIOMEDICAL SCIENCE

On Poliomyelitis Vaccine

Simon Flexner, Director of the Rockefeller Institute for Medical Research, was quoted in an article in the *New York Times* in 1911, which said (2):

The Rockefeller Institute ... believes that its search for a cure for infantile paralysis is about to be rewarded. Within six months, according to Dr. Simon Flexner, definite announcement of a specific remedy may be expected. "We have already discovered how to prevent the disease," says Dr. Flexner, "and the achievement of a cure, I may conservatively say, is not now far distant. ... We have learned where it [the germ] resides, how the disease is spread, how the germ enters the body, the main sources of infection and the means of combatting the disease."

Sir Macfarlane Burnet (Nobel Laureate 1960) wrote in 1949 (3):

The natural way to prevent paralytic poliomyelitis is to ensure that infants are repeatedly infected with strains of virus of low paralytic potentialities. ... In a present day community, any use of living virus for immunization would be unthinkable. ... A killed virus is a theoretical possibility, ... but there is in sight no solution of the practical difficulties of producing it. Until someone can find a means of producing relatively large amounts of pure or nearly pure virus free of foreign nervous tissue, even experimental immunization of children would be absolutely unjustifiable. I can see no hope at present of such a vaccine being produced. ... I have adopted a frankly defeatist attitude toward the problem of poliomyelitis and I hope that future developments will prove me wrong. ... No means of controlling poliomyelitis is at present visible.

If only these two predictions had been switched in time—if Burnet's 1949 words had been spoken by Flexner in 1911 and vice versa—both predictions would have been correct, for it was in 1949 that Enders, Weller, and Robbins learned to grow large quantities of poliovirus in non-neural tissue. Successful polio vaccine came a few years later.

On Cardiovascular Diagnosis
In 1905 (the year that Korotkoff published his new noninvasive method for measuring both systolic *and* diastolic blood pressure, a method that at last permitted objective study of the natural course of hypertension and of methods to treat it) the *British Medical Journal,* official organ of the British Medical Association, argued that by sphygmomanometry "we pauperize our senses and weaken clinical acuity" (4).

James Mackenzie, England's great cardiologist, was antagonistic toward both the use of X-rays and the electrocardiogram because he was convinced that such aids would "blunt the senses and the acute perception of the clinical observer" (5).

The senior cardiologists of Great Britain strongly opposed and censured McMichael and Sharpey-Schafer in their pioneer efforts to use cardiac catheterization as a diagnostic tool (6). Nevertheless, by April 1945, the two had performed 353 cardiac catheterizations in humans without complications, apart from local venous thrombosis, and proved that all dire predictions of disaster were unwarranted.

On Cardiac Surgery
Sir Stephen Paget, author of the authoritative text, *The Surgery of the Chest,* predicted in 1896 (7):

Surgery of the heart has probably reached the limits set by Nature to all surgery: no new method and no new discovery can overcome the natural difficulties that attend a wound of the heart. It is true that heart suture has been vaguely proposed as a possible procedure, and that it has been done on animals, but I cannot find that it has ever been attempted in practice.

On September 9 of that same year, Ludwig Rehn of Frankfurt performed the first successful suture of a human heart wound! A little later, Samways (1898), Brunton (1902), and Carrel (1912) all proposed methods to open the narrowed valve in patients with mitral stenosis. Sir Lauder Brunton (8) suggested that, before attempting this in man, surgeons should perform experiments on animals to develop a suitable technique. He himself obtained the necessary license and certificates for animal investigation and did a few preliminary experiments. However, his limited time prevented him from carrying on, and he decided to try to stimulate interest of fellow surgeons in continuing the work. His brief communication to the *Lancet* was followed the next week by an editorial in the same journal castigating him for suggesting such a highly dangerous procedure that might actually make a patient worse, even if he survived the operation.

Little more was done about the mitral valve until Cutler and Levine (1923) and Souttar (1925); each report dealt with one patient. After another long hiatus, Bailey performed a successful mitral commissurotomy in 1949, and surgery on cardiac valves began its spectacular journey.

Munro, in 1907, proposed ligating a patent ductus arteriosus, but as late as 1939, Robert

Gross's professor cautioned him against performing such an operation. Despite this advice, Gross was bold enough to ligate such an artery and overnight became the father of modern cardiac surgery. Yet shortly thereafter, when a pediatric cardiologist named Helen Taussig proposed to Gross that he perform an aortic-pulmonary artery shunt to relieve cyanosis in "blue babies" with a type of congenital heart disease known as tetralogy of Fallot, he turned her down. Gross's crystal ball was working only 50% of the time in 1940, but he was then America's leading cardiac surgeon and would certainly have been chairman of a 1940 NIH Committee to advise on cardiac surgery.

According to Medawar (9), Lord Moynihan, Britain's great surgeon, said in 1930, "Surgery as a craft has reached its peak" and, in 1932, "We can surely never hope to see the craft of surgery made much more perfect than it is today. We are at the end of a chapter." Medawar noted in 1975 that Moynihan remarked that operations could be carried out (in 1932) of a kind that even Lister would not have dreamed possible, but the thought never entered Moynihan's head that in the future, operations could be done that even he considered impossible in 1932. Medawar commented that Moynihan was a very great surgeon and a man of very great gifts, but these did not include clairvoyance!

John Gibbon, who spent 19 years bringing the pump-oxygenator (artificial heart lung) from a "mission impossible" idea to a practical device now essential for much of modern cardiac surgery, was fortunate enough to get laboratory space in which to work and funds for technical help, first at the Massachusetts General Hospital and then at the University of Pennsylvania. But Gibbon recalls that "Churchill [in Boston] was not enthusiastic about my project but raised no objection to my pursuit of my goal. Still less enthusiastic was my friend, Walter Bauer.... Eugene Landis was my only medical friend who did not discourage me ... he said that if I thought I could succeed, it was worth giving it a try" (10). Landis recalls encouraging Gibbon, all the while thinking (silently, thank heavens), "what a long, hard, impossible road to choose" (11).

When Gibbon worked in Ravdin's Department of Surgical Research at Penn (1936 to 1942), I was an instructor in Pharmacology working on the floor below Jack and Mary Gibbon. I know that they were well liked and also respected for their intense dedication to their project, but I don't recall any faculty member, old or young, who had much interest in it or expectation that anything would come of it. I can't think of any Presidential Advisory Panel, appointed in 1936 to 1942, that would have recommended "full speed ahead" on Gibbon's work.

On the Discovery of Insulin

Many scientists in the 30 years preceding 1921 tried to learn the function of the islets of Langerhans in the pancreas. So it is not remarkable that when a young small town surgeon, Frederick Banting, who had done *no* research (let alone research in the baffling field of endocrinology-metabolism) had an idea and took it to J. J. R. Macleod (Professor of Physiology at the University of Toronto, Canada's scientific leader in this field), Macleod did not roll out the red carpet. It appears that Macleod in fact did his best to discourage Banting. What did Banting know about the anatomy, histology, and physiology of the pancreas, about the chemistry of blood sugar, about clinical diabetes, and what could Banting hope to accomplish that highly trained physiologists had not succeeded in achieving, establishing, or proving? Banting replied that all he wanted was 10 dogs and an assistant for eight weeks. Macleod was about to go on vacation in Europe and against his better judgment provided Banting with 10 dogs and an assistant, Charles Best, who was a medical student. Banting started to work on May 16, 1921, and on July 27 (10 weeks later) administered the first crude preparation of insulin into a dying depancreatized dog. By early 1922, the purification and commercial preparation of insulin, and the saving of lives of dying diabetic patients, had become the full-time occupation of Banting, Best, Macleod, Collip (a chemist), and scores of others. In 1923 Banting and Macleod won the Nobel Prize.

Harry Eagle has stated that he has "more confidence in the collective judgment of 10,000 independent investigators than in that of 10 wise men sitting around a table" (12). In this case, Banting and Best were two of 10,000 scientists with special imagination, conviction, and determination, and Macleod was one of 10 wise men.

On Heparin

No one predicted an important use for heparin (discovered by McLean in 1916) until the 1940s. William Howell, McLean's professor, presented a Harvey Lecture in 1916–17; his only prediction with respect to the clinical importance of heparin was that hemophilia might be due to excessive amounts of heparin in circulating blood (13). It is surprising that he did not suggest that heparin be purified and used to replace hirudin in the artificial kidney (vividiffusion) reported by Abel, Rowntree, and Turner in 1913 and 1914; the best explanation is that no one in 1916 predicted any clinical use of the artificial kidney!

Best, co-discoverer of insulin in 1921, put Charles and Scott to work in 1933 to prepare pure heparin for laboratory use. Best also gave a Harvey Lecture on heparin; this one was in 1940 (14) after the Toronto group had pioneered in the clinical use of heparin. Best did "hope that some day the technique [of exchange transfusions] may be perfected by which kidneys or perhaps some other organ of normal subjects may be made available, as it were, to patients in whom there is a serious *but presumably transient* deficiency in some physiological function." He also said that "heparin is a valuable adjuvant in certain types of vascular surgery ... on the substitution of veins for arteries in certain cases of arterial aneurysm, the removal of emboli, ... and the repair of severed arteries." He also suggested carefully controlled clinical studies of the value of heparin in treating patients with coronary artery thrombosis.

Best, in 1940, was both cautious and accurate in most of his predictions, and from his association with Murray's surgical group in Toronto made some that didn't occur to Howell in 1916. But Best still did not predict one major use of heparin—as an anticoagulant for pump-oxygenators—although Gibbon had been at work on his artificial heart-lung for six years and had published papers in 1937 and 1939 mentioning his use of heparin.

On the Artificial, Implanted Heart

In mid-1964, one of America's most eminent scientists wrote to the Director of the National Heart Institute:

For sometime I have been puzzling why an artificial heart has not yet been made available as a fruit of our technological developments. . . . I believe the problem is technically difficult but easily manageable within the framework of our present scientific knowledge and technical proficiency. We have however permitted it to remain a subject of fragmentary scientific studies rather than of a unified engineering program. We do ourselves a great disservice to neglect the opportunity of a systems response to what is now a well-defined technical problem, which is so much a matter of engineering design, material development and empiric testing and should not be confused with the basic research that was needed at its foundation.

The NHI had indeed been supporting research and development on the artificial heart, but following this "we know all we need to know; it's time to apply it" letter from a Nobel Laureate, the National Heart Institute drew up a master plan for a systems approach to the artificial heart that called for the signing of contracts by July 1, 1965 and implantation of artificial hearts in patients by February 14, 1970. It asked for Congressional appropriations of $270,000 for fiscal year 1965, about $8,000,000 for 1966, and a little more than $100,000,000 in 1967—in true "moon shot" style.

By mid-1976, a clinical practical device was still not on the horizon and the NHI (now the NHLBI) had long since decided to emphasize support of short-term ventricular-assist devices rather than the more dramatic implanted plutonium-powered mechanical heart. Why? Some may say, "because Congress never appropriated the 'moon shot' type of money for an all-out systems approach for the plastic heart." Could it have been because we really did *not* know all we needed to know and that we needed more than a group of engineers to glue the parts together?

On the Management of Infection

Oliver Wendell Holmes, Professor of Anatomy and Physiology at Harvard Medical School, presented evidence in 1843 that childbed fever was contagious and was frequently carried from patient to patient by physicians and nurses. He was attacked by C. L. Meigs, Professor of Midwifery at Jefferson Medical College in Philadelphia and by Hodge, Professor of Obstetrics at the University of Pennsylvania:

Hodge begged his students to divest their minds of the dread that they could ever carry the dreadful virus. Meigs scorned Holmes's deductions as characteristic of the "jejune and fizzenless vaporings of sophomore writers" and added that he preferred to attribute the deaths to "accident, or providence, of which I can form a conception, rather than to a contagion of which I cannot form any clear idea, at least as to this particular malady." (See 15, 16)

Undoubtedly, Holmes had antagonized mem-

124

bers of the medical profession by suggesting that they were carriers of death, and his scientific observations further drew scorn because he was "a sophomore writer."

In 1847, Ignaz Semmelweiss of Vienna independently proposed that childbirth fever was contagious. He stated that it was carried to women in the city's obstetrical wards by "cadaveric material" on the hands of physicians and students coming directly from the postmortem room to the delivery room. He instituted a strict routine that all hands about to touch patients must first be thoroughly washed in a solution of chlorinated lime. Mortality from puerperal sepsis fell at once from 12 to 3 per cent and later to one per cent. But his revolutionary doctrine, like that of Holmes, incriminated obstetricians as the carriers of disease and death and aroused fierce opposition from medical authorities, including the great pathologist, Virchow (16). Semmelweiss, ostracized, denounced and ridiculed, died 18 years later in an insane asylum. If there had been a Viennese Imperial task force on puerperal sepsis, would it have given Semmelweiss a chance to prove his theory?

Lord Lister's acceptance of Pasteur's germ theory of disease and his vigorous attempts to achieve antisepsis in surgical operating rooms met with fierce opposition partly by hospital administrators who saw the reputations of their hospitals being destroyed, and partly by physicians who still disbelieved the germ theory of infection. It is interesting that one physician most influential in disparaging Lister was James Simpson, who, when he introduced chloroform into obstetrics and surgery only a few years earlier, was denounced by the clergy, both from the pulpit and in pamphlets, on the grounds that anesthetics were decoys of Satan (see 17). Apparently, being attacked without reason does not deter one from attacking another without reason!

In 1938, the Medical Research Council of England turned down Ernst Chain's request for very modest support of his research project on the chemical and biochemical properties of antibacterial substances produced by microorganisms (now known as *antibiotics*), which a few years later (with support from the Rockefeller Foundation) led to the purification of penicillin and a Nobel Prize; Medawar (9) recalls Lord Florey's telling him that wise old gray heads in England shook (or wobbled) regretfully from side to side, pronouncing that the future of antibacterial therapy lay not with extracts of fungi and other medieval-sounding concoctions but with synthetic organic chemicals of which sulfanilamide was the paradigm. We must flunk the MRC of England in clairvoyance on this decision; fortunate indeed that not *all* funds are controlled by one agency with one set of advisers!

SOME PREDICTIONS IN OTHER SCIENCES

Any scientist—not only biomedical scientists—can have a clouded crystal ball. Neils Bohr, Danish atomic physicist and Nobel Laureate, is reported to have said, "It is very difficult to predict—especially the future"; Mark Twain remarked that "the man with a new idea is a crank until the idea succeeds"; and Peter Medawar entitled one of his articles "Some Follies of Prediction."

Francis Bacon could not believe that the earth goes around the sun; Galileo could not accept Kepler's evidence that planets move in ellipses; Maxwell in 1879 said, "Atoms . . . continue to this day as they were created, perfect in number, measure and weight"; Pasteur at the height of his fame stated that scientific methods could never be applied successfully to the study of emotions (at a time when Pavlov and Cannon were waiting in the wings); Lord Kelvin, throughout a very distinguished life in science, never discarded the concept that the atom is an indivisible unit (18, 19).

In 1845, J. J. Waterston submitted a paper on the molecular theory of gases to the Proceedings of the Royal Society. Although Waterston's work anticipated much of the later work of Joule, Clausius, and Maxwell, the referee entrusted with evaluating the manuscript said, "This paper is nothing but nonsense." The paper lay in oblivion until rediscovered 45 years later. According to Trotter (20), after the rejection Waterston lived on disappointed and obscure for many years and then disappeared, leaving no sign.

Thomas Edison, one of the world's greatest and most prolific inventors (he had almost 1,300 patents in all), could not predict any practical use for his only discovery in "pure" science. It was the ability of electrons, under certain conditions, to travel unimpeded through a vacuum. This "Edison effect" later was used by J. A. Fleming to develop a "current rectifier" and that, in turn permitted Lee deForest to invent the first radio tube (see 21).

Western Union Telegraph Company and its experts looked into a very murky crystal ball at a young voice teacher named Alexander Graham Bell who devised a new-fangled gadget that he claimed could transmit the human voice (and not just dots and dashes) from one place to another through wires. In 1876 or 1877, he offered to sell all patents and rights to it to Western Union for $100,000. Western Union turned down the offer (22).

Western Union's blunder became such a classic that it inspired circulation of a number of reports of "Commissions" appointed to advise the company on the potential use of the telephone. One of these "reports" advised:

These fanciful predictions, while they sound very rosy, are based upon wild-eyed imagination and a lack of understanding of the technical and economic facts of the situation, and a posture of ignoring the obvious technical limitations of his device, which is hardly more than a toy, or a laboratory curiosity. Mr. A. G. Bell, the inventor, is a teacher of the hard-of-hearing, and this "Telephone" may be of some value for his work, but it has too many shortcomings to be seriously considered as a means of communication.

And William Orton, President of Western Union, is reputed to have said to Bell, "What use could this company make of an electrical toy?"

These stories cannot be substantiated by written records or correspondence and are no doubt apocryphal. However two facts remain: (1) The Western Union Telegraph Company *did* receive, consider and decline an offer to buy all of Bell's telephone patents in 1876-77 for $100,000. (2) AT&T today has assets in excess of $80 billion, Western Union slightly in excess of $1 billion.

Professor Simon Newcomb, famous American astronomer, professor of mathematics and astronomy at Johns Hopkins University and editor of the *American Journal of Mathematics,* said (23):

"Human flight is not only impossible but illogical." A new metal or a new force in nature would have to be discovered before man could fly. Even if by some miracle a man should invent a power-machine that could get off the ground, it would inevitably crash and kill its pilot. "Once he slackened his speed, down he begins to fall. Once he stops, he falls a dead mass."

His views were published in 1903. On December 17 of that year, Orville and Wilbur Wright made their first flight in a heavier-than-air plane, at Kitty Hawk, North Carolina.

Stern (24) points out that:

Most steel men knew that Henry Bessemer's ideas of making steel by blowing air through molten iron was absurd. Despite universal ridicule Bessemer built his own plant, and revolutionized steel making. The ridiculers are lost to history. William Siemens knew that his open-hearth process for making steel was fundamentally sound. No one else believed it until he had demonstrated its success in the steel plant he built himself. After the steel makers had all climbed on the wagon with him, many of them contended that they had thought of it first. Hadfield discovered that steels containing 13 per cent of manganese were strong, tough, and very desirable. He couldn't convince even his own father, a foundry owner, that this was true. Eventually, Hadfield's work led to the opening of the entire field of alloy steels. Not many years ago all electronic experts knew that chromium plating could never be practical—all but one or two. Millions of automobile bumpers show evidence of the experts' errors. Before 1908 it was known that it was impossible to make ductile tungsten wire, but in that year Dr. W. D. Coolidge, of the General Electric Laboratory, forced that tradition out of the window.

SUCCESS IN PREDICTING

Some decisions that involved large sums of money and changed the directions of many scientists have been very wise ones. The decision of the National Foundation for Infantile Paralysis to put much of its resources into basic studies in virology rather than into specific applied programs is credited with speeding the work of Enders and his associates and the development of a successful and safe polio vaccine. The scientific advice that led the United States into the Manhattan project and the atomic bomb was correct and greatly increased the respect of Congress and the Administration for scientific consultants. As Senator Tydings admitted to Dr. Leo Szilard in 1945 (25):

Doctor, if in 1939 we had been conducting a hearing like we are conducting today, and men like yourself had come before our committee and projected the possible development of the bomb up to now with reasonable accuracy, I imagine they would have been called a lot of crackpots and . . . visionaries who were playing with theories. I certainly would not have had the receptivity that I have today to say the least.

The decision in the early 1940s of the Committee on Medical Research of the Office of Scientific Research and Development to proceed

126

with a crash program for mass production of penicillin had far-reaching effects, and part of its success must be attributed to Roosevelt's decision to activate these advisory committees long before America entered World War II.

Many cooperative clinical trials, such as those for penicillin and antituberculosis drugs, were also highly successful. The decision of the Armed Forces Epidemiological Board to create a Streptococcus Disease Laboratory in 1948 resulted in the prophylactic treatment of acute rheumatic fever. It appears that special Task Forces, Panels, or Commissions can work very well when all the basic information is at hand, when the goal is clear cut, and when the time is ripe to wrap up a problem. They are less effective when the basic information is not at hand and one needs whole new ideas and concepts and methods for scientific advance.

No one has yet made a long-term, serious attempt to study the factors that make for successful predictions (26), although a recent Ciba conference, "The Future as an Academic Discipline," suggests the possibility that departments dealing with the Future may stand side by side with departments of History in the structure of universities (27).

CONCLUDING REMARKS

(1) This look into the Retrospectroscope makes no pretense at being a scientific, quantitative analysis of clairvoyance. But it does produce examples of prominent scientists who were sometimes deficient in this attribute—enough examples to justify a study of the fallibility or infallibility of scientists eminent enough to become advisers to Congress and institutes. Such a study is needed because leading scientists today control not only the direction that their own research takes, and maybe that of their immediate staff, but also the direction of research of many, perhaps the great majority, of biomedical scientists in the United States. How? Simply because Presidents, Congress, Institutes, and Foundations, eager to cure dread diseases as quickly as possible, have appointed Councils, Panels, Task Forces, Commissions, and Committees and asked the members of these to look into their crystal ball and find specific programs guaranteed to eliminate these diseases promptly. Quite often such panels recommend significant changes in federal research budgets that in effect decrease the free choice of scientists to do what they and

their peer review groups consider to be good science.

(2) Producing examples of errors in predicting the future requires naming names. Naming scientists was certainly not the prime purpose of this Retrospectroscope, nor was it intended to lessen the stature of the named scientists. Obviously, this look backward would have been pointless if it dealt only with unheard of, unsuccessful scientists. As my kindly old professor of surgery said repeatedly in his quiz sections with students, "Boys, everyone makes mistakes; that's why they always put erasers at the end of lead pencils." Science progresses by continuously revising, extending, or completely overturning existing "facts" to create new concepts that may become "facts" and in turn be revised or discarded; it rarely progresses by producing "breakthroughs" on demand.

(3) This look has concerned itself with official clairvoyance at the national (Congressional or NIH) level that can alter the flow of vast amounts of research funds and so direct many scientists into fewer and more restricted channels. It has not concerned itself with *speculation* that, I believe, should be an important part of every oral or written scientific presentation. Such speculation, in my view, *broadens* the choice of individual scientists who are exposed to it because they are quite free to ignore it, verify it, or demolish it.

References

1. This volume, How to delay progress without even trying, pp. 114-119.
2. New York Times, March 9, 1911, quoted by Paul, J. R.: A History of Poliomyelitis, Yale University Press, New Haven, 1971, p. 116.
3. Burnet, F. M.: Some aspects of the epidemiology of poliomyelitis, Proc R Australasian Coll Physicians, 1949, 4, 95–100.
4. British Medical Journal, 1905, quoted by Wakerlin, G. E.: From Bright toward light: The story of hypertension research, Circulation, 1962, 26, 1–6.
5. McMichael, J.: A Transition in Cardiology: The Mackenzie-Lewis Era. The Harveian Oration of 1975, Royal College of Physicians, London, 1976.
6. Cournand, A.: Cardiac catheterization, Acta Med Scand [Suppl], 1975, 579, 3–32.
7. Paget, S.: The Surgery of the Chest, J. Wright & Co., Bristol, 1896, p. 121.
8. Brunton, L.: Preliminary note on the possibility of treating mitral stenosis by surgical methods,

Lancet, 1902, *1*, 352.

9. Medawar, P. B.: Some follies of prediction, Hosp Practice, 1975, *10* (4), 73–74.

10. Gibbon, J. H., Jr.: The development of the heart-lung apparatus, Rev Surg, 1970, *27*, 231–244.

11. Landis, E. M.: Personal communication, October 17, 1970.

12. Eagle, H.: Minutes of the Committee on Science Policy for Medicine and Health, Institute of Medicine, National Academy of Sciences, Washington, D. C., June 22, 1973.

13. Howell, W. H.: The coagulation of the blood, Harvey Lect, 1916–17, *12*, 272–323.

14. Best, C. H.: Heparin and thrombosis, Harvey Lect, 1940–41, *36*, 66–90.

15. Cannon, W. B.: The Way of An Investigator. A Scientist's Experiences in Medical Research, Hafner, New York, 1968 (facsimile of 1945 edition).

16. Stern, B. J.: Historical Sociology. Selected Papers of Bernhard J. Stern, Citadel Press, New York, 1959, pp. 363–365.

17. *Ibid.*, p. 368.

18. Barber, B.: Resistance of scientists to scientific discovery, Science, 1961, *134*, 596–602.

19. Stevenson, I.: Scientists with half-closed minds, Harper's, November 1958, *217*, 67–71.

20. Trotter, W.: The Collected Papers of Wilfred Trotter, Oxford University Press, Humphrey Milford, London, 1941, p. 186.

21. Asimov, I.: Introduction. Of what use, in *The Greatest Adventure: Basic Research That Shapes Our Lives*, E. H. Kone and H. J. Jordan, ed., Rockefeller University Press, New York, 1974.

22. Bruce, R. V.: Bell. Alexander Graham Bell and the Conquest of Solitude, Boston, Little Brown, 1973, p. 229.

23. Untermeyer, L.: Makers of the Modern World. Wilbur Wright and Orville Wright. Simon and Schuster, New York, 1955, pp. 360–367.

24. Stern, p. 97 (see reference 16).

25. Atomic Energy: Hearings before the Special Committee on Atomic Energy, U. S. Senate, 79th Congress, 1st Session, U. S. Government Printing Office, Washington, D. C., 1945, p. 290.

26. Lilley, S.: Can prediction become a science?, Discovery, November 1946, pp. 336–340, reprinted in *The Sociology of Science*, B. Barber and W. Hirsch, ed., Free Press of Glencoe, New York, 1962, pp. 142–152.

27. The Future as an Academic Discipline, Ciba Foundation Symposium No. 36 (New Series), Elsevier, Amsterdam, 1975.

Who's Who in World History

A few nights ago I watched a rerun on television of one of Groucho Marx's quiz shows, "You Bet Your Life." Groucho's standard format is first to interview a pair of contestants, slyly insulting each in his inimitable way, and then giving them a chance to make a little money. All they must do is answer correctly four questions, in a category they themselves have selected. The first round of questions is pretty easy and most contestants win a few hundred dollars and so qualify for a chance at the big money, either $2,000, $5,000, or $10,000, depending on the turn of a wheel. Now the contestants must provide the right answer to a single but not-so-easy question. This time the question was, for me, elementary—"Who discovered penicillin?" The contestants hadn't the foggiest idea and left the stage without the big prize, and dejected.

I wondered and kept on wondering why they didn't know. Certainly the discovery of penicillin has resulted in saving more lives than most any other single event since the beginnings of history. I turned to the F's in an unabridged dictionary (1) to see if Fleming's name was there; it was indeed—"Sir Alexander, Scottish bacteriologist and physician; co-discoverer of penicillin, 1929." I then turned to the same dictionary's "Major Dates in World History," a special supplement of 21 oversize pages containing, in all, 1,770 entries. The first entry was 3200 B.C. (the first dynasty in Egypt) and the last was Pope Paul VI's ecumenical council at the Vatican in 1965.

I found the year 1929, when Fleming discovered penicillin. There were four entries for 1929: the reign of Zogu (King of Albania), the acceptance of the Young reparations plan by the Germans and the Allies, the crash of the New York Stock Market, and the inauguration of Herbert Hoover as President. The discovery of penicillin was not there. I wondered whether Roentgen's 1895 discovery of x-rays was a "major date in world history"; it was not, though the entries for 1895 included the Sino-Japanese War, the Dreyfus case, the reign of Nicholas II of Russia, and "Far Eastern Crises." Surely, I mused, Harvey's

discovery of the circulation of the blood must have made it. But although the year 1628 included the reign of Philip IV of Spain, the reign of Charles I of England, the signing of the Petition of Right by Charles I, and the chartering of the Massachusetts Bay Company, it did not include William Harvey.

I then thought that it would be interesting to see whether any of the 56 discoveries honored by Nobel prize awards in medicine or physiology between 1901 and 1965 (the dates of the first Nobel award and the compilation of Random House's list) were included in "Major Dates in World History." I didn't expect to find Crick, Watson, and Wilkins's discovery of the double helical structure of DNA (too esoteric) but I thought I might find von Behring (who discovered diphtheria antitoxin), or Ross (who found that malaria was transmitted by mosquitos), or Koch (who identified the tubercle bacillus as the cause of tuberculosis), or Banting and Macleod (who extracted insulin from the pancreas and initiated the treatment of diabetes), or Domagk (who inaugurated modern chemotherapy with the discovery of Prontosil®, forerunner of sulfanilamide), or Theiler (who prepared vaccines effective against yellow fever), or Enders, Weller, and Robbins (who made polio vaccine possible). No; none made the list. Neither did any pre-Nobel biomedical scientist such as Claude Bernard, Gregor Mendel, Louis Pasteur, Edward Jenner, or Charles Darwin.

With the single exception of the discovery of "blue galaxies" in 1960, physics, chemistry, astronomy, and mathematics also struck out—not a single line for Aristotle, Copernicus, Galileo, Kepler, Newton, Cavendish, Lavoisier, Volta, Dalton, Thomson, Hertz, Curie, Einstein, Bohr, or Lawrence, and not a single word about electricity, atomic structure, or radioactivity.

Engineering and invention fared better. Lucius Tarquinius Priscus (616-578 B.C.) made the list for building the "great sewer" (Cloaca Maxima). Prince Chen (259-210 B.C.) got in by standardizing weights and measures. The Tennessee Valley Authority (1933) is there, as is the use of pilotless jet missiles (1944), the dropping of the first atomic bomb (1945), the launching of Sputnik (1957), and the U-2 high altitude reconnaissance plane (1960). Indeed, the atomic bomb and its more powerful derivatives received 11 separate entries and space•vehicles racked up 15 (7 more than all of the earlier explorers of the then-unknown world—Ericson, Columbus, da Gama, Vespucci, de Leon, Drake, Raleigh, and Hudson). But invention and engineering completely ignored the printing press, the steam engine, the airplane, radio, television, and radar; it even skipped the whole Industrial Revolution.

Art? Music? Painting? Architecture? Literature? No—not even Homer or Leonardo or Shakespeare. Only three of the 1,770 entries mention a museum (Ptolemy's in Alexandria about 300 B.C.), a library (Pope Nicholas V's in the Vatican about 1450), or a book (the King James version of the Bible in 1611).

Law made it 5 times for legal, judicial, or constitutional reforms: Hammurabi, Babylon, eighteenth century B.C.; Solon, Greece, about 590 B.C.; Roman law, 451 B.C.; Magna Carta, 1215 A.D.; and systemization of English law, about 1280 A.D.

Social reform had 3 entries: prohibition of slavery in British colonies (1833), restrictions on child labor in England (1834), and Lincoln's Emancipation Proclamation (1863).

Because these account for only 50 of the 1,770 entries, I began to wonder "What *is* history? What were the other 1,720 entries?" I haven't categorized and tallied them but most of them deal with who ruled whom, when, and how; how rulers met their death or meted it out to others (beheading—old style, guillotine—modern style, assassination, poisoning, suicide); invasions, wars, battles, massacres, and the number of casualties; treaties and when they were broken; burning, sacking, razing, looting, inquisition, and excommunication. (This isn't much different from Ambrose Bierce's definition of history: "An account mostly false, of events mostly unimportant, which are brought about by rulers mostly knaves, and soldiers mostly fools." [2])

Back to Groucho Marx and "Who discovered penicillin?" If the Random House supplement is representative of modern teaching of world history, Groucho's contestants didn't really have a chance at their $10,000. *Is* it representative? I tracked down about 10 history texts now in use in our high schools and colleges and leafed

through them. Some, I'm glad to say, do devote a fair number of pages to the arts and sciences; one even traces science from its beginnings in Greece (great science) through Rome (little science), to the intellectual revolution of the 17th and 18th centuries and the new intellectual revolution of the 19th and 20th centuries, and it does indeed mention Banting, Salk, Sabin, Waksman, Fleming, and Domagk—right in the middle of a history text! Others give only a nod to the arts and sciences. Most treat art and science in separate chapters—not really part of the real ongoing history of kings, princes, czars, emperors, presidents, popes, wars, and treaties, and easy to omit if the instructor chooses to skip about.

One interesting presentation was not in a history text but in J. B. Conant's *Harvard Case Histories in Experimental Science* (3). Conant was an eminent chemist and educator who was President of Harvard University between 1933 and 1953. He believed it important for future voters and those they elect to office to understand the "tactics and strategy" of science and how science fits in with all other fields of human activity. His method was to show when, how, and why great scientific discoveries came about.

His Chapter Two deals with the great Chemical Revolution of 1775-1789 (ushered in by the discovery of oxygen), and he intertwines its events with those of three other revolutions: the Industrial Revolution, the Declaration of American Independence, and the French Revolution. On the next page, slightly abridged, is *his* table of what mattered between 1760 and 1799.

Conant might have gone beyond interweaving four revolutions into one chronological table; he might, from his vantage point almost two centuries later, have analyzed critically the influence of each on the quality of life throughout the world in mid-20th century. The American Revolution might have received first place with the Industrial and Chemical Revolutions (and the Revolution in Physics that followed just a few years later) close behind. Two hundred years from now, the order may be reversed. Or the Revolution in Biomedical Sciences may take top place. In any case, I fervently hope that Random House, if space prevents *additions* to its "Major Dates in World History," will be willing to delete "Reign of Zogu, King of Albania" from its 1929 listings and substitute "Fleming discovers penicillin."

CONANT'S CHRONOLOGICAL TABLE

Table 1. Starred (*) events are also listed in Random House's Supplement (1).

1760	Smeaton improves blast furnaces for producing cast iron.
1760	Bridgewater canal completed; halves cost of coal in Manchester.
1760	Factory system and use of water-driven machinery firmly established in English silk industry.
1764	Hargreaves' spinning jenny introduced into English textile industry.
*1765	Stamp Act.
1766	Cavendish (London) isolates and describes hydrogen gas (inflammable air).
1769	Watt's first steam engine.
1772	Lavoisier's experiments with sulfur and phosphorus. Priestley publishes his test for the "goodness" of air.
1774	Death of Louis XV.
1775	Lavoisier's "Easter Memoir" on calcination. ["Calcination" here refers to the heating of metallic mercury in air to yield mercuric oxide; the latter, heated to much higher temperatures, decomposes into metallic mercury and oxygen gas.] Priestley's effective discovery of oxygen.
*1776	Declaration of American Independence.
1776	Publication of Adam Smith's *Wealth of Nations*.
1778	Lavoisier's revised memoir on calcination [and discovery of oxygen].
*1781	Capitulation of British at Yorktown.
1782- 1783	Composition of water established; spread of Lavoisier's ideas; last stand of phlogiston theory.
1783	Lavoisier and Laplace determine large number of specific heats.
*1783	Peace between Great Britain and the United States.
1784	Cort's puddling process for making malleable iron from cast iron using coal as fuel.
1784	Watt's improved steam engine.
1785	Watt proposes bleaching textiles with chlorine gas.
*1787	Constitutional convention at Philadelphia.
1789	Publication of Lavoisier's *Traité Élémentaire de Chimie* setting forth results of the chemical revolution in clear and systematic form.
*1789	Fall of the Bastille (July).
1791	Birmingham mob burns Priestley's house.
*1792	Attack on the Tuileries, Louis XVI a prisoner; French Republic proclaimed.
*1793	War between Great Britain and France, continues with only short truces until 1815.
1794	Execution of Lavoisier (May 8); fall and death of Robespierre (July); end of [the Reign of] Terror.
1796	Production of cast iron in Great Britain 125,000 tons, double the figure of a decade earlier.
*1798	Battle of the Nile. Nelson's victory ensures supremacy of British fleet.
1798	Publication of *Essay on Population* by Malthus.
*1799	Napoleon becomes First Consul.

References

1. The Random House Dictionary of the English Language, Unabridged Edition, Random House, New York, 1966.
2. Bierce, Ambrose: The Devil's Dictionary. Dover Publications, New York, 1958 (republication; original publication, 1906).
3. Conant, J. B.: Harvard Case Histories in Experimental Science, Harvard University Press, Cambridge, 1957 (Volume 1, pp. 113-114).

The Courage to Fail

I recently read a book, *The Courage to Fail*, written by two sociologists with a considerable interest in medicine (1). In one section they analyzed the character of the "transplant surgeon." They interviewed a number of surgeons dedicated to transplanting human organs (the "transplanters"), who emphasized how important it is to have what they term *courage* and particularly the *courage to fail*. This sent me to several dictionaries to find some definitions of courage. The search didn't help much. I got involved in similarities and differences between "courageous" and "fearless," "brave," "bold," "daring," "audacious," and "intrepid," and finally decided that there is no single definition but that courage comes in different sizes, each with its own definition.

Courage, Size 1. This, the largest size, means to me that the person voluntarily involves himself in an action (or sometimes inaction) that places *himself* in grave peril such as loss of life, liberty, or pursuit of happiness. Courage, Size 1, by my definition, also bars as a motive any possible gain, material or otherwise, to the individual should he fail or succeed, and postulates that, if he succeeds, he wants the gain to be for someone else. Unintended gain during life or posthumous recognition does not diminish the magnitude of Courage, Size 1.

Good examples of Courage, Size 1, in this century were the volunteers who allowed mosquitoes to bite them repeatedly, after the insects had recently feasted on the blood of patients with yellow fever. Yellow fever had killed 10 per cent of the population of Philadelphia in 1793, killed 7,000 persons in New Orleans in 1853, and in 1878 hit 74,000 Americans, of whom 15,932 died. It also aborted the first attempt, by de Lesseps, to build the Panama Canal in the late 1800s.

In 1900 there was an epidemic of yellow fever among the U.S. Army troops stationed in Havana after the Spanish-American War. Because no one knew the cause of the disease or how it spread, the Secretary of War appointed a 4-man board on May 24, 1900, to "pursue scientific investigations with reference to the infectious diseases prevalent on the island of Cuba." The four men were Major Walter Reed and Acting Assistant Surgeons James Carroll, Aristides Agramonte, and Jesse Lazear (2).

They decided to tackle first the proposal, made by Charles Finlay of Havana 15 years earlier but largely ignored, that mosquitoes carried the disease from man to man (3). The Army team hatched mosquitoes from eggs, induced the insects to bite patients with known yellow fever, and then maintained colonies of presumably infected mosquitoes for future experiments. Some of these bit Carroll, Lazear, and Private William Dean (a volunteer); all three contracted yellow fever. Carroll and Dean made uneventful recoveries; Jesse Lazear, however, died. Final proof that yellow fever was transmitted *only* by the bite of an infected mosquito came when three additional volunteers, never exposed to Cuban mosquitoes, slept for 20 nights in a room free of mosquitoes, but filled with mattresses, pillows, towels, sheets, underwear, pajamas and blankets soiled with blood and a variety of discharges from patients with known yellow fever; none became sick. Eradication of mosquitoes eliminated yellow fever (and malaria) from Cuba and Central America and a few years later permitted the building of the Panama Canal.

The volunteers' reward? James Carroll died of myocarditis in 1907; his widow and Jesse Lazear's widow each received $125 per month appropriated year by year in the Army appropriation bill (2); several other volunteers received a donation of $100.

Carroll, Lazear, and Dean fit my definition of Courage, Size 1: all were volunteers; all endangered their own lives; none received any personal gain; others benefited immeasurably.

Another who deserved the Courage, Size 1, medal was Werner Forssmann, who introduced a catheter into his own right atrium in 1929, not knowing whether the tip might cause ventricular fibrillation, but hoping that the procedure might eventually be useful in diagnosing or treating certain disorders. He received no acclaim, fame, or reward in his own country, although very much later, in 1956, the Nobel Prize Committee recognized his courage.

Courage, Size 2. Size 2 (by my definition) differs from Size 1 in that the investigator (the recipient of our medal) is not the subject who takes the risk (as was the case with Lazear and Forssmann); in initial experiments the subject is usually a close member of his family, even one of his children when the experimental design precludes the use of an adult. One who fits this definition is Lady Montagu, who, after surviving an attack of smallpox, had her children inoculated with pus from patients suffering from virulent smallpox; this was in the early 1700s, long before Jenner thought of using cowpox, instead of smallpox itself, to confer immunity. Another is Edward Jenner himself, who was so convinced from his careful observations that the mild disease, cowpox, provided lasting immunity against the deadly disease, smallpox, that he vaccinated his first son Edward, and then proved that the child was immune to smallpox by injecting into him pus from smallpox patients on five or six different occasions. He also vaccinated his second son, Robert, when the boy was only eleven months old. Jenner's discovery received a cool reception from London physicians but an enthusiastic one from Professor Benjamin Waterhouse in Boston, who promptly vaccinated his own children and then notified then-Vice President Thomas Jefferson, who in turn vaccinated his whole household of 60. It was not long thereafter that vaccinated persons numbered millions instead of hundreds.

Courage, Size 3. This is similar to Size 1 in that the individual puts his own life at risk instead of that of another (as in Size 2), the risk is a grim one, and considerable benefits to mankind would surely accrue if his mission should be successful. It ranks below Sizes 1 and 2 because his act is motivated by assured fame and fortune if he succeeds. I have not found an instance of Size 3 Courage in medicine so I turn to aviation for my example.

A Courage, Size 3 medal goes to Charles Lindbergh, who in 1927 flew solo across the Atlantic Ocean in a single engine plane and in so doing convinced many of the public that the airplane might well become a safe form of travel. Why only a Size 3 medal for Lindbergh instead of Size 1? After all, he did risk his own life and not that of another, and the risk was not an insignificant one; between 1927 and 1930, only 10 of 31 transatlantic flights succeeded and 16 men and three women died in the 21 failures.

Size 3 because, though he had everything to lose if he failed, he had everything to gain if he won. The flight was not made on an impulse. A number of pilots and their planes were lined up in the 1927 transatlantic derby with the $25,000 Raymond Orteig prize for the first to make the nonstop crossing; in addition, there was bound to be a hero's welcome abroad and at home and as much fame, honors, medals, and riches as the winner wanted.

Courage, Size 4. Size 4 medals go to patients who, informed by specialists that they have advanced disease and statistically have only weeks, months, or a year to live, elect to undergo a previously untested operation or other form of therapy (or even one that has failed repeatedly). It might benefit them or might lead to earlier death; neither the physician nor the patient can know which because (1) though the mortality rates for conservative treatment are reasonably correct for a thousand patients, they are not precise for any individual, and (2) there are no data on life or death following the new procedure.

One who gets a Size 4 award was the first patient (a 33-year-old man, name or initials not reported) to have a bilateral sympathectomy (4) to lower his very high arterial blood pressure in 1925, in an era when hypertension was considered to be compensatory and essential to drive sufficient blood through narrowed renal vessels to maintain life. The operation by Dr. A. W. Adson was successful and opened the door to active surgical and then medical treatment of malignant and essential hypertension.

Another is Dr. James Gilmore, who in 1933 was the first patient to have one whole lung removed surgically at a single operation (5). He was 48 years old and had a squamous-cell carcinoma of his left upper lobe bronchus, very close to the bifurcation of the main bronchus. His surgeon was Evarts Graham. When Graham, on the basis of bronchoscopy and biopsy, was certain that the tumor was malignant, he told Gilmore and described the operation he planned to do. Gilmore asked to go home for a few days to arrange his affairs. In those few days, he quite naturally bought a cemetery lot, but, to Graham's amazement and delight, Gilmore also paid a visit to his dentist to fill some cavities that had been bothering him! Graham said, in 1957, "The visit to the dentist by this patient gave me great assurance!" (6). The pneumonectomy went well and the patient lived until 1963, when he died at age 78 of cardiorenal disease. He outlived his surgeon by 6 years; Graham died of inoperable cancer of the lung in 1957 (7).

Others with Courage, Size 4 were the first patient to receive Prontosil® (Hildegarde Domagk, the daughter of its discoverer), the family of the first patient to receive insulin (the patient was in a coma), the first to receive penicillin, and the family of the first "blue baby" operated upon by Blalock.

Courage Sizes 1 to 4 for surgeons? Many have said that cardiac surgery eventually succeeded only because some pioneers had the "courage to fail." One such pioneer was Ludwig Rehn, a German surgeon. Billroth, the Geheimrat of European surgery, had stated flatly in 1883: "A surgeon who tries to suture a heart wound deserves to lose the esteem of his colleagues." And in the face of this edict, it undoubtedly took courage on the part of Rehn, who, in 1896, did indeed try to suture a stab wound 1.5 cm long in the right ventricle of a young man, and not only tried but succeeded (8). This marked the beginning of modern cardiac surgery. Since a surgical Geheimrat is reputed to be a wrathful and even vengeful god, I'm inclined to give Rehn a Size 4 award because, even though his patient was sure to die without surgical intervention, Rehn's future as a German surgeon might have been at an end had he failed.

What about cardiac surgeons after Rehn? For decades thereafter, cardiac surgeons largely limited themselves to treating traumatic injuries of the heart—suture of stab wounds, removal of bullets and shell fragments—and pretty much avoided operations on cardiac valves and congenital defects. True, between 1913 and 1928, six surgeons had operated on 12 patients with stenotic valves (10 mitral, one pulmonic and one aortic) in the hope of enlarging the narrowed openings. Nine of the twelve patients died within six days of the operation: two recovered and improved, and a third lived for 4½ years after the operation. Although Cutler and Beck, who reviewed these twelve cases in 1929 (9) concluded that "the mortality figures alone should not deter further investigation, both clinical and experimental, since they are to be expected in the opening up of any new field for surgical endeavor," no

surgeon tried again for fifteen years. It was as though cardiac surgeons respected the subtitle of the Cutler-Beck review, "*Final* report on all surgical cases" (italics added), and rejected the conclusions.

In November 1945, Dr. Charles Bailey decided that the time had come to try again (10). Patient No. 1 died on the operating table; 7 months later patient No. 2 died 60 hours after the operation; 21 months later, patient No. 3 died 6 days after the operation.

Time to quit? Not for Bailey. He had two more patients who had consented to the operation. Bailey planned to do both operations in late May, but he became ill and rescheduled No. 4 and No. 5 for the same day, June 10, 1948. No. 5 was a 24-year-old woman, Claire Ward; during the reprieve (between late May and June 10), her family physician advised her not to go ahead with the proposed operation, but she returned to Philadelphia and agreed that Bailey operate as planned.

On the morning of June 10, Bailey operated on patient No. 4 at Philadelphia General Hospital; the patient died on the operating table before Bailey even reached the mitral valve. Bailey and his team drove directly to Episcopal Hospital in Philadelphia where Patient No. 5 was confidently waiting in the operating room. I don't know whether she learned the outcome of operation No. 4 before she actually became No. 5. The operation on Claire Ward went well and she survived. She survived not only the operation, but a train ride from Philadelphia to Chicago nine days later (to be presented to the American College of Chest Surgeons meeting there on June 20), two subsequent pregnancies, and (when last noted in 1971) 23 more years of active life. Bailey operated on 10 more patients in the next 9 months. Of the total of 15, 10 died; of the 8 in whom he had divided (or planned to divide) the commissures ("mitral commissurotomy"), 4 lived and 4 died. Bailey concluded that "commissurotomy is a simple, direct, effective and *safe* procedure" (italics added) (11). No one knows whether, on the basis of Bailey's figures, his surgical colleagues would have judged the operation to be "safe" (for the surgeon perhaps, but for the patient?) but they never had to decide on this basis. Six days after Bailey's successful operation, Harken in Boston performed a successful commissurotomy (12) and three months after that Brock had success in London (13). During the next decade, surgeons performed thousands of similar operations on stenotic pul-

134

monary and aortic as well as mitral valves. Eventually, commissurotomy was upstaged by complete excision of the badly diseased valve and replacement by an artificial valve, implanted during an open heart operation.

This is a story of a great surgical advance that was due in large part to courage. But *whose?* Courage of the surgeon to risk his professional career by failing over and over again? Or courage of Patient No. 5, Claire Ward, who knew that at least patients No. 1, 2, and 3 had died but, nevertheless, decided to risk her life? I vote to give a Courage, Size 4 award to the *patient*.

Why not to the surgeon who had "the courage to fail" in operations 1 to 4? Largely because this story—of early failures crowned by a single success—was a pretty common one (though not many physicians today remember this). And so far I can't find instances of surgeons who suffered professional disgrace and poverty by failure in their bold, daring, audacious, innovative surgical procedures. If I could find such cases, I'd give them all courage Size 4 or maybe even Size 2 awards. But the evidence of professional obloquy is not be found in their published accounts, reminiscences, or biographies.

Trendelenberg, the famous German surgeon, wrote in 1912: "Twelve times we have done it [pulmonary embolectomy in man] at the clinic, my assistants oftener than myself, and not once with success. And yet, I would continue trying" (14). He did and continued to be respected. Cutler and Beck remained respected physicians after six consecutive patients with mitral stenosis died postoperatively; Streider did not suffer disgrace when his patient died after his pioneer attempt to close her patent ductus arteriosus. Clarence Dennis was the first to try open heart surgery in man using a pump-oxygenator, about a year before Gibbon; his patient died (15). John Gibbon, the great pioneer in surgical research who almost single-handedly developed the heart-lung apparatus, was the first to use it successfully, for the repair of a large interatrial septal defect in an 18-year-old girl. But his first report told of operations in *four* patients, three of whom died (16). Harken and his associates were the first to replace a diseased aortic valve with an artificial valve, but of the first five patients, only No. 2 survived (17).

Their colleagues continued to respect these men despite failures. It is for this reason that I prefer to call them innovative, bold, daring, resolute, persevering, determined, obstinate, stubborn, or dogged, rather than courageous. The surgeon working at the frontier of his specialty, usually on poor-risk patients, seemed to lose little by failure except the instant fame of success.

This assessment may not be correct. Sociologists Fox and Swazey believe that to a "transplant" surgeon the most devastating form of defeat is the death of a patient. Some quotes are, "I realize I can't win every time. But emotionally, I want to. So when a patient dies, I feel terribly dejected" and "Whenever we lose someone on the operating table, the old man is devastated. He . . . goes to his office and locks the door. It's as if it were some sort of personal defeat." A tortured mind and soul, if it persists for long, may well be worse than outright loss of professional prestige or privileges.

Perseverance, Size 1. Some can't qualify for a Courage award of any size but do deserve a Perseverance, Size 1 award. These are the physicians who have nothing to lose because they are involved with restoring to life one who, at the time of their intervention, was already legally dead. Persevering, determined, and dauntless describe Claude Beck's attempt after attempt to use electrical defibrillation in patients with an open chest and ventricular fibrillation and Zoll's attempt to convert ventricular fibrillation to normal rhythm in patients with a closed chest. Beck had five failures in a row before his first success (18); Zoll had three failures before his first success (19). Both get the Perseverance, Size 1 award. But those who stubbornly keep *parts* of patients alive although the whole patient will never function again get no award from me, even for perseverance.

Awards for cardiac transplanters? What about Christiaan Barnard and his followers in the field of cardiac transplantation? Because this is a special case, I prefer to let surgeons speak, as they did in a book review (20) of *The Courage to Fail:*

. . . the "transplant surgeon" . . . is seen as something of a superman pioneering the therapeutic unknown. He has "the courage to fail." A long discussion of the problems of heart transplants follows with, apparently, little recognition of the fact that the 1968-69 development of heart transplantation was an unfortunate period in the history of American surgery. A group of surgeons, experienced in cardiac surgery but unaware of the problems of organ transplantation and immunosuppression, took up, without suitable laboratory background, an operation that had previously been performed only once or twice in South Africa. Although the book builds up the physician and surgeon as having the "courage to fail" he can also misunderstand the nature of biologic and biochemical science, and abuse or exploit the power of persuasion that physicians have in dealing with patients.

Looking into my Retrospectroscope, it seems certain that great medical and surgical advances have often resulted from the unique combination at the right moment of a courageous subject or patient and an innovative, persevering, dogged physician, surgeon, or even layman (such as Lady Mary Montagu). Ethical considerations require that the subject (or his or her parents) be fully informed; scientific considerations require that the dogged physician or surgeon also be maximally informed in the totality of knowledge pertaining to his innovation—*before* he persists, and not *after*.

References

1. Fox, R. C., and Swazey, J. P.: The Courage to Fail: A Social View of Organ Transplants and Dialysis, University of Chicago Press, Chicago, 1974, 395 pp.
2. Agramonte, A.: The Inside History of a Great Medical Discovery, Havana, Cuba, 1915.
3. Finlay, C.: Yellow fever: Its transmission by means of the culex mosquito, Am J Med Sci, 1886, 92, 395-409.
4. Rowntree, L. G., and Adson, A. W.: Bilateral lumbar sympathetic neurectomy in the treatment of malignant hypertension, JAMA, 1925, 85, 959-961.
5. Graham, E. A., and Singer, J. J.: Successful removal of an entire lung for carcinoma of the bronchus, JAMA, 1933, 101, 1371-1374.
6. Graham, E. A.: A brief account of the development of thoracic surgery and some of its consequences, Surg Gynecol Obstet, 1957, 104, 241-250.
7. Eloesser, L.: Milestones in chest surgery, J Thorac Cardiovasc Surg, 1970, 60, 157-165.
8. Rehn, L.: Ueber Penetrierende Herzwunden und Herznaht, Arch Klin Chir, 1897, 55, 315-329.
9. Cutler, E. C., and Beck, C. S.: The present status of the surgical procedures in chronic valvular disease of the heart, Arch Surg, 1929, 18, 403-416.
10. Bailey, C. P.: The surgical treatment of mitral stenosis, Dis Chest, 1949, 15, 377-397.
11. Bailey, C. P., Glover, R. P., and O'Neill, T. J. E.: The surgery of mitral stenosis, J Thorac Surg, 1950, 19, 16-49.
12. Harken, D. E., Ellis, L. B., Ware, P. F., and Norman, L. R.: The surgical treatment of mitral stenosis. I. Valvuloplasty, N Engl J Med, 1948, 239, 804-809.
13. Baker, C., Brock, R. C., and Campbell, M.: Valvulotomy for mitral stenosis: Report of six successful cases, Br Med J, 1950, 1, 1283-1293.
14. Meyer, W.: The surgery of the pulmonary artery, Ann Surg, 1913, 58, 188-205.
15. Dennis, C., Spreng, D. S., Nelson, G. E., Karlson, K. E., Nelson, R. M., Thomas, J. V., Eder, W. P., and Varco, R. L.: Development of a pump oxygenator to replace the heart and lungs: An apparatus applicable to human patients, and application to one case, Ann Surg, 1951, 134, 709-721.
16. Gibbon, J. H., Jr.: Application of a mechanical heart and lung apparatus to cardiac surgery, Minn Med, 1954, 37, 171-180.
17. Harken, D. E., Soroff, H. S., and Taylor, W. J.: Partial and complete prostheses in aortic insufficiency, J Thorac Cardiovasc Surg, 1960, 40, 744-762.
18. Beck, C. S., Pritchard, W. H., and Feil, H. S.: Ventricular fibrillation of long duration abolished by electric shock, JAMA, 1947, 135, 985-986.
19. Zoll, P. M., Linenthal, A. J., Gibson, W., Paul, M. H., and Norman, L. R.: Termination of ventricular fibrillation in man by externally applied electric countershock, N Engl J Med, 1956, 254, 727-732.
20. Moore, F. D., Goldman, M., and Gates, C.: "The Courage to Fail" (book review), N Engl J Med, 1975, 292, 654.

Frankenstein, Pickwick, and Ondine

In 1816, Percy and Mary Shelley were on holiday in Switzerland and became the neighbors of Lord Byron and his friend Polidori. Incessant rain kept them indoors for days; to relieve the tedium, Byron suggested that each write a ghost story. All four accepted the assignment but only one, Mary Shelley, completed it; she produced a story, published in 1818, "Frankenstein or, the Modern Prometheus."

Over the years, some interesting errors have crept into the telling and retelling of her story. One of these concerns the answer to "Who was Frankenstein?" Another concerns the answer to "Who created the destructive monster?" If there were a Gallup poll on these questions, I would estimate that half of those queried would answer that Frankenstein was the monster that was created by a scientist (name unknown), and the other half would answer that Frankenstein was a scientist who created a destructive monster (name unknown). Of my dictionaries, most give two answers (that Frankenstein was a student who created a monster, and that Frankenstein was the man-made monster). One dictionary simply labels Frankenstein as the monster; only one states that the name Frankenstein is often *incorrectly* employed to denote the monster itself.

If you will go to the original story (and that is one of my themes today)—Mary Shelley's book, rather than latter-day entertainment "based on" her novel—you will soon see that Frankenstein was neither the monster nor the creator of a destructive monster. Victor Frankenstein was a brilliant student of "natural philosophy" (medicine?) at Ingolstadt University, then in central Bavaria. But Victor Frankenstein did *not* create a *destructive monster*; create he did, but the "monster" was a gentle, intelligent man who longed for the affection of his fellow man.*

* Frankenstein "succeeded in discovering the cause of generation and life and . . . became capable of bestowing animation upon lifeless matter." But he worked long before the advent of microsurgery, and because he could not handle certain minute parts,

Mary Shelley went to great lengths to tell her readers that it was cruel treatment by his fellow man that turned him into a destructive monster.

As the "monster" later recounted to his creator: "Everywhere I see bliss from which I alone am irrevocably excluded. I was benevolent and good; misery made me a fiend . . . my soul glowed with love and humanity; but am I not alone, miserably alone? Your fellow creatures . . . they spurn and hate me." Again, "I had hardly placed my foot within the door, before the children shrieked, and one of the women fainted. The whole village was aroused; some fled, some attacked me, until, grievously bruised by stones and many other kinds of missile weapons, I escaped. . . . I retreated from the barbarity of man. . . . There was none among the myriads of men that existed who would pity or assist me."

Finally, upon rescuing a young girl from drowning, he was shot by her friend. He *then* became a destructive monster. "This was then the reward for my benevolence! I had saved a human being from destruction, and, as a recompense, I now writhed under the miserable pain of a wound, which shattered the flesh and bone. Inflamed by pain, I vowed eternal hatred and vengeance to all mankind."

he was forced to work on a larger-than-human scale. As a result, he put together a man about eight feet tall. Although he took infinite pains over several years to collect appropriate materials from dissection rooms and slaughter houses, and although he was a master in his new art of transplantation, he was not a genius in cosmetic surgery and his product was not the thing of physical beauty that he had hoped for. Frankenstein recalls: "His yellow skin scarcely covered the work of muscles and arteries beneath; his hair was lustrous black and flowing; his teeth a pearly whiteness; but these luxuriances only formed a more horrid contrast with his watery eyes, that seemed almost of the same colour as the dun white sockets in which they were set, his shrivelled complexion and straight black lips. . . . The beauty of the dream vanished, and breathless horror and disgust filled my heart."

Mary Shelley is long dead and Victor Frankenstein and his monster were fictional, so does it matter who was who and who created what? I believe it does matter a bit and for several reasons.

One is that today's public is concerned with the effects on society of unrestricted scientific experimentation and wonders whether the world would be better off without knowledge of nuclear physics and the genetic code. Maybe it's worth noting here that it was a scientist, Frankenstein, who created the *man*—a scientist whose goals were to "pour a torrent of light into a dark world," to create better beings with "happy and excellent natures" and "to renew life where death had apparently devoted the body to corruption." To be sure, the scientist did create an oversize man (except for a basketball team) whose physical features were somewhat less pleasing than those of Paul Newman, but the man he created glowed with love and humanity. It was others (nonscientists) whose lack of love and humanity changed him from an unattractive giant into a destructive monster. (It is interesting that the role of the scientist was a matter for discussion when Mary Shelley wrote her book in 1816–1818; she has one of Frankenstein's professors saying: "The labours of men of genius, however erroneously directed, scarcely ever fail in ultimately turning to the solid advantage of mankind.").

Another reason to keep authors and characters straight is that errors pop up over and over whenever medical scientists decide to draw from literature to "enrich" medical terminology. Two literary errors in the field of pulmonary medicine are the "Pickwickian Syndrome" and "Ondine's Curse"; such errors rarely advance and usually retard medical science.

The "Pickwickian Syndrome" (1). In 1836–1837, Charles Dickens wrote *The Posthumous Papers of the Pickwick Club,* usually referred to as the *Pickwick Papers;* the members of this club were called Pickwickians. And so we have every right to expect that these Pickwickians suffered from the classic symptoms that today's physician associates with the Pickwickian Syndrome. But neither Samuel Pickwick nor any of his fellow Pickwickians, as far as one can tell, was either unusually plump or pathologically sleepy. Joe, who sometimes drove Mr. Wardle's barouche, ran errands for him, and waited at table, was indeed fat and unbelievably sleepy—even dozing off while running errands and snoring while serving at table. Dickens sometimes

called him "Joe" but more often "the fat boy." Dickens' descriptions of Joe's combination of excessive obesity and unique somnolence are probably better-than those entered into medical records by medical residents or into medical journals by medical authors. But "the fat boy" (or Joe) was simply *not* a "Pickwickian"; labeling Joe's condition the "Pickwickian Syndrome" creates both literary and scientific errors. Scientists who are painfully wounded by scientific errors that find their way into medical journals actually seem to be amused—even delighted—by literary errors and happily accept and perpetuate them. For example, James and associates (2) call it a "charming sobriquet more justified by poetic license than by literary history," but then go right ahead and title their paper, "Pickwickian Syndrome." I believe that dubbing "the fat boy" a Pickwickian is much like calling the transformation of Lot's wife into a pillar of salt the "Biblical Syndrome" because she was a minor character who appeared in a well-known book called the Bible.

Let's pass over the "charming" literary error and go on to the clinical errors in the title "Pickwickian Syndrome." Dickens' description of Joe does serve nicely as a prototype for patients with coexisting obesity and somnolence. But nowhere in *The Posthumous Papers of the Pickwick Club* does Joe have apnea, irregular respiration, slow breathing, or cyanosis. Once Dickens says that Joe "breathed heavily," but this is scarcely evidence for hypoventilation. Once Dickens refers to the fat boy as "red faced," but this is scarcely evidence of cyanosis; indeed, we Americans assume that most nineteenth century Englishmen were red faced, either from living in underheated quarters or from being overtoasted by an open fire! And at the end of *Pickwick Papers*—two years later—Joe is much the same as at the beginning, fat and sleepy, but no better and no worse.

One essential feature of Burwell's "Pickwickian Syndrome" (1) is hypoventilation; another is extreme obesity. The title gives no clue as to what causes either of these. Since Burwell's patient lost his hypoventilation when forced to lose weight, the patient's disorder was a specific one: hypoventilation due to obesity. Such a label would have identified the disorder, its cause, and treatment and avoided confusion with hypoventilation that occurs in thin, lively patients or thin lethargic patients with either healthy lungs or with one of many diseases of the lungs and thorax.

"Ondine's Curse" (3) also suffers from both literary and clinical errors. There were indeed ondines and from time to time one fell in love with a man and longed to be transformed into human form (female) and acquire a soul. But the King of the Ondines (4b), sometimes called the "King of the sea" (4a), "the old one" (4a), or Uncle Kühleborn (5), warned his school of mermaids that an ondine who went the mortal route was on a risky course: a disagreeable ending was in store for someone if an ondine married a mortal and was then jilted for an ordinary human female. This warning was referred to as "the pact" and everyone (except the mortal husband) knew the rules.

However, each author who wrote about ondines concocted different rules. The original rule —way back—was that, if deserted, the jilted ondine must give up her lower limbs, take back her fishy tail, and return forever to the sea (and since ondines lived about 300 years, this wasn't too severe a penalty). However, Hans Christian Andersen (6), in "The Little Mermaid," was tougher and ruled that she would suffer a broken heart and return to the sea as foam. Actually, Andersen relented and agreed to save her if she killed her unfaithful husband ("either he or you must die before the sun rises"). She refused to make a deal and Andersen relented again and changed her to a special kind of angel ("daughter of the air").

De La Motte-Fouqué (5) ruled that the jiltee must return forever to the sea and the jilter must forfeit his life. Giraudoux (4) changed the rules again by specifying the manner of the jilter's death: he had to command himself to perform voluntarily all of his body functions that normally went on automatically (one, but *only one*, of these was breathing). It was Giraudoux's pact that inspired the appellation "Ondine's Curse" (more later).

The literary error is that no ondine ever "cursed" her unfaithful husband—no matter who wrote the story or in what century. "The Little Mermaid" (6) was incapable of killing her husband and her last act as a human was to kiss her husband as he slept with his lovely bride! Undine (5) kissed her errant husband "with a heavenly kiss... pressed him ever closer and closer to her and wept as if she would weep away her soul. The tears flooded the eyes of the knight, and in a sweet agony of woe they so whelmed his bosom that at length they bore his breath away...." Ondine (4) pleaded with her King to save her Hans. Failing at that, she

then concocted a story that it was *she* and not Hans who was unfaithful. Failing again, she conceded that Hans had made her unhappy but argued, "Just because I'm unhappy, it doesn't mean that I'm not happy as well. . . . The more you suffer, the happier you are. And I'm happy; I'm the happiest woman in the world. ... Save him!" And as Hans was dying, he said, "We can only talk or kiss, Ondine, we can't do both," and Ondine replies, "Then I'll be quiet." Ondine would turn over in her watery grave if she could read in medical journals, "Rebuffed by the man she loved, in revenge she cursed him ... ," or, "shunned by her lover, she placed upon him a curse," or, "jilted by her mortal husband, (she) took from him all automatic functions."

The scientific error in "Ondine's Curse" is that it was meant to describe a patient with a single disorder—a specific type of respiratory failure in which the patient breathes inadequately or not at all unless commanded to ventilate normally. The first well-studied case (7) was that of a 63-year-old man who had only one medical problem. He was *not* obese. He was *not* somnolent. He had *nothing* wrong with his lungs or thorax; his pulmonary function tests were completely normal (imagine a 63-year-old man with a maximal breathing capacity of 194 liters per min!). His only problem was that he lapsed into hypoventilation (and hypoxemia and CO_2 retention) unless paced by his physician. Contrast that with Hans' syndrome in *Ondine* (4a):

ONDINE: Try to live, Hans. You will forget too.

HANS: Try to live! That's easy to say, isn't it. If only I cared about living! Since you went away, I've had to force my body to do things it should do automatically. I no longer see unless I order my eyes to see. I don't see the grass is green unless I tell them to see it green. And it's not much fun, black grass, I can tell you. I have five senses, thirty muscles, even my bones to command; it's an exhausting stewardship. If I relax my vigilance for one moment, I may forget to hear or to breathe. He died, they'll say, because he could not longer bother to breathe. He died of love ...

By no stretch of the imagination did Hans suffer from a single disorder of hypoventilation. He had lost his color vision, his vision, his hearing, and indeed all five senses; and he couldn't move nonrespiratory muscles unless he commanded that they function properly.

A generalized clinical disorder such as this—

involving all sensory and motor systems (and therefore loss of all reflexes), and yet reversible by willing that it be reversed—may exist in the annals of neuropsychiatry, but no one has yet described hypoventilation or apnea as part of such a widespread disaster.

Mellins and associates (8), in reviewing the published cases of "Ondine's Curse" titled their paper, "Failure of Automatic Control of Ventilation." Doesn't that say everything that need be said without invoking both literary and clinical errors?

CONCLUDING REMARKS

(1) Those who quote literature should first read it. An "Ondine's Curse" (in its entirety) on writers who fail to read original accounts!

(2) It's nice to have a short name for a long syndrome but not if it makes more work for the reader. To make my point, I will label a highly specific and rare syndrome "The Angels' Curse" and refer you to Genesis 19:17–26. When you find your Bible and read the proper chapter and verse, you will wonder why I didn't call it directly by its scientific name (hypersalinic rigor) and save you the trouble of reading the Bible.

(3) There are many causes of hypoventilation, such as stiff lungs and thorax, obstructed small airways, extra work of breathing imposed by excessive obesity, disorders of the motor system (spinal cord, anterior horn cells, motor nerves, neuromuscular junction, and respiratory muscles), diminished sensory input to the reticular activating system or medulla, depression of the brain or brain stem, deep sleep, and obstructed upper airways. Burwell and associates (1) described hypoventilation coupled with obesity and somnolence; Auchincloss and co-workers (9) wrote about hypoventilation coupled with obesity but not somnolence; Ratto and associates (7) described hypoventilation without obesity, without somnolence, and without lung disease. Obviously, a lot of specific disorders must still be sorted out of a bag called hypoventilation; good terminology might help.

(4) Someone once wrote: "Scientists who introduce new terminology should, by law, be required to post a $1,000 bond, to be forfeited if the terminology is both misleading and used." (10a). Not a bad idea at all except that the author repeated the same statement nine years later (10b)—without making allowances for inflation!

References

1. Burwell, S., Robin, E. D., Whaley, R. D., and Bickelman, A. G.: Extreme obesity associated with alveolar hypoventilation; A Pickwickian Syndrome, Am J Med, 1956, 21, 811–818.
2. James, T. N., Frame, B., and Coates, E. O.: De Subitaneis Mortibus. III. Pickwickian Syndrome, Circulation, 1973, 48, 1311–1320.
3. Severinghaus, J. W., and Mitchell, R.: Ondine's Curse—Failure of respiratory center automaticity while awake, Clin Res, 1962, 10, 122.
4. Giraudoux, Jean: Ondine. 1939 (French).
   (a) English adaptation by Maurice Valency, Random House, New York, 1954.
   (b) English translation by Roger Gellert, Oxford University Press, New York, 1967.
5. De La Motte-Fouqué, F. H. K.: Undine, 1811 (German); English translation by Edmund Gosse, Limited Editions Club, New York, 1930.
6. Andersen, Hans Christian: Fairy Tales, English translation by L. W. Kingsland, Oxford University Press, Oxford, 1959 and 1961.
7. Ratto, O., Briscoe, W. A., Morton, J. W., and Comroe, J. H., Jr.: Anoxemia secondary to polycythemia and polycythemia secondary to anoxemia, Am J Med, 1955, 19, 958–965.
8. Mellins, R. B., Balfour, H. H., Jr., Turino, G. M., and Winters, R. W.: Failure of automatic control of ventilation (Ondine's Curse), Medicine, 1970, 49, 487–504.
9. Auchincloss, J. H., Jr., Cook, E., and Renzetti, A. D.: Clinical and physiological aspects of a case of obesity, polycythemia and alveolar hypoventilation, J Clin Invest, 1955, 34, 1537–1545.
10. Comroe, J. H., Jr.: Physiology of Respiration, Year Book Medical Publishers, Chicago.
    (a) ed. 1, 1965, p. 179.
    (b) ed. 2, 1974, p. 212.

Premature Science and Immature Lungs

Part I. Some Premature Discoveries

When I was a medical student, we studied the tenth edition of Holt's *Diseases of Infancy and Children*. I still have my copy, 45 years later. The tenth edition, as were its predecessors, was authoritative and up to date; published in 1932, it contains references to many articles published in 1931 or 1932. But among its 1,240 pages there is no mention of hyaline membrane disease or respiratory distress syndrome. There are three pages on asphyxia of the newly born and another three on congenital atelectasis; when these conditions occurred in premature babies, the authors thought it likely that they were due to lack of development of the respiratory center.

Three years earlier, a Swiss respiratory physiologist, Kurt von Neergaard, had published a now-classic paper (1); its title (translated from German into English) is "New notions on a fundamental principle of respiratory mechanics: the retractile force of the lung, dependent on the surface tension in the alveoli." Much more about Neergaard later, but in that 1929 paper he demonstrated clearly that surface forces at the interface of moist alveolar walls and alveolar gas caused a strong retractile force (even stronger than that of stretched elastic tissues) tending to collapse alveoli and he speculated that atelectasis of the newborn might be due to the considerable retractile force of surface tension that opposes the first expansion of the lungs.

It's too much to expect that the two pediatricians responsible for the tenth edition of Holt's text had noticed and read Neergaard's 1929 article in a German journal of experimental medicine in time to have included it in their 1932 revision, so I looked in the medical physiology texts of the 1930s, then those of the 1940s and then those of the 1950s for a discussion of surface forces. They contained little or nothing on surface tension and nothing at all on a possible role that surface tension might play in expansion and retraction of the lungs.

What is surface tension? Figure 1 explains it well. Possibly there are better definitions but I have selected this one because it keeps me humble; it comes from pages 2 and 3 of the text (2) that I used as a second-year college student in 1929 in L. V. Heilbrunn's stimulating course in general physiology at the University of Pennsylvania! Indeed, all of Chapter 1 (24 pages) was devoted to surface action and ways of measuring surface tension. Much later in life, I became a pulmonary physiologist and was even associated briefly with a pediatrician who measured pressure-volume curves of atelectatic lungs from babies who had died from hyaline membrane disease. But I had total *lack* of recall of Ponder's Chapter 1 and the thought never occurred to me that forces at an air-liquid interface might be keeping alveoli closed. I had lots of very good company in failing to make this association and in failing to appreciate a few small voices that did make it. Fortunately, a series of events in the mid- and late 1950s led to the discovery of pulmonary surfactant, a unique substance formed and secreted by pulmonary Type II alveolar cells, that decreases surface tension to very low values at low alveolar volume and so serves as an anti-collapse factor. Absence of this surfactant (as in the lungs of some newborn babies, particularly premature ones) favors collapse of the lungs and puts an almost impossible burden on the weak inspiratory muscles of newly born premature babies. Because the key to understanding, to diagnosing before birth, and to managing respiratory

Surface tension. In order to appreciate the forces acting on a molecule at the air-water surface or phase boundary in our simple system, let us first consider the forces acting on a molecule of water situated in the interior of the system itself. The molecule A, situated in the interior of the water (Fig. 1) is attracted by all the other molecules around it with considerable forces known as the forces of molecular attraction; this attraction is similar to that exerted by every portion of matter on every other portion, and generates a pressure upon the molecule A of thousands of atmospheres. Since the attractions take place from all sides, however, their effects cancel out, and the molecule A is not constrained to move in any particular direction. Now consider the molecule B at the surface of the water. There are no water molecules above it, but only molecules of gas, which attract it very little; it is accordingly pulled down by the water molecules beneath it, and so tends to be drawn into the interior of the water. It cannot move, however, unless the mass of water becomes smaller in volume, and so the effect of the attraction from below is that the surface layers of the water become compressed. In addition to this, as every molecule within this surface layer is strongly drawn towards the interior of the fluid, the surface tends to become as small as possible. In fact, the surface behaves as if it were a stretched elastic membrane, always tending to contract, and just as we speak of the tension of stretched elastic membrane, so do we speak of a *surface tension* at the phase boundary under consideration.

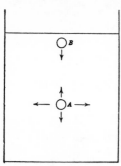

Fig. 1.

Fig. 1. Definition of surface tension by Eric Ponder.

distress syndrome before and after birth is a knowledge of surface tension and the behavior of surface films, let's start at the beginning—with the discovery of surface tension.

Pierre Simon Laplace and Surface Forces

The Marquis de Laplace, sometimes called a latter-day Newton, was a brilliant French mathematician, physicist, and astronomer. His genius was recognized early and he became professor of mathematics in the École Militaire de Paris. One of his students there was Napoleon Bonaparte. Certainly Laplace benefitted from this association, because Napoleon richly rewarded Laplace with estates and a Ministry, forgave him his administrative ineptitudes, and continued to favor Laplace during Napoleon's 100 days' return to France (even though Laplace was among those who had signed the earlier order banishing Napoleon). Laplace had an amazing talent not only for mathematics but also for political survival, for although his friend Lavoisier went to the guillotine during the Reign of Terror in 1794, Laplace not only kept his head but his estates and wealth as well.

Laplace devoted his scientific career to a profound theoretical analysis of the solar system and between 1798 and 1827 published five huge tomes—more than 2,000 pages in all—entitled *Traité de Mécanique Céleste* (3). It dealt with the general laws of mechanics, gravitation, and motions of celestial bodies. Certainly it was a sequel to Newton's *Principia* and some rated it as intellectually on par with it.

What does Laplace's study of the heavenly bodies have to do with surface forces? In Tome IV of *Mécanique Céleste* are two supplements on "La théorie de l'action capillaire"—read before the French Academy and published in 1806 and 1807. On page 689 of Volume IV of Bowditch's translation (4) is Laplace's presentation of his general law in words:

> From these results, relative to bodies terminated by sensible segments of a spherical surface, I have deduced this general theorem. *"In all the laws which render the attraction insensible at sensible distances, the action of a body terminated by a curve surface, upon an infinitely narrow interior canal, which is perpendicular to that surface, at any point whatever, is equal to the half sum of the actions upon the same canal, of two spheres which have the same radii as the greatest and the least radii of curvature of the surface at that point."*

On page 823 is Laplace's equation (figure 2). It contains his formulation of the relationship between force, surface tension, and radii of curvature of surfaces.

Two questions call for answers: *(1) What does capillary action have to do with surface tension?*

One of the simplest and earliest methods of measuring (statically) the surface tension of fluids of biological interest was to observe the height to which a column of fluid rises in a capillary tube. Actually, this was one of the methods used by Neergaard in 1929. A tube with an internal diameter of about 0.5 mm is dipped into the liquid; provided the liquid "wets" the internal wall of the tube, the meniscus rises above the flat surface of the water outside the tube, and it is pulled upward by surface forces (that tend to contract the surface) until balanced by the downward force of gravity on the column of liquid. Laplace (see p. 1,009 of Volume IV of Bowditch's English translation) gives his explanation of why fluid rises in a capillary tube above its expected level:

$$K + \tfrac{1}{2}H \cdot \left(\frac{1}{R} + \frac{1}{R'} \right),$$
$\qquad$ [Pressure at the point O.] $\qquad$ [9845]

---

formulas of the author, with his values of H, K, supposing them always to be those which are [9842k] obtained from observation, and therefore such as would arise from the action of a fluid of a variable density.

We shall suppose, in fig. 143, page 820, that the line OT is drawn tangent to the surface NOM, in the point O, and from any point S of the surface there is let fall upon this tangent [9842l] the perpendicular $ST=z$. We shall also suppose that the cylindrical column $O'O$ is continued below the surface NOM, so as to form the canal $O'OVSU$, which, in its upward direction SU, meets the surface NOM at S, in a perpendicular direction, and passes on, in the same direction, to the external surface in U. Putting $R_{,}$ and $R'_{,}$, respectively, for the [9842m] greatest and the least radii of curvature of the surface NOM at the point S, we shall have, in like manner as in [9842g],

$$K + \tfrac{1}{2}H \cdot \left(\frac{1}{R_{,}} + \frac{1}{R'_{,}} \right) = \text{the pressure on the base } S \text{ of the column } US \text{ of a variable density.} \qquad [9842n]$$

If the line $ST=z$ be vertical, it will express the elevation of the point O above the point S; and the pressure of a column of fluid of that height will be gz. If this line be inclined to the horizon by an angle whose cosine is represented by $\frac{u}{z}$, the vertical pressure will [9842o] become $gz \times \frac{u}{z}$, or simply gu; u being the vertical elevation of the point O above the point S. Adding this quantity gu to the pressure at O [9842g], we get the whole pressure at S, which ought to balance the pressure in the canal US, given in [9842n], upon the principle of the equilibrium of the canals, which is so frequently used in this work; hence we have

$$K + \tfrac{1}{2}H \cdot \left(\frac{1}{R} + \frac{1}{R'} \right) + gu = K + \tfrac{1}{2}H \cdot \left(\frac{1}{R_{,}} + \frac{1}{R'_{,}} \right). \qquad [9842p]$$

If we suppose the situation of the point S to be successively varied, by infinitely small intervals, along the surface $NOSM$, while the point O remains the same, we shall have K, H, R, R', g, constant; and u, $R_{,}$, $R'_{,}$, variable; and then the differential of [9842p] [9842q] will become, by transposing the term gdu,

$$\tfrac{1}{2}H \cdot d \cdot \left(\frac{1}{R_{,}} + \frac{1}{R'_{,}} \right) - gdu = 0, \qquad [9842r]$$

which is of the same form as [9811], changing H into H, as in [9842e'], and placing an additional accent on R, R', as in [9842m], to conform to the notation which we have here used. This equation may also be deduced from the same principle which is employed in [9842s] [9808]; for the quantity g being multiplied by the element $-du$, is the same as in [9307"]

Fig. 2. Laplace's law. This states that force is proportional to the mathematical expression in line 1, in which K = "intrinsic pressure," H = surface tension, and R and R′ are the radii of curvature. Figure 2 is p. 823 of Volume IV of Bowditch's translation (4). Laplace's contribution to p. 823 consists of only the first line; the remainder of the page is filled with Bowditch's annotation and explanation of the preceding page.

At the surface of a fluid, the attraction of the particles, modified by the curvature of the surface and of the sides of the vessel which contains it, produces the capillary attraction. Therefore these phenomena, and all those which chemistry presents, correspond to one and the same law, of which now there can be no doubt. Some philosophers have attributed the capillary phenomena to the adhesion of the fluid particles, either to each other, or to the sides of the vessels which contain them; but this cause is not sufficient to produce the effect. For, if we suppose the surface of water, contained in a glass tube, to be horizontal, and upon a level with that of the water in the vessel into which the tube is dipped by its lower end; the tenacity of the fluid, and its adhesion to the tube, would not curve this surface and render it concave. To produce that, it is necessary to suppose that there is an attraction in the upper part of the tube, which is not immediately in contact with the fluid.

(2) *Why do two supplements dealing with capillary action (and surface forces) belong in a treatise on the movements of planets and stars?* Let Henri Poincaré (5) answer that:

The astronomic universe is formed of masses, very great, no doubt, but separated by intervals so immense that they appear to us only as material points. These points attract each other inversely as the square of the distance, and this attraction is the sole force which influences their movements. But if our senses were sufficiently keen to show us all the details of the bodies which the physicist studies, the spectacle thus disclosed would scarcely differ from the one the astronomer contemplates. There also we should see material points, separated from one another by intervals, enormous in comparison with their dimensions, and describing orbits according to regular laws. These infinitesimal stars are the atoms. Like the stars proper, they attract or repel each other, and this attraction or this repulsion, following the straight line which joins them, depends only on the distance. The law according to which this force varies as function of the distance is perhaps not the law of Newton, but it is an analogous law; in place of the exponent—2, we have probably a different exponent, and it is from this change of exponent that arises all the diversity of physical phenomena, the variety of qualities and of sensations, all the world, colored and sonorous, which surrounds us; in a word, all nature.

Such is the primitive conception in all its purity. It only remains to seek in the different cases what value should be given to this exponent in order to explain all the facts. It is on this model that Laplace, for example, constructed his beautiful theory of capillarity; he regards it only as a particular case of attraction, or, as he says, of universal gravitation, and no one is astonished to find it in the middle of one of the five volumes of the Mécanique céleste.

Nathaniel Bowditch

Laplace's *Mécanique Céleste* came to the attention of English-speaking scientists largely through Bowditch's translation (4). Bowditch in some ways is more remarkable than Laplace himself. Bowditch, an American with no formal schooling beyond the age of 10, signed on as a clerk on a sailing vessel in 1795 at the age of 22 and was at sea for most of the next 9 years. During that time, he made his own studies of navigation that resulted in his correcting more than 8,000 errors in the then-bible of navigators, Moore's *Practical Navigator*. His great interest in the planets and stars led him to Laplace's *Mécanique Céleste* and he devoted more than 30 years of his life to translating it into English. He never completed Tome V, but his translation of the first four Tomes (10 "Books") occupies more than 3,700 pages.* More remarkable than his translation are his annotations and explanations of Laplace's work and his corrections of Laplace's many errors. His annotations were helpful even to expert mathematicians because Laplace's mathematics was highly sophisticated and difficult to follow; Bowditch's corrections were essential because previously Laplace's errors went unnoticed. Figure 2 shows the extent of Bowditch's contributions to Laplace's work; of Bowditch's 3,700 pages, about half are a translation of Laplace's French edition and the remaining half are Bowditch's annotations. All of this from an unschooled young man in a rough new world!†

Bowditch had other accomplishments. A son, Henry Ingersoll Bowditch, was a professor of clinical medicine at Harvard (1859–1867) and an early specialist in diseases of the chest. A grandson, Henry Pickering Bowditch, who established the first physiological laboratory in

---

* Only 500 copies of Bowditch's original translation were printed, and most of these are held in "rare books" collections, but the Chelsea Publishing Company, Bronx, New York, reprinted the four volumes in 1966 ($125 per set in 1976).

† For a 168-page biography of Bowditch, written by his son Nathaniel, see Volume IV of Bowditch's translation (4) or Volume I of Chelsea Company's reprint (4).

America (1871), was one of the three founders of the American Physiological Society, a co-editor of the new *American Journal of Physiology*, first president of the American Physiological Society, and a Dean of the Harvard Medical Faculty.

Thomas Young

As so often happens in science, the first was not the first. Laplace read his paper to the Institute of France in 1805 and it was published in 1806 as a supplement to *Mécanique Céleste*. Young read *his* paper, "An essay on the cohesion of fluids," before the Royal Society of London December 20, 1804, and it was published in the Philosophical Transactions for 1805 (6). Young's paper contained, in words, most of what Laplace presented a year later in elaborate, formidable, and impressive mathematical terms. Notorious for borrowing from the work of others (and giving little or no credit to them), Laplace made no reference to Young in his first supplement and discussed Young's work in one brief paragraph in his second supplement a year later. Young, in some "additional remarks" added to an 1807 reprint of his 1805 article (6), took exception to Laplace's behavior in the following nicely composed paragraph.

> In an essay read to the Institute of France in December 1805, and published in 1806, as a supplement to the Mécanique Céleste, Mr. Laplace has advanced a theory of capillary attraction, which has led him to results nearly similar to many of those which are contained in this paper [Young's 1805 paper]. The coincidence is indeed in some respects so striking, that it is natural, upon the first impression, to inquire whether Mr. Laplace may not be supposed either to have seen this essay, or to have read an account of its contents in some periodical publication; but upon further reflection, we cannot for a moment imagine a person of so high and so deserved a reputation as Mr. Laplace, to wish to appropriate to himself any part of the labours of others. The path which he has followed is also extremely different from that which I had taken; several of the subjects which I had considered as belonging to the discussion, have not occurred to Mr. Laplace; and it is much more flattering than surprising, that, to an assembly of philosophers not extremely anxious to attend to the pursuits of their contemporaries, investigations should be communicated, by the most distinguished of their members, as new and important, which had been presented, a year before, to a similar society in this country.

S. M. Tenney ("The Tangled Web," unpublished manuscript) has proposed that the name of Laplace's law be changed to the "Young-Laplace law." Whether it ever will be or not, Young's fame is secure without it. While a medical student, he established the mechanism by which the lens of the eye accommodates for far and near vision. He later formulated a theory of color vision (the Young-Helmholtz theory), he discovered the principle of interference of light, proposed the wave theory of light transmission, contributed to the theory of tides, and established a coefficient of elasticity (Young's modulus). Most fascinating of all his accomplishments was his contribution to deciphering the Rosetta stone. Young provided the important clue necessary for unlocking the Egyptian system of writing; it was his idea that, in the transliteration of non-Egyptian names, hieroglyphic symbols with phonetic values would be used. The credit for the full translation in 1822 goes to Champollion the Younger, but Young's 1819 article persuaded Champollion to drop his conviction that hieroglyphic symbols were never phonetic.

The Long Quiet Period

It took almost 100 years after Bowditch's translation for Laplace's law to become of interest to biomedical scientists. Neergaard's work on the lung came in 1929. And Burton, who applied Laplace's law to the stability of small blood vessels in 1951 (7), stated that the only previous application he found to a vascular problem was that of Woods in 1892 (8). Woods, a throat surgeon at the Richmond Hospital in Dublin demonstrated that the pressure in the cardiac ventricles depended not only on the tension developed by the contracting muscle but also on the size and shape of the heart (i.e., the principal radii of curvature).** In 1960 Burton devoted six pages of his chapter in Ruch and Fulton's textbook of medical physiology (9) to applications of Laplace's law to the heart and vessels; the same book contained no mention of any role of surface tension in the lungs, although Neergaard's 1929 experiments had been discovered, repeated, confirmed, and published in 1954 by Radford (10).

However, the long quiet period in which mam-

** Woods also applied Laplace's law to the urinary bladder, uterus, and to arteries and veins.

malian physiologists and biophysicists failed to become interested in surface forces was a very busy one for physicists and chemists. Lord Rayleigh, 1904 Nobel laureate in physics, used surface physics to prepare monomolecular films of liquids and to determine the dimensions of molecules (11). Langmuir, working in General Electric's Research Laboratory, developed a more precise method in 1917 (12) for measuring molecular dimensions and orientation using technics of surface physics and chemistry. He must have had his eye on a Nobel prize in chemistry (which he won in 1932) because he devoted two and a half pages of fine print at the beginning of his 1917 article to establishing in great detail his priority in the experiments he was about to report; he opened with the statement that, "The fundamental idea of the orientation of group molecules in the surfaces and in the interior of liquids as a factor of vital importance in surface tension and related phenomena occurred to me in nearly its present form in June and July, 1916."

Other physicists developed methods that were suitable for measuring surface tension under dynamic conditions; these were eventually used by biologists. Maxwell devised his frame (13), Wilhelmy his surface balance (14), Langmuir his balance (12), and Adam his improved Langmuir balance (15). And Ms. Agnes Pockels (insensitively referred to as *Miss* Agnes Pockels by Lord Rayleigh) "described a simple method for increasing or diminishing the surface of a liquid in any proportion, by which its purity may be altered at pleasure" (16). Ms. Pockels apologized for her boldness, not being a professional physicist, in writing about her experiments to Lord Rayleigh, who promptly had her paper published in *Nature*.

And beginning in the 1920s, numerous monographs and reviews appeared on interfacial phenomena, surface chemistry, soap films, foams, surface physics, and monomolecular layers; a World Congress on Surface Active Agents was held in 1954.

These subjects were also of great interest to general and cellular physiologists and especially to those interested in membranes. William Bayliss' first edition of *Principles of General Physiology*, published in 1915, devoted Chapter III to surface action (17). J. B. Leathes, who gave the Croonian Lectures in 1923 (18) on "Role of Fats in Vital Phenomena," described experiments on compressing and enlarging surface films of phospholipids (lecithin) and palmitic acid using Adam's surface balance. Leathes was coming very close to what we now call pulmonary surfactant.

But the mammalian physiologists didn't become interested in alveolar surface tension until 1929, and then only one did—Neergaard.

Back to Neergaard

Neergaard was born in Schleswig-Holstein in Germany. Because he was in poor health as a child, his mother brought him to Davos, the famous Swiss health spa. He remained in Switzerland, became a Swiss citizen, and was graduated from the University of Zurich in 1917. In 1922 he moved to Basel where he worked with a well-known internist, Professor Staehelin. But he spent little of his time in the medical clinic in Basel and most of it with physiologists. There he met Dr. Karl Wirz. The Swiss physiologists had been unusually active and innovative in the study of pulmonary mechanics. Rohrer had done his now-classic study on airway resistance in 1915 (19), and Fleisch had devised an excellent apparatus for continuous measurement of inspired and expired air flow in 1925 (20). Wirz, a pupil of Rohrer's, had measured changes in pleural pressure during respiration in 1923 (21). Neergaard joined forces with Wirz to study first lung elasticity, and then flow resistance in air passages of normal humans and those with asthma or emphysema (22, 23).

Shortly thereafter, Neergaard had a novel idea about lung elasticity that had eluded all previous physiologists. He said (1):

> The lung is probably unique among tissues in its extraordinary ability to expand and retract. So far, this has been regarded as due to the elasticity of the tissue itself, and particularly that of the elastic fibers. Although attempts have recently been made to determine the elasticity of the elastic fibers directly with the aid of a micromanipulator (Redenz), this does not prove that the entire retractility of lung can be attributed to these structures. . . .
>
> So far, one force has not been taken into account that definitely merits consideration in this context. This is *surface tension*. It is active at the boundary between alveolar epithelium and alveolar air. Wherever the surface of an aqueous solution touches upon a gaseous space, the influence of molecular attraction on the marginal layer of molecules gives rise to tensions in the solution that are described as surface tension. All the phenomena of capillary chemistry, the rise of liquids in

146

fine capillaries, the pressure of soap bubbles, and numerous other phenomena, are based on surface tension. Considerable forces are involved which also play a role in other aspects of respiratory mechanics (as previously pointed out in the evaluation of the so-called adhesion of the pleural surface). The surface tension partly depends on the nature of the solution that constitutes the bordering medium and particularly on the curvature of the boundary. The smaller the radius of curvature, the stronger the force of surface tension, which is like a taut rubber membrane attempting to retract like a rubber balloon. Such deeply curved boundaries between fluid or an aqueous gel (the cellular membrane of the alveolar epithelium) and a gaseous space exist in countless numbers in the pulmonary alveoli. . . .

To visualize the mechanism even more clearly, one should imagine a thin capillary tube at the end of which a soap bubble has been blown. As soon as blowing is discontinued and the inside of the soap bubble is allowed to communicate with the atmosphere via the capillary, the bubble immediately becomes smaller and retracts owing to the influence of surface tension. The smaller the diameter of the capillary in this situation and the smaller the radius of curvature of the bubble, the more rapid and more energetic the retraction. Such small bubbles, which communicate with the atmosphere via narrow capillaries, can be compared to the alveoli of a lung.

In view of the almost complete saturation of expired air with water vapor, we can imagine the alveolar epithelium as covered by a thin film of fluid. The surface tension attempts to make the alveoli smaller, and therefore exerts an influence in the same direction as the retractive force of the entire lung. There can be no doubt, therefore, about its *qualitative* significance, but the quantitative aspects are not known.

Neergaard then set out to obtain quantitative values for pulmonary surface tension. He reasoned as follows:

To measure the influence of surface tension on retractility, the total retractile force must first be measured by known methods; that is, the so-called elasticity curve in relation to lung volume must be obtained. Since it is impossible to measure surface tension by itself independent of tissue elasticity, our only alternative was to eliminate surface tension in a second series of determinations, thus measuring tissue elasticity separately. The difference between total retraction and the retraction remaining after elimination of surface tension is a measure of surface tension at the same lung volume.

To eliminate surface tension, the lungs had to be filled with a fluid down to the alveoli to remove the effect of the air-tissue interface. . . . *the lung was finally emptied of air by a pressure difference method and then immediately filled with an isotonic gum solution.* By the addition of about 7 percent gum arabic to the Tyrode solution, the oncotic pressure was adjusted so that no edema occurred. The solution thus obtained met physiological requirements to a very high degree [see figure 3].

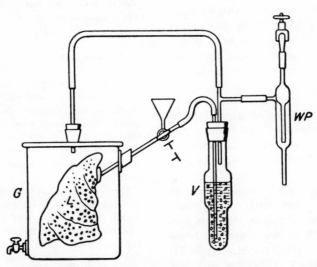

Fig. 3. Apparatus for evacuation of air from the lung. G = glass vessel; L = lung, the main bronchus of which has an airtight connection with the lateral support; V = water valve to obtain a difference between intrapleural and extrapleural pressure; WP = water jet pump. Between WP and V, a mercury manometer is used to determine total retraction on filling with air. From Neergaard (1).

Neergaard divided each experiment into two parts. First he measured the pressure-volume curve with the lung air-filled, and then again with the lung fluid-filled, to eliminate the air-fluid interface and the effects of surface tension; the second curve must then represent the force exerted by elastic tissues. By subtraction, he calculated the force exerted by surface tension. He found, in all states of expansion, that surface tension was responsible for more of total lung retraction than was tissue elasticity. To put it in another way, the pressure needed to distend the lung to a given volume was always higher when the lungs were air-filled and always lower when they were saline-filled. Thus Neergaard, using a direct, simple, unequivocal method, found that the Laplace (or the Young-Laplace) law held for pulmonary alveoli and that surface effects were important forces to be reckoned with in inspiration and expiration.

He went further in his experiments, reasoning, and speculation. He reasoned that the surface tension of alveoli may be lower than that of other body fluids, by the accumulation of surface-active substances, according to the Gibbs-Thomson law, and that "it is also conceivable that this [lower tension] would be useful for the respiratory mechanism because without it pulmonary retraction might become so great as to interfere with adequate expansion." He tried to measure surface tension of aqueous extracts of lungs and found unexpectedly low values of 35 to 41 dynes (water was 73, serum 60-65, and extracts of muscle, spleen, liver, and heart were between 47 and 53 dynes). He was not satisfied with his methods†† and suggested that the question (of surface tension as a force counteracting the first breath of the newly born) be investigated further. Unfortunately, he himself did not do so, and no one repeated or extended his experiments for more than 25 years.

In 1929, the year in which his now-famous report was published, he moved from Basel back to Zurich to become head physician at the Institute of Physical Therapy there. He never wrote another paper on the lung and did no further scientific investigations. Instead he immersed himself in subjects such as the interrelationship of medicine with philosophy, politics, and social problems (again, ahead of his time). In 1940 he was appointed Director of his clinic and Professor of Physical Therapy in Zurich. He died in 1947, at least a decade before Clements demonstrated clearly, by direct measurement, that lungs contain a unique surfactant and a dozen years before Avery and Mead published direct evidence linking its absence to the respiratory distress syndrome of the newly born.

Why did Neergaard leave Basel and research shortly after making his most important discovery? No one knows for sure. He must have known that it was important because he used the word "Grundbegriff" (fundamental or basic principle) in the title of his article. But he received no recognition for his discovery, then or later in his life. Few of his obituaries in 1947 even mentioned that he had ever done research on the lung (just as Paul Bert's obituary told of his work on skin grafting but said little of his momentous study of the effects of high and low atmospheric pressures on man). Dr. Joan Gil has learned that Professor Böni, who was Neergaard's disciple, daily collaborator for his last 18 years in Zurich, and finally his successor, never heard Neergaard mention his work in Basel on pulmonary physiology or express any particular interest in the lung.

Apparently, Neergaard's work fell into the category described by Gunther Stent in his article "Prematurity and Uniqueness in Scientific Discovery" (26); according to Stent, a discovery is premature if its implications cannot be connected by a series of simple logical steps to canonical, or generally acceptable, knowledge. Von Neergaard by temperament was neither a fighter nor a scientific entrepreneur. As a result, his work, which could have led to saving lives of premature babies in the 1930s, suffered a premature death.

Neergaard's work ends Part I of this story. Part II (for the most part) begins 25 years post-Neergaard—in the mid-1950s.

---

†† Unfortunately, Neergaard worked with the equilibrium methods of Jäger (24) and Lenard (25) instead of methods that permitted changing the area of a surface film so as to alter the concentration of water-insoluble molecules such as lipids; Neergaard must have regarded the moist surface alveolar layer as water-soluble.

Acknowledgment

I acknowledge with thanks valuable assistance from Dr. Joan Gil, who made careful inquiries into Neergaard's career in Basel and Zurich, from Dr. John

148

Clements, who reviewed Part I, and from Drs. Alan Burton and Marsh Tenney.

References

1. von Neergaard, K.: Neue Auffassungen über einen Grundbegriff der Atemmechanik. Die Retraktionskraft der Lunge, abhängig von der Oberflächenspannung in den Alveolen, Z Gesamte Exp Med. 1929, *66*. 373–394. English translation in *Pulmonary and Respiratory Physiology*, Benchmark Papers in Human Physiology, J. H. Comroe, Jr., ed., Part I; Dowden, Hutchinson & Ross, Stroudsburg, Pa., 1976, pp. 214–234.

2. Ponder, E.: Essentials of General Physiology, Longmans, Green, New York, 1929, pp. 2, 3.

3. Laplace, P. S.: Traité de Mécanique Céleste, 5 vols., Crapelet, Courcier, Paris, 1798–1827.

4. Bowditch, N.: Mécanique Céleste by the Marquis de Laplace, translated and with a commentary by Nathaniel Bowditch, 4 vols., Little and Brown, Boston, 1829–1839. Reprinted by Chelsea Publishing Co., New York, 1966, 3,939 pp.

5. Poincaré, H.: The Foundations of Science, G. B. Halsted, trans., The Science Press, Lancaster, Pa., 1946, p. 298.

6. Young, T.: An essay on the cohesion of fluids, Philos Trans R Soc Lond, 1805, *95*, 74–87. Reprinted with alterations and additions in *Miscellaneous Works of the Late Thomas Young*, John Murray, London, 1885; see vol. 1, p. 436.

7. Burton, A. C.: On the physical equilibrium of small blood vessels, Am J Physiol, 1951, *164*, 319–329.

8. Woods, R. H.: A few applications of a physical theorem to membranes in the human body in a state of tension, J Anat Physiol, 1892, *26*, 362–370.

9. Burton, A. C.: in *Medical Physiology and Biophysics*, T. C. Ruch, and J. F. Fulton, ed.; Howell's Textbook of Physiology, ed. 18, W. B. Saunders, Philadelphia, 1960, pp. 660–666.

10. Radford, E. P., Jr.: Method for estimating respiratory surface area of mammalian lungs from their physical characteristics, Proc Soc Exp Biol Med, 1954, *87*, 58–61.

11. Rayleigh, J. W. S.: On the theory of surface forces, I & II, Philos Mag, 1890, *30*, 285–298, 465–475.

12. Langmuir, I.: The constitution and fundamental properties of solids and liquids. II. Liquids, J Am Chem Soc, 1917, *39*, 1848–1906.

13. Maxwell, J. C.: Capillary action, in *The Scientific Papers of James Clerk Maxwell*, vol. II, W. D. Niven, ed., Cambridge University Press, 1890, pp. 541–591.

14. Wilhelmy, L.: Ueber die Abhängigkeit der Capillaritäts-Constanten des Alkohols von Substanz und Gestalt des benetzten festen Körpers, Ann Phys Chem, 1863, *119*, 177–217.

15. Adams, N. K.: Thin films, Proc R Soc Lond [A], 1922, *101*, 516–531.

16. Pockles, A.: Surface tension, Nature, 1891, *43*, 437–439.

17. Bayliss, W. M.: Surface action, in *Principles of General Physiology*, ed. 1, chapter III, Longmans, Green, London, 1915, pp. 48–73.

18. Leathes, J. B.: Croonian lectures. On the role of fats in vital phenomena, Lecture II, Lancet, 1925, *1*, 853–856.

19. Rohrer, F.: Der Strömungswiderstand in den menschlichen Atemwegen und der Einfluss der unregelmässigen Verzweigung des Bronchialsystems auf den Atmungsverlauf in verschiedenen Lungenbezirken, Pfluegers Arch Gesamte Physiol, 1915, *162*, 225–299.

20. Fleisch, A.: Der Pneumotachograph: ein Apparat zur Geschwindigkeitsregistrierung der Atemluft, Pfluegers Arch, 1925, *209*, 715–716.

21. Wirz, K.: Das Verhalten des Druckes im Pleuraraum bei der Atmung und die Ursachen seiner Veränderlichkeit, Pfluegers Arch Gesamte Physiol, 1923, *199*, 1–56.

22. von Neergaard, K., and Wirz, K.: Über eine Methode zur Messung der Lungenelastizität am lebenden Menschen, insbesondere beim Emphysem, Z Klin Med, 1927, *105*, 35–50.

23. von Neergaard, K., and Wirz, K.: Die Messung der Strömungswiderstände in den Atemwegen des Menschen, insbesondere bei Asthma und Emphysem, Z Klin Med, 1927, *105*, 51–82.

24. Jäger, G.: Über die Abhängigkeit der Capillaritätsconstanten von der Temperatur und deren Bedeutung für die Theorie der Flüssigkeiten, Sitzungsber K Akad Wissen Wien, Math-Wissen Klasse, Abt. 2a, 1891, *100*, 245-270.

25. Lenard, P., Dallwitz-Wegener, R. v., and Zachmann, E.: Über Oberflachenspannungmessung, besonders nach der Abreissmethode, und über die Oberflachenspannung des Wassers, Ann Phys, 1924, *74*, 381–404.

26. Stent, G. S.: Prematurity and uniqueness in scientific discovery, Sci Am, 1972, *227* (6), 84–93.

Note: Translations of references 19, 21, 22 and 23 from German into English are available in *Translations in Respiratory Physiology*, West, J. B., ed., Stroudsburg, Pa., Dowden, Hutchinson & Ross, 1975.

Premature Science and Immature Lungs

Part II. Chemical Warfare and the Newly Born

In Part I I gave an account of the beginnings of the quantitative approach to surface tension (Laplace's law [1806], Bowditch's remarkable translation of it into English, with annotations and corrections [1829–39], and Young's work on cohesion of fluids [1804–05] which antedated Laplace's law) and of the considerable interest of physicists, chemists, and general physiologists in surface tension and interfacial phenomena. However, the discovery of surface forces was premature for mammalian physiologists; 123 years elapsed before Neergaard did his now-famous studies on surface forces generated by alveolar tissue-air interfaces. Neergaard's work was also premature for pulmonary physiologists who came after him, and another 25 years elapsed before his work was rediscovered. Part II tells some highlights of the 30-year post-Neergaard period up to the 1959 paper of Avery and Mead.

"Hyaline Membranes"

Not because of Neergaard's paper, but coincidentally with its publication, pediatricians and obstetricians became increasingly interested in the diagnosis and treatment of atelectasis of the newborn and in the pathologic state of lungs of infants who died with this syndrome. Curiously, they centered their interest on "hyaline (or hyaline-like) membranes" that pathologists, depending on the intensity of their convictions, found in the alveoli of all, most, many, or some newborn infants that had severe respiratory distress at birth and died shortly thereafter. These "membranes" had been described as early as 1903. They were the subject of three papers in the 1920s, nine in the 1940s, thirteen in the 1940s, and many more in the 1950s. In retrospect, they were not really membranes at all (in the sense of being a thin sheet covering or lining a tissue); they were merely a translucent, homogeneous something that stained with eosin. And they were the *result,* not the cause, of severe asphyxia and the consequent process of deterioration of cells, tissues, and the baby. More important, the "membranes" diverted the attention of most investigators away from atel-

ectasis and away from new concepts that might have led to finding the cause of the disorder; in retrospect they were red (eosinophilic) herrings drawn across the trail and distracted the scientific hounds.

The history of science contains many examples of investigators who considered a problem solved because they had named it (or renamed it); it seems that this happened in the case of "hyaline membrane disease."* The history of science also includes more scientists whose goal was to find the *presence* of something rather than the *absence* of something. Thus, in the late nineteenth century, when new pathogenic bacteria were discovered almost monthly and the *presence* of each was associated with a disease, nutritionists had a hard time selling the medical public that the *absence* of specific sub-

---

* At one time or another, the syndrome was called by 13 different names. The abundance of names and the paucity of evidence linking the name and the cause of the disease is another example of the "law" that the amount of knowledge of the *cause* of a disease is inversely proportional to the square of the *number of names* acquired by the disease.

stances, called vitamins, could also cause disease. Fascination with the *presence* of hyaline membranes may well have delayed the discovery of the *absence* of surfactant.

Not everyone concentrated his attention on hyaline membranes. Wilson and Farber in 1933 (27) emphasized the importance of "cohesion of the moist surfaces in collapsed and airless lungs." This "stickiness," they wrote, offers considerable resistance to the entry of air, and a relatively great force

> ... is required to overcome it and to separate the bronchiolar and alveolar walls during the initial expansion. The first breath of every new-born baby may thus be its most difficult one, and especially vigorous inspiratory efforts must be maintained for a variable period after birth until the normal atelectasis is finally overcome. This initial resistance of the atelectatic lungs to expansion is always present and contributes to the maintenance of atelectasis to a pathologic extent....

> It is believed that this initially lessened distensibility of the lungs after they have stood for several hours in a state of passive collapse or after they have been entirely exhausted of air by forceful suction is due to the cohesion of the moist surfaces of the air passages, and that this is an important factor in the maintenance of the fetal state of atelectasis after birth; it is a factor that is always present, and when combined with any of the other conditions to be discussed, it causes the state of atelectasis to persist to a pathologic extent.

Wilson and Farber in their report referred neither to Neergaard's research nor to Thomas Young's 1806 paper on cohesion. They noted that lungs that were collapsed and contained neither air nor liquid required considerable force to expand them initially and then less on subsequent breaths. They realized that babies born with atelectasis continued to have it for variable periods after birth but didn't connect it with the continued absence of something in the alveoli (other than the absence of air).

In 1947, Gruenwald (28), also not knowing of Neergaard's work, determined, first using saline and then air, the smallest pressure needed at autopsy to expand nonaerated lungs of stillborn infants and those dying shortly after birth. In 15 infants, the pressure was 9 cm H_2O for filling with saline and 18 for filling with air. This difference he attributed to the existence of surface tension at the tissue-air interface and its absence at tissue-saline interface. He decided to see whether anything could be done to decrease surface tension at the tissue-air interface. He introduced amyl acetate into the lungs by two methods; one consisted of forcing in air containing amyl acetate vapor and the other of rinsing the lung with 0.25 per cent amyl acetate in saline before introducing air. He reported his findings:

> There was a marked reduction in the pressure necessary to introduce air when amyl acetate was used by either of the two methods. The reduction amounts to nearly one-half the difference between the values for pure saline and air. This correlates well with the reduction of surface tension by amyl acetate, as shown roughly by the height of a fluid column in a capillary (33 mm for saline, and 21 mm for amyl acetate solution).

> Another change was noted when amyl acetate was used. The aeration was more diffuse than usual, affecting larger portions of a lobe at the same time without immediately expanding them completely. In this respect, too, the condition was intermediate between normal aeration and expansion with saline. It is thus demonstrable that surface tension is a major factor in the resistance of the lung of the newborn to aeration but does not interfere with the aspiration of fluid.

He then concluded by suggesting that the addition of surface active agents to the infant's inspired air or oxygen might be helpful in relieving initial atelectasis of newborn infants. Gruenwald, being a pathologist, could not put his suggestion into action; the pediatricians and obstetricians continued to debate the origin of hyaline membranes (29, 30).

Macklin and the Pneumonocytes

Staub, Clements, Permutt, and Proctor have recently written a brief biography and an appreciation of Macklin's work (31). Macklin spent most of his academic career as Professor of Histology and Embryology at the University of Western Ontario in Canada. Much of it was occupied studying the airways, the pulmonary circulation, and macrophages; some of it was devoted to speculation on surface forces in alveoli. Macklin, like others, was unaware of Neergaard's work and reasoning. Macklin's first reference to surface tension was a brief sentence in 1946 in a long paper describing epicytes (32). In it he stated that epicytes ("residual alveolar epithelial cells") may be in the class of a secretory cell and play a useful role in conditioning the surface fluid film of alveoli. "It may be," he wrote, "that it [the epicyte] contributes something to the circumscribing fluid film of the alveolar capillary wall which is advantageous in external respiration." In this 1946 statement he neither defined the "something" nor explained how it was "advantageous," but obviously he realized that it might be physiologically important, though he didn't specify how.

In 1954, Macklin (33) published his well-known paper on the alveolar mucoid film and the epicytes, which he had now renamed "pneumonocytes." In it he first noted that on September 4, 1953 (at the International Physiological Congress in Montreal) he had elaborated on his 1946 views and had suggested that a watery mucoid film, a hydrated secretion of granular pneumonocytes, provided a noncellular interface between alveolar air and the thin alveolar epithelium. He then elaborated on his 1953 suggestion by making a clear statement of his concept that a thin, aqueous, mucoid, cohesive flexible film, about 0.2 μm thick, covers alveolar walls and, as he put it:

. . . [performs] vital functions, such as assisting in the removal of fine living and dead particulate matter, the maintenance of a constant favourable alveolar surface tension, the facilitation of gaseous exchange, the protection of the underlying tissue from desiccation, and the suppression of invading micro-organisms. Its mechanism of production normally insures a constancy of volume, thickness, water and solid content, and other features.

There is evidence pointing to the granular pneumonocytes as the originators of the secretion which composes this film. . . .

It may be causally related to the myelin figures (Leathes 1925) which are seen by phase-contrast microscopy to emerge in great abundance from the surfaces of the alveolar walls in sections of fresh lung mounted in water or in physiological saline solution, for they are generated in hydrophilic material (Frey-Wyssling 1953b). It may have something to do with the inhibition of bubble formation, for in life no air-bubbles are normally formed in the alveoli. If they were so formed, in quantity, the effect would be disastrous.

Staub and associates (31) wrote:

Although Macklin did not overtly state that the granular pneumonocytes secrete surfactant, it is obvious that he recognized "myelinogens" (phospholipids) in the alveolar lining and knew that they were connected with the osmiophilic lamellar bodies of the granular pneumonocytes. He also recognized the aqueous, mucopolysaccharide-rich nature of the alveolar surface and the need to regulate alveolar surface tension.

Although the "aqueous, mucopolysaccharide-rich" film *is* indeed there, Macklin did not appreciate that on top of it is a monomolecular layer of phospholipid-containing surfactant and that this lowers surface tension of the film when alveoli become smaller. Macklin thought that the function of the film was to maintain a *"constant* favorable alveolar surface tension" (italics added); if he had written "constant*ly* favorable" he would have been correct—but instead he wrote "constant . . . tension." And so direct, tangible evidence of the existence of pulmonary surfactant was still a few years away.

The Role of Chemical Warfare Research

Macklin's work on the pneumonocytes was supported by the National Cancer Institute of Canada, but his earlier work on alveolar size was supported by the Canadian Chemical Warfare Laboratories (34, 35). Next in our highlights come the studies of Radford, Pattle, and Clements. Before going on to the research of each, it's worth recording in the history of science that their papers—ones that were crucial to the discovery of surfactant—were supported by the chemical warfare laboratories of the United States and England. Radford worked at Harvard supported by a contract from the Medical Research Laboratories of the U. S. Army Chemical Center; Pattle was a physicist-physiologist working full time for the British Chemical Defence Experimental Establishment at Porton, England, and Clements was a full-time clinical physiologist working at Edgewood, Md., in the U. S. Army Chemical Center. All had the over-all mission of preventing, diagnosing, and treating damage to personnel by a variety of war gases, such as the new nerve gases that cause neuromuscular block and respiratory paralysis, and phosgene, which causes pulmonary edema.

During World War II, the U. S. laboratories had an all-star uniformed staff including Alfred Gilman, Oscar Bodansky, George Koelle, Maurice Strauss, Hale Ham, Richard Bing, Clarke Wescoe, Timothy Talbot, Frederick Crescitelli, Frederick Phillips, and James Whittenberger; the staff at Porton included Sir Charles Lovatt Evans (physiology), J. H. Gaddum (pharmacology), and G. R. (later Sir Roy) Cameron (pathology). When peace came, medical research to combat the effects of chemical warfare continued on both sides of the Atlantic, both intramurally in government laboratories and extramurally supported by contracts at universities.

Chemical warfare has never been a popular wartime weapon and, except for isolated instances, has not been used since World War I. In a sense then, the input of dollars and manpower and the output of research for chemical defense have not been applied to the military needs for which they were intended. But somehow or other, though never planned that way by any general staff or commission or task force, research supported by chemical warfare dollars led to our first real understanding of the nature and cause of the respiratory distress syndrome in the newborn; that, in turn, proved essential for the first effective management of a disorder that, until a few years ago, caused the death of at least 20,000 newborn babies each year in this country alone. If you had known this when the Mansfield amendment (which prohibited Department of Defense scientists from doing basic research) was being debated by Congress, you might have testified that a lot of good science can come out of "military" research when the right commanding officer, the right scientific director, and the right scientists come together at the right moment. Basic research on alveolar surfactant never won any military battles, but it largely won the war against atelectasis of the newborn.

So much for this aside. Now for the work of Radford.

Radford and Alveolar Surface Area

At last we come to someone writing in English who knew of Neergaard's work.† Radford, before receiving his M.D. degree at Harvard (1946), went to Massachusetts Institute of Technology and had an excellent background in the physical sciences when he joined the physiology department first at Harvard Medical School (1949–52) and then at Harvard's School of Public Health (1952–55). Not only that but he

---

† Christie and McIntosh (1934) list Neergaard and Wirz (1927) and Neergaard (1929) in their bibliography but refer to the 1929 paper in their text only once, and incorrectly, in a listing of previous workers who had measured intrapleural pressure; Neergaard in 1929 reported only his work on excised lungs, distended either with air or fluid.

had an unusual dual knack of knowing how to apply physical knowledge to physiology and medicine and how to teach; when I organized a Medical Faculty Training Program at the University of Pennsylvania in 1956–57, designed to acquaint or reacquaint faculty members with both basic sciences and basic medical sciences, I turned to Radford (then at DuPont's Haskell Research Laboratories in Delaware) to give a course on "The Physical Basis for Analysis of Biological Processes" for the group, and a splendid course it was.

Radford didn't set out in his research to find the cause and treatment for atelectasis of the newborn. What he wanted to do in the early 1950s was to estimate the total surface area of the alveoli of mammalian lungs. The Harvard group of Whittenberger, Mead, and associates, at the School of Public Health, had a deep interest in pulmonary physiology, and alveolar surface area was an important number to those interested in diffusion and gas exchange between alveoli and pulmonary capillary blood. Radford believed that the estimates of this area that had been made using histologic methods (on lungs scarcely in a physiologic state) tended to result in overestimates of the number of alveoli and of the total alveolar surface. So he decided to use a physical method based on surface tension and energy. His work, which began in 1952, was published in 1954 (his first published paper) (36). In it he wrote:

> The method of estimating lung surface described in this report is based on physical measurements of the lungs and avoids any assumption of size or configuration of respiratory structures. The calculation depends on consideration of the changes in free energy of the lungs as they are deflated. During inflation, energy is stored by deforming elastic elements, and by the creation of a large air-liquid interface. If the lungs are deflated by allowing volume equilibrium at successive pressure decrements, the stored energy released during deflation can be measured. . . .
>
> As will be shown below, it is possible to estimate the contribution of elastic energy to the total free energy and obtain the surface free energy by difference. . . .
>
> Gas-free animal lungs are prepared by allowing the pulmonary blood flow to absorb the alveolar gases, after initially hyperventilating the lungs with pure oxygen. These completely deflated lungs are removed, filled with isotonic NaCl solution while suspended in a saline bath, and the "elastic" curve is obtained during deflation by allowing the volume to reach equilibrium at each pressure.

This curve is then compared with the deflation curve subsequently obtained in the same way after air inflation at the same temperature.

Here is another example of the Lost and Found Phenomenon (37). Radford did his initial experiments completely independently of Neergaard's work and did not know of Neergaard's paper until later in his experiments, when Mead found it in searching the literature. However, Radford's rediscovery provided a necessary confirmation of Neergaard's conclusions on the importance of surface tension in alveolar expansion and retraction. Radford then set out to calculate alveolar surface area. Using a figure of 50 dynes per cm (that of human serum) as that of the interfacial layer between tissue fluid and air in alveoli, he calculated that the total alveolar surface area was about one-tenth that calculated by those who had used histologic methods. He then commented on the difference in numbers obtained by the new and the old methods:

> The striking difference between the estimate for human lungs of 5 to 10 m2 by the method discussed in this report and the estimates of 50 to 100 m2 obtained from histologic measurements, deserves additional comment. None of the assumptions on which the surface energy method depends could account for this difference unless the lung surface were a semi-solid phase or consisted of a highly surface-active substance. *Neither of these possibilities is at all likely* [italics added].

Radford had come to a fork in the road and had to decide which fork to take: one, that his theory, assumptions, and calculations were correct, or the other, that his assumed value for surface tension was wrong and that instead, the "lung surface consisted of a highly surface-active substance." He chose the former, and missed the opportunity to be the first to find and identify pulmonary surfactant.

We might speculate why Radford had more faith in his values than in the estimates of histologists. In the 1950s and earlier, anatomists did not concern themselves with studying lungs under physiologic conditions and their data were suspect on this account. Histologists who studied lungs closer to their physiological state got smaller values for alveolar area; other got the higher figures. It was logical for Radford to question the histologists' data; it would have been illogical in 1954 to have assumed the existence of a biologic substance that could lower surface tension

to extremely low values. Radford therefore accepted a value of 50 dynes per cm for the surface tension of the alveolar film. Why wasn't he influenced more strongly by Neergaard's measurements of surface tension? Radford said in his paper (36):

> Neergaard . . . measured the surface tension coefficient of lung tissue extracts, using the method of Lenard *et al.* His results varied from 35 to 41 dynes/cm; in view of errors of the method and the presence of intracellular substances, these values cannot be applied to intact lungs. von Neergaard found no conclusive evidence for a surface-active film in the lung, and concluded that the interfacial layer is probably an aqueous solution having a surface tension coefficient near that of serum.

There were no published translations of Neergaard's German into English in 1954. Now there are two (38 a, b). The translators agree that what Neergaard wrote was as follows:

> In such extracts [aqueous extracts obtained from the lung parenchyma] . . . I found consistently unexpectedly low values of 35-41 dynes. From a physicochemical point of view, it would be understandable that surface-active substances gradually accumulate at the alveolar surface. . . . The uncertainty about our results, arising from the fact that we do not know the exact surface tension in the alveoli, cannot therefore be fundamental, because the surface tension of the gum solution is very low, and that in the alveoli must also be very low, that is, at the lower biological limit. . . . the error cannot be great; it is probably less than individual and species differences. Our main findings and their order of magnitude remain unchanged; nevertheless, the question should be further investigated.

I interpret Neergaard's words (in these translations) as an expression of his conviction that the surface tension at the alveolar-air interface must be very low, but that scientific caution compelled him to call for further investigation. Radford may have interpreted Neergaard's words as an expression of uncertainty about his method and that the surface tension must be near that of plasma. Further, Radford knew that lung tissue contained lipids that mixed with real lung tissue (alveolar walls), could give a misleadingly low value. Actually to a "fat and soap" scientist of Neergaard's time (and Neergaard consulted with Professor Scherrer of Zurich Federal Technological College who was quite sophisticated in surface chemistry), the difference between 50 dynes per cm (the value for plasma) and 35 (Neergaard's lowest value for lung extracts) was enormous; as Neergaard put it, 35 was "at the lower biological limit." However, Radford may have interpreted this difference as being within experimental error. We now know that pulmonary surfactant is unique in lowering surface tension far below 35 dynes per cm, to 10 dynes per cm or less.

Sometimes, an incorrect assumption or conclusion holds back scientific advance. In this case, Radford's did not, for it served as an important stimulus to others, including Clements a few years later, to reopen the issue. More of Clements soon; but first we should discuss Pattle and his noncollapsing foam.

Pattle and Pulmonary Edema Foam

Pattle became interested in science at an early age, "six or possibly earlier . . . particularly chemicals and such things as frogs and beetles." He went to Westminster School at the age of 14, started with the usual classical curriculum (which he didn't think did any harm), but switched to science a year later. He read the literature thoroughly for a prize essay on surface tension; he didn't win the prize because he never wrote the essay, but he acquired a good knowledge of surface forces at an early age.

Pattle received first class honours in physics at Oxford at 1940, then worked on medical aspects of the war effort from 1941 to 1943 with the British neurophysiologist, Weddell; his research dealt largely with clinical electromyography, denervated muscle and human pain fibers. In 1943, he joined the Royal Electrical and Mechanical Engineers, concerned mainly with radar, becoming a Captain in 1946. In 1947, while in Germany, he saw an advertisement for biophysicists, and applied and received a post, now in civil service, at the Chemical Defence Experimental Laboratory at Porton, England.

He worked in the Physics Department under H. L. Green and W. R. Lane, noted authorities on particulate clouds, dust, smokes, and mists, and they assigned him the task of studying surface tension in certain liquids intended to be used as aerosols. In the course of this work, he devised a simple method of producing a "raft" of equal-sized bubbles on the surface of a liquid. This "raft" could be measured and manipulated to yield useful information on the properties of the liquids. In 1950, he published a note on mutually immiscible layers, and two full papers, one on the production of small bubbles and the other on the mechanism of action of anti-foams. Though no one then knew it, this was the best possible groundwork for his later, completely unrelated, research.

However, in 1952, after several years of administrative assignments in London, Pattle returned to Porton to work under Dr. Kenneth Wilson in Porton's Physiology Department. (Wilson is now at the U. S. Army Chemical Center in Edgewood and Assistant Professor of Anesthesia at Johns Hopkins.) No one at Porton was then thinking about surface tension in pulmonary alveoli. From November 1952 to July 1953, John Clements joined Wilson's group as an exchange scientist from the U. S. Army Chemical Center— to do collaborative work on the treatment of nerve gas casualties. Johns and Cooper at Edgewood had just introduced mask-to-mask resuscitation for treating patients with respiratory paralysis, and the group at Porton frequently discussed pulmonary compliance and factors affecting it. Clements brought word of Radford's work-in-progress at Harvard and of the influence of surface tension on lung compliance; Neergaard's name had now reached England via Boston and Edgewood.

At this time, Pattle was still interested more in improving preamplifiers and electrodes for electromyography than in pulmonary physiology. But, even though a neurophysiologist, bubbles continued to intrude into his work. As he put it, "the curse of these microelectrodes was that small bubbles of air kept getting into them, and the only thing you could do was to wait until the bubble had disappeared under the influence of surface tension. This gave me the idea of measuring surface tension by the rate of contraction of a bubble." He became involved in pulmonary research in 1953— not because he wanted to find the cause and treatment of respiratory distress in newborn babies, but because of practical problems, again associated with bubbles. Phosgene kills by producing pulmonary edema so severe that foam fills alveoli and airways and causes asphyxia. One afternoon, Wilson was talking to Pattle over tea when the "Chief," Harry Cullumbine, and Professor Cameron dropped in. Cameron had been full-time at Porton during World War II and became so interested in pulmonary edema that he continued working part time at Porton for years after the end of the war. Cameron was studying experimentally-produced pulmonary edema in goats and losing most of them when foam welled into the airways. Cullumbine had learned of the work of Curry and Nickerson (39), who claimed that antifoam agents were effective in breaking up the foam of pulmonary edema, and Cameron remarked, "Pattle, I hear that you're an expert on foams." Pattle averred that he knew something about them. So Cameron continued, "Can you do something to break the foam in my goats?" Pattle thought he could, and started by repeating the work of Curry and Nickerson. However, when he added several powerful antifoams to a sample of tracheal foam from a rabbit suffering from pulmonary edema, the foam remained unaffected (40). Pattle knew then that the air bubbles of foam originating in alveoli must be covered with the lining layer of the alveolar surface, a unique material that conferred great stability on the bubbles.

Though he concluded that using silicone antifoams was an ineffective way of treatment of phosgene-induced edema, he became intensely interested in stable bubbles. In 1955, he published a note in *Nature* (41); it occupied only a little more than one column, but he packed a lot into it. Here are some excerpts from it:

> In acute lung oedema in the rabbit, fluid and foam are found in the trachea. This foam has an altogether peculiar property, in that it is unaffected by silicone anti-foams; these rapidly destroy the foams produced by shaking oedema fluid or blood serum with air. . . . Similar foams are obtained from healthy lung by cutting and squeezing under water, or after introduction of saline into the trachea. The stability of such foams is due to an insoluble surface layer on the bubbles; this layer can be attacked by pancreatin or by trypsin.
>
> Oedema foam is thus not produced by agitation of the oedema fluid with air during respiration; it can only have been formed by air originally contained in the fine air spaces of the lung being broken up into bubbles and afterwards expelled into the bronchi and trachea. The lining layer of the bubbles cannot have come from the oedema fluid, and must therefore have formed the original lining layer of the fine air spaces. . . .
>
> In air-saturated water, bubbles (say 40 μ in diameter) from foam from the lung usually remain unchanged in size for long periods (60 min.), whereas similar bubbles from serum and other foams, owing to their internal excess pressure, dissolve and disappear within a few

minutes. The surface tension of the lung bubbles is therefore zero; or, to put this another way, the surface pressure of the layer is equal to the surface tension of the underlying liquid. . . .

> 40-μ bubbles squeezed from a fragment of the artificially inflated lung of a mature foetal rabbit (within a few seconds of inflation) and kept in air-saturated saline usually contract by about 30 per cent in diameter and then remain stable. The layer is therefore initially formed by rapid surface adsorption from a substance already present in the foetal lung. It probably matures somewhat during the first few hours after birth. . . .
>
> By none of the many methods tried have small bubbles stable in air-saturated saline been regularly produced from blood or from amniotic fluid. The layer is thus not formed from either of these liquids, or from a transudate from the blood. Such bubbles have been formed from nasal (but not, so far, from tracheal) mucus: they are easily formed from a solution of an extract of hog gastric mucosa ('gastric mucin'), and from this solution also a foam resistant to silicone anti-foams has been prepared. These findings suggest that a layer of some form of mucus [Macklin in 1954 had referred to it as a mucoid film], secreted in the depths of the lung, is the source of the insoluble alveolar lining layer.

Pattle also proposed that a very low surface tension was essential if an alveolar lining layer was to prevent continuous transudation into alveoli and consequent pulmonary edema. He wrote:

> Published calculations on the pressure balance between the lung capillaries and the alveoli have disregarded the surface tension at the sharply curved, and probably moist, alveolar wall. If the surface tension were that of an ordinary liquid, enough suction would be exerted to fill the alveoli with a transudate from the capillaries. Means for keeping the surface tension low must therefore be part of the design of the lung. It is thus evident that the alveoli are lined with an insoluble protein layer which can abolish the tension of the alveolar surface.

This concept has not yet been susceptible to direct experimental proof.

Because the Porton laboratories became involved in a study of atmospheric pollutants (as a result of the Great London Smog of December 1952, in which 4,000 people died), Pattle published no more on the subject until 1958 when a full paper, with the same title as the 1955 paper, appeared in the Proceedings of the Royal Society of London (42). This contained a paragraph well worth adding to the above excerpts:

> The finding that the lung lining substance appears only late in the foetal life of the guinea-pig suggests that absence of the lining substance may sometimes be one of the difficulties with which a premature baby has to contend; such a defect may possibly play a part in causing some cases of atelectasis neonatorum. The appearance of a hyaline membrane might possibly be due either to a defective lining layer causing transudation from the blood or to excessive secretion of lining substance. These matters need experimental investigation.

In the meantime, Clements, working in the Chemical Warfare Medical Research Laboratories on the other side of the Atlantic (at Edgewood, Maryland) began to worry seriously about Radford's data and Pattle's statement on zero surface tension.

Clements and Quantitative Studies of Surfactant

Clements, very much like Pattle, decided on his career at an early age. Clements decided to be a scientist when 8 or 9 years old and announced the decision to the world (or at least to his neighborhood) by cutting the letters S-C-I-E-N-T-I-S-T out of the front of a heavy cardboard box, then lining the inside of the box with red paper, installing a flashing light behind the letters and finally placing the completed sign in the front window of the family's house, advertising his wares (figure 1). (I hope that the neighbors got close enough to read SCIENTIST instead of standing off and recognizing only a red light.) He didn't know what kind of scientist he wanted to be and debated a bit between chemical engineering and medicine. His father helped him to decide by sending him on a tour of industrial chemical engineering plants; that tour settled him on medicine.

His decision to go into medical research was reinforced by the state of medical knowledge when he was a medical student between 1943–1947. He found so much in each patient that was unknown that he felt it impossible to have a satisfying career in the practice of medicine. Therefore, after receiving his M.D. in 1947, he skipped the internship and went directly into the department of physiology at Cornell Medical College, headed by Eugene DuBois. Clements thought that he would like to study neurochemistry, especially the intermediary metabolism of brain tissue. But two years later, James Forrestal, Secretary of Defense, issued an appeal to physicians to volunteer for Army service. It is said that his nationwide appeal netted three volunteers, one of whom was Clements, who had been in the Army Specialized Training Program while in medical school.

Fortunately for science (although not for Clements' later income), Clements, having no internship and no license to practice, was assigned for two years to the Army Chemical Corps Medical Research Laboratories at Edgewood, Maryland. At the end of this hitch, Captain Clements decided that he liked the scientific environment at Edgewood and the freedom that he had there to follow his own ideas,** and he stayed on as a scientist in civil service. Edgewood did have some unique aspects: the Research Laboratory's military commander was Colonel John Wood, a highly respected and beloved man, and its civilian Director of Research was D. Bruce Dill, one of America's leading physiologists. And Edgewood was close to Baltimore and Hopkins (where Clements had a part-time appointment as Lecturer in Anesthesiology) and to Philadelphia and Penn (where he was a Research Associate in Physiology).

Clements' first years at Edgewood were spent working on a continuous method for measuring oxygen tension in flowing blood, studying nerve-gas poisoning and methods of treating it

---

** That he was not completely free from administrative work is attested to by this letter:

Dear Doctor Comroe:

    In order to comply with current Army Regulations and directives from the Office of Chief Chemical Officer re proposed publications, manuscripts of scientific papers pertaining to research performed under contractual agreement with these Laboratories must be forwarded in sextuplicate to these Laboratories for clearance prior to submission to the publisher. Present experience indicates that about four weeks are required for action on clearance.

    Your cooperation in this matter is appreciated.

           Very truly yours,

14 July 1952   John A. Clements

           Contract-Project Officer

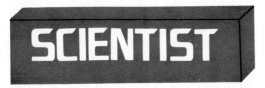

Fig. 1. A Madison Avenue concept of Clements' window ad.

(including artificial respiration) and measuring respiratory dead space, airway and pulmonary tissue resistance, and lung compliance.

When Radford submitted the report on his research to Edgewood (1953), Clements thought a great deal about it, and became increasingly unhappy with Radford's conclusion that the histologic estimates of lung area could be so bad as to be ten times too high. Clements applied Laplace's equation to the data and found that calculated surface tension was not 50 dynes per cm at low volumes but fell to values far lower than that, and changed with changing lung volume.

At this point, Elwyn Brown, an anesthesiologist, received a "Greetings" letter and came to Edgewood for a 2-year hitch to work in Clements' lab. At Clements' suggestion, he repeated and extended Radford's work, but he used 50 dynes per cm as the upper limit for surface tension (maximal inspiration) and a calculated value of 15-20 dynes per cm at maximal expiration. Calculated alveolar area now agreed well with histologic estimates of surface area (43). Radford visited Clements and Brown at Edgewood in 1955 and discussed ongoing work on surface tension; he became convinced at this time that lung surface tension was not necessarily fixed at 50 dynes per cm (that of plasma) and that the values he had assumed in 1954 to be correct were not.

Clements, impressed by Pattle's observations on pulmonary edema foam and stable bubbles but unhappy with the fact that they were qualitative estimates, decided the time had come to be quantitative about pulmonary surface tension. Of crucial importance was Clements' decision *not* to use methods that provided a single static value of surface tension (especially of stretched film, as Neergaard had done). Instead he used a dynamic method that provided continuous measurements while he altered the surface area in which molecules of surfactant were contained; this permitted him to measure surface tension in a compressed film as well. He constructed a modified surface balance, combining features of both Wilhelmy's balance and the Langmuir-Adam film balance. He was now able to mince whole lungs, place extracts in the balance, and measure continuously the surface tension while alternately compressing and expanding the surface layer. At the 1956 fall meetings of the American Physiological Society, he reported his remarkable findings (44):

The force-area behavior of surface films prepared from rat, cat and dog lungs has been studied. Surface tension falls from 46-44 to a limiting value of 10-1 dynes per centimeter upon compression of the surface to 30% of its area, with a minimum compressibility of 0.015 to 0.020 cm/dyne. Upon extension the surface shows extreme hysteresis, 10% expansion returning the tension to the upper limit of 46.

In 1957, he published his results more fully (45). Figure 1 from his 1957 paper (see figure 2) shows the close correspondence between the surface tension of plasma and that of lung extract when the surfaces on the Wilhelmy balance were expanded and the marked deviation when they were compressed. Here indeed was a unique surface active material in that it had a variable effect on surface tension such that surface tension decreased to as little as 10 dynes per cm when the surface film was compressed. This obviously was the antiatelectasis factor that was necessary for alveoli to remain open during

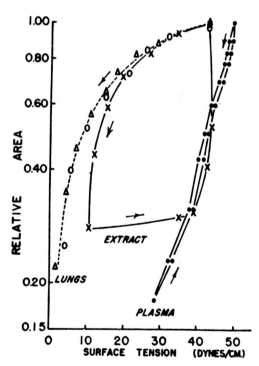

Fig. 2. Variation of surface tension with surface area. Upper curve (lungs) calculated on the basis of relative area from Brown's data. Large loop constructed from measurements on lung extract in Wilhelmy balance. Narrow loop constructed from measurements on blood plasma in Wilhelmy balance. (Clements, figure 1, 1957)

158

complete expiration. A few others had toyed with the idea previously, but here was proof. The flood gates were now open for all types of applications to physiology and medicine.

Before going on to further developments, I want to make two comments. The first is that Neergaard's work went unappreciated for 25 years (was "premature") because recognition of its significance required that it come to the attention of scientists who were both trained in physics and mathematics and interested in the lungs. Radford was well trained in physics and Pattle was a physicist. Clements had no mathematics in college and no special training in physics, but a friend taught him rudiments of calculus when both were medical students together and Clements took advanced courses in math at Columbia's night school as soon as he became a physiologist by day at Cornell; physics and physical chemistry, he taught himself. The second point relates to the importance of good communication among scientists. Afternoon tea in British laboratories is not merely a social rite but a way of getting scientists together who, without tea, might never have known of the others' existence. In addition, the close ties between Edgewood, Porton, and Harvard scientists also speeded the exchange of information and ideas. You may read of highly secretive, competitive scientists who clutch their data close to their breasts until their report is published, but Radford, Clements, Pattle, Avery, and Mead were not of this type; each knew what the other was doing long before formal publication. There were no lags here that could be attributed to poor communication.

Avery; Lungs without Surfactant

When Clements constructed his first surface balance in 1955 from sealing wax, chewing gum string, and other odds and ends, it was probably the only such balance in use in biomedical laboratories. Today, to keep up with the demands of researchers on surface tension, surface balances are made commercially, not by one mechanic working in his garage on weekends, but by at least seven widely known instrument companies. The boom began when Avery and Mead proved that something was wrong with pulmonary surfactant in babies born with respiratory distress syndrome—i.e., what was wrong was that it wasn't there.

Mary Ellen Avery received her M.D. degree from Johns Hopkins in 1952. Within a few months, she received a discouraging blow—she learned that she had pulmonary tuberculosis, and she was shipped off to Trudeau Sanitarium. When she got there and was labeled "complete bed rest" (chemotherapy of tuberculosis was just in its infancy) with the prospect of two years in bed, she began to do what every good scientist does—she doubted the rationale of established regimens. Why, she thought, does lying on one's back for two years have any beneficial effect on the course of pulmonary tuberculosis? Not getting any good answer, she checked out of Trudeau after two days, went home for a year, then abroad for six months and then started her internship at Hopkins. But the experience was probably critical in her choice of career. One can't be laid up with pulmonary disease for a year or more without thinking and reading and then thinking some more about lungs, and so she became a pediatrician with a subspecialty in pulmonary disease.

During her residency in pediatrics, over and over again she watched newborn babies either taking their first breath or not taking it and she couldn't get answers to penetrating questions about why *yes* and why *no*. Worse yet, she saw clinicians treating respiratory failure in the newborn with the Bloxsom apparatus which at best produced two breaths per minute. So she decided that absolutely essential to good diagnosis and care of the newborn was *new knowledge* (to replace hallowed customs) and if she was ever to contribute some herself, she needed advanced training in research. She consulted Richard Riley at Hopkins and he suggested several centers. She received a two-year special traineeship from the N.I.H. and chose the Boston Lying-in Hospital because Clement Smith was there, making physiological measurements of respiration in newborn babies, and Whittenberger and Mead worked across the street in the School of Public Health. Thus she had the best of both worlds: she could work with the physiologists between 9 and 5 and go across the street to observe the newly born in the early mornings and evenings.

Mead was interested in studying pulmonary edema in dogs (again supported by a contract from the Army Chemical Center) and he asked her to do some thinking about where the foam originates. So she went to the M.I.T. library and read about foam and surface chemistry and ran into Pattle's article on stable bubbles. She didn't like the idea of using a microscope to measure the diameter of bubbles in foam as a quantitative approach to research on edema so she asked Whittenberger about alternative methods. An Edgewood alumnus himself (from World War II), Whittenberger sent her to Clements to learn how to use a surface balance. Clements recalls that she probably didn't think much of his home-made balance but she went back to Boston where she and Mead made a better balance and went to work. Having a clinical traineeship at the Lying-in Hospital gave her access to lungs of babies who had just died of respiratory distress syndrome and, in no time, before cells could deteriorate, extracts of these lungs were in her surface balance.

Avery and Mead studied the lungs of individuals without "hyaline membrane disease": 35 were infants, 5 were children who died between 9 weeks and 4 years of age, and 4 were adults. The mean minimal surface tension (on compression of the surface film) was 7.6, 6.7, and 7.2 dyne per cm, respectively, in these three groups. The minimal surface tension of lung extracts from nine infants who died of hyaline membrane disease was 30.4 dynes per cm. They concluded (46):

> The results show that without exception the surface behavior of lung extracts of the nine infants with hyaline membrane disease was different from that of infants dying from other causes and the same as that of infants smaller than 1,200 gm. This suggests that the disease is associated with the absence or delayed appearance of some substance which in the normal subject renders the internal surface capable of attaining a low surface tension when lung volume is decreased.
>
> It is of interest to attempt to relate the results obtained to the pathogenesis of the disease. In all lungs with the first breath, large pressures are necessary to create an air-liquid interface. In this respect the normal lung would not differ from the lung without the surface-active material since surface tension on extension of the surface is similar in both cases. Thereafter, during expiration, the alveolar surface of the normal lung would have diminished tension thus reducing the tendency of the air spaces to collapse. On the other hand, in a lung lacking this lining material, surface tension would tend to remain high during expiration; the air spaces would be unstable, and some would collapse. Once a sufficient number had closed, others would remain open inasmuch as the interpleural pressure at end-expiration would be sufficiently negative to prevent further closure. (46)

This explains clearly why the early explanation of atelectasis by Wilson and Farber (1933) based on cohesion (or stickiness) of the alveolar surfaces was an unsatisfactory one beyond the first inspiration of the newborn. Something had to be operating over a longer period of time to explain collapse of the lungs over and over again with each breath; it was the absence of surfactant instead of the presence of stickiness.

The measurements of Avery and Mead also provided the rationale for continuous positive airway pressure (CPAP) as a physiological method for managing the respiratory distress syndrome, though this was not accepted until the work of Gregory and associates in 1971.

Two asides here in connection with Avery's paper: (1) If you look at its credit line at the bottom of the first page, you will see that the work was supported by a special traineeship from the National Institute of Neurological Diseases and Blindness. I'm sure you're aware that a few congressmen (such as Senator—I forget his name, but he's the one who had transplant surgery [an unusual kind—external instead of internal]) scan the titles of projects to determine the appropriateness of support by a particular institute or indeed by any of the National Institutes of Health. In Avery's case, they might have been disturbed by finding that the Institute of Neurological Diseases and Blindness was supporting a youngster who wanted to learn about the mechanical properties of the lungs. I can't find the original application (applications were then only two pages, with five lines allowed to describe the training plan) but I suspect that the body of the grant pointed out that the respiratory difficulties in the newborn might be due to damage to the respiratory center and hence be appropriate for support by a Neurological Institute. It's hard to judge a book (or a Retrospectroscope article) by its title and even harder to know the importance of a grant proposal by its title. (2) Inexplicable events occur in the transmission of scientific knowledge. In 1961, Jere Mead wrote his classic *Physiological Reviews* article, "Mechanical Properties of Lungs" (47). It included a ten-page scholarly discussion of pulmonary surface tension and 258 references; among these were a 1959 paper by Avery, Frank, and Gribetz and a 1960 paper by Avery but *not* the Avery and Mead paper of 1959 proving that the minimal surface tension of extracts was invariably high when prepared from the lungs of babies who died of hyaline membrane disease. Let this be a warning to those who depend upon review articles to find *every* important published article!

The Attack on Immature Lungs

Avery and Mead's discovery ended Phase 2 of this story. No longer were discoveries premature; each now reached receptive and perceptive basic and clinical scientists. But Phase 3 had now begun and a tremendous amount still had to be learned: the chemical composition of surfactant; its source: factors regulating its release and replenishment; how to detect its absence in the fetus; how to hasten maturation of the lungs; how best to ventilate immature lungs that contain little or no surfactant. Part III considers these matters.

References

27. Wilson, J. L., and Farber, S.: Pathogenesis of atelectasis of the new-born, Am J Dis Child, 1933, *46*, 590-603.

28. Gruenwald, P.: Surface tension as a factor in the resistance of neonatal lungs to aeration, Am J Obstet Gynecol, 1947, *53*, 996-1007.

29. Miller, H. C., and Jennison, M. H.: Study of pulmonary hyaline-like material in 4117 consecutive births. Incidence, pathogenesis and diagnosis, Pediatrics, 1950, *5*, 7-20.

30. Tran-Dinh-De, and Anderson, G. W.: Hyaline-like membranes associated with diseases of the new-born lungs. A review of the literature, Obstet Gynecol Survey, 1953, *8*, 1-44.

31. Staub, N. C., Clements, J. A., Permutt, S., and Proctor, D. F.: Charles Clifford Macklin; 1883-1959: An appreciation, Am Rev Respir Dis, 1976, *114*, 823-830.

32. Macklin, C. C.: Residual epithelial cells on the pulmonary alveolar walls of mammals, Trans R Soc Canada, 1946, *40*, 93-111.

33. Macklin, C. C.: The pulmonary alveolar mucoid film and the pneumonocytes, Lancet, 1954, *1*, 1099-1104.

34. Macklin, C. C.: The size of pulmonic alveoli based on measurements of their outlines in 25-μ microsections of human and common laboratory animal lungs fixed in the state of expansion, Report to Section of Physiology, Chemical Warfare Laboratories, Ottawa, Canada, June 30, 1943.

35. Macklin, C. C.: The alveoli of the mammalian lung. An anatomical study with clinical correlations, Proc Inst Med Chicago, 1950, *18*, 78-95.

36. Radford, E. P., Jr.: Method for estimating respiratory surface area of mammalian lungs from their physical characteristics, Proc Soc Exp Biol Med, 1954, *87*, 58-63.

37. McDowell, R. S., and McCutchen, C. W.: The Thoreau-Reynolds Ridge, a Lost and Found Phenomenon, Science, 1971, *172*, p. 973.

38. Neergaard, K. v.: (a) New interpretations of basic concepts of respiratory mechanics. Correlation of pulmonary recoil force with surface tension in the alveoli, Rattenborg, C., trans., in *Translations in Respiratory Physiology*, West, J. B., ed., Dowden, Hutchinson & Ross, Stroudsburg, Pa., 1975; (b) New notions on a fundamental principle of respiratory mechanics: The retractile force of the lungs, dependent on the surface tension in the alveoli, Arnhold, R., and Hahn, H., trans., in *Pulmonary and Respiratory Physiology*, Part I, Comroe, J. H., Jr., ed., Dowden, Hutchinson & Ross, Stroudsburg, Pa., 1976.

39. Curry, C. F., and Nickerson, M.: Control of pulmonary edema with silicone aerosols, J Pharmacol Exp Ther, 1952, *106*, 379-380.

40. Pattle, R. E.: A test of silicone anti-foam treatment of lung oedema in rabbits, J Pathol Bacteriol, 1956, *72*, 203-209.

41. Pattle, R. E.: Properties, function and origin of the alveolar lining layer, Nature, 1955, *175*, 1125-1126.

42. Pattle, R. E.: Properties, function and origin of the alveolar lining layer, Proc R Soc Lond B, 1958, *148*, 217-240.

43. Brown, E. S.: Lung area from surface tension effects, Proc Soc Exp Biol Med, 1957, *95*, 168-170.

44. Clements, J. A.: Dependence of pressure-volume characteristics of lungs on intrinsic surface active material, Am J Physiol, 1956, *187*, p. 592.

45. Clements, J. A.: Surface tension of lung extracts, Proc Soc Exp Biol Med, 1957, *95*, 170-172.

46. Avery, M. E., and Mead, J.: Surface properties in relation to atelectasis and hyaline membrane disease, Am J Dis Child, 1959, *97*, 517-523.

47. Mead, J.: Mechanical properties of lungs, Physiol Rev, 1961, *41*, 281-330.

Acknowledgment

I thank Drs. M. E. Avery, J. A. Clements, R. E. Pattle, E. P. Radford, and K. M. Wilson for their kindness in reconstructing events of 20-25 years ago.

Premature Science and Immature Lungs

Part III. The Attack on Immature Lungs

In Part I, I gave an account of the discovery of surface forces by Laplace and by Young (1805-1806) and of its first application to the lung by Von Neergaard in 1929. Part II told some highlights of the rediscovery of surface forces, the discovery of pulmonary surfactant and of its unique properties, and the finding that the lungs of babies who died of respiratory distress syndrome ("hyaline membrane disease") lacked this remarkable substance; part II dealt largely with the work of Radford, Pattle, Clements, Avery, and Mead. Part III tells of the multidisciplinary attack on immature lungs; it concludes this series, but not the story, because, as is almost always true in science, many questions still need answers.

Introduction

Thus far, the cast of characters—from 1805 to 1959—can be counted on the fingers of two hands. From here on, it numbers hundreds, perhaps thousands. The post-1959 cast is large because many important questions had to be answered: What is surfactant? Where does it come from, where does it go and what regulates its formation and movements? Can it or a similar substance be prepared synthetically and used as replacement therapy? Can the physician, instead of nature, make an immature lung become mature? Can the physician not only maintain the life of a newly born baby until the lung matures but also ensure normal postnatal function of all organs?

Fortunately, as often happens in science, pediatricians and pulmonary scientists were ready for new fields, and study of the newly born was one of the most challenging of these. And new technics, concepts, and knowledge discovered for other purposes, or just for the sake of knowing, were ready at the proper time to rescue the baby with immature lungs; these included the modern technics of lipid and protein chemistry (e.g., differential ultracentrifugation, a large number of chromatographic methods, electrophoresis, immunological methods, and the use of radioactive isotopes), high resolution electron microscopy, cell culture, and cell biology in general, the concept of intensive care units, and the ability to examine amniotic fluid.

It would take a scholarly monograph or two

to tell of the contributions from many scientists in many disciplines that made the respiratory distress syndrome one of the best studied of all disorders, and it would take most of the pages in this long article just to list those involved. All I can do is to tell of a few.

What Is Pulmonary Surfactant?

As biochemical technics became more and more powerful, knowledge of the chemical composition of surfactant became more and more exact. Macklin, who had only light microscopic and histochemical technics at his command, suggested that the surface lining of alveoli contained mucopolysaccharides and myelinogens and spoke of it as a "mucoid film" (48). Pattle in his 1955 report (49) noted that his bubbles owed their stability to an insoluble surface layer that was attacked successfully by protein-splitting enzymes such as pancreatin or trypsin. He said, "It is thus evident that the alveoli are lined with an insoluble protein layer" and "findings suggest that a layer of some form of mucus (Macklin 1954), secreted in the depths of the lung, is the source of the insoluble lining layer." In his 1958 paper (50) he suggested that the "lining layer is ... of similar thickness to a monolayer of protein spread on the surface of water, and very much thinner than any recorded membrane or anatomical structure."

Clements in his 1957 paper noted that surfactant was "saline-extractable" and "probably mucoprotein" (51). But in 1961, three groups, each using different methods, characterized it as a lipoprotein. Pattle and Thomas (52) forced water down the main bronchus of the excised lung of a cow, allowed the water to well out, laden with bubbles, washed and dried the material, and analyzed it spectrophotometrically; it had all of the characteristics of a lecithin-protein complex. Buckingham made extracts of sheep lungs, put them in a Langmuir trough, compressed the surface, and harvested folded films of surface material; she too found it to be a lipoprotein (53). And in the same year, Klaus, Clements, and Havel (54), using Bondurant and Miller's newly developed technic (collecting thick white foam from the trachea of beef lungs ventilated with intermittent positive pressure and perfused with saline through the pulmonary artery) (55), isolated a phospholipid fraction that decreased surface tension as much as extracts of whole lung; the material closely resembled dipalmitoyl lecithin.* The chemical analysis suggested that a matrix of protein was an essential component of functioning surfactant. A year later Brown isolated dipalmitoyl lecithin from saline washings of alveoli (56).

It is interesting that in 1946 Thannhauser and his associates (57) analyzed various organs for what was then called hydrolecithin or dipalmi*tyl* lecithin (but none other than our new friend DPL, or even newer, DPPC) and found that lung contained more of it than did other large-animal organs except brain. Thannhauser remarked that the physiological significance of the compound was unknown; I don't believe that he or anyone else ever made any attempt to find out why it was there even though Leathes in 1925 (58) had studied the behavior of hydrolecithin (DPL, DPPC) in surface films. In the 1940s, it was believed that the lung was an organ designed for gas exchange and the fewer cells there to get in the way of gas exchange the better. This is another example of premature science. Today, if someone found a new chemical substance in high (or even low) concentration in lung tissue, it would excite the interest of many scientists.

But DPL or DPPC wasn't the end of the story.

---

* The term *lecithin* is gradually disappearing from textbooks of biochemistry and is being replaced by the more specific *phosphatidyl choline*. Instead of the DPL (dipalmitoyl lecithin) of the 1960s, you will now see DPPC (dipalmitoyl phosphatidyl choline). I am reminded of the Swedish scientist working in America who said rather plaintively: *"Just as I learn to say jam, you change it to yelly."*

King summarized present knowledge of the lipid composition of the lung in 1974 (59); his table 1 contains 14 different lipid compounds isolated from the total lipids of whole lung—some in easily separated fractions of lung and some in fractions isolated by more sophisticated technics.

What about the protein fraction of surfactant? It is now certain, by use of immunologic technics, that surfactant contains one or more *specific* apoproteins that come neither from plasma nor from bacteriological contamination of lung tissue. Their function may be to accelerate the extracellular transport of surfactant from its intracellular origin to the alveolar interface (60). Mephistopheles in Goethe's *Faust* remarked that "blood is a super extraordinary juice"; it appears that surfactant, when fully characterized, will also be a "super extraordinary juice."

But chemical characterization of the phospholipids and apoproteins in surfactant did much more than just that. It opened a whole new field of biochemistry of the lung so that by 1976 it was possible for one to read a monograph of 534 pages entitled *The Biochemical Basis of Pulmonary Function* (61). And this was not merely biochemical analysis of whole lungs put through a meat grinder but separation of lung tissue into individual cell types, attempts to produce pure *in vitro* cultures of these, and the beginnings of examining the intracellular components of each. The alveolar Type II cell is one of these and is now known to be the source of surfactant.

Where Does It Come From?

Just as the development of new and more powerful methods provided answers to the question, "What is surfactant," so the use of the electron microscope provided answers to "Where does it come from," and the answers now included not only what *cell* but what parts of what cell.

Macklin, the first to propose the existence of surfactant, pointed to what we now call the alveolar Type II cell. This cell has had a lot of names. Macklin called it first the epicyte and then the pneumonocyte and more specifically the granular pneumonocyte. Others have called it the Type B cell; the Type II pneumonocyte; the great, large, or cuboidal alveolar cell; the secretory alveolar cell; and the niche, septal, or wall cell. Pattle was sure that surfactant came from deep in the lung and noted that "there seems very little [deep] in the lung except these alveolar cells which could possibly produce the complex" (62).

In 1954, Low (63) and Schlipköter (64), pioneers in studying the lung by electron microscopy, found mitochondria in the alveolar epithelial cells and also some unusual inclusion bodies with lamellar forms. Between 1956 and 1959, Schultz saw what he called mitochondrial transformations into lamellar forms, and for a while, histologists thought that at least some mitochondria turned into lamellar inclusion bodies.

The first connection between structure and function came a few years later. Woodside and Dalton (65) used the electron microscope in 1958 to study these forms in the lungs of mice and noted that they were absent until the seventeenth or eighteenth day of gestation (full term in mice is 19 to 21 days). Four years later, Buckingham and Avery (66) found that they could not detect surfactant in the lungs of fetal mice until the seventeenth or eighteenth day of gestation; the appearance of lamellar forms and surfactant at about the same time led them to propose that the lamellar forms secrete surfactant.

In the same year, Klaus and associates (67) studied structure and function (surface activity) in the same lungs and concluded that "the surface active lining of the lung develops during the process of lamellar transformation of mitochondria in the alveolar epithelial cell." Pattle (62), in his 1965 *Physiological Reviews* article, questioned whether their mitochondrial fraction was pure or whether this fraction contained a number of discrete organelles, and he placed the subcellular origin of surfactant in his list of unanswered questions.

In 1965 Campiche (68), fixing lung tissue with potassium permanganate (which binds to saturated lipids) rather than osmium tetroxide (which does not), believed that he could safely say that the lamellar inclusion bodies were similar to myelin figures and were composed largely of phospholipids, possibly similar to saturated lecithin, then known to have powerful surfactant properties.

But not everyone believed that the answers were all in. Some suggested that surfactant was assembled, wholly or in part, in cells that were not part of the alveolar wall; two candidates that were proposed were the Clara cells in terminal bronchioles and alveolar macrophages. Eventually, overwhelming indirect evidence and convincing direct evidence, based on developmental, cytochemical, and autoradiographic studies, pointed only to the lamellar inclusion bodies of the alveolar Type II cell as the sur-

factant factory and eliminated its mitochondria and other non-alveolar cells (see Gil and Reiss [69]).

But cell biologists had now committed themselves to the study of alveolar cells, and a modern cell biologist is not satisfied with a static picture of what a cell looks like at one moment (no matter how great the magnification and resolution), but wants to visualize and reconstruct dynamic events in the daily life of the cell. Surfactant, which means phospholipids and proteins, must come from somewhere within the cell, be assembled into lamellar inclusion bodies, and, when so directed, move out of the cell— through the cell membrane into the alveolar air space and by some magic become a monomolecular layer covering everything in sight.

Dr. Mary C. Williams has kindly selected from her vast collection some electron micrographs that show the birth of a lamellar inclusion body, its coming of age, and finally its leaving its home to venture out into the air spaces.

Figure 1 shows part of an alveolar Type II cell. At the top left is just a bit of the cell nucleus. In the center is a lamellar body. It bears a strong resemblance to the layers (lamellae) of an onion except for the dense center of the lamellar body. It also resembles the arrangement of long-known myelin layers, noted in 1854 by Virchow, and later shown to consist of bimolecular leaflets, or lamellae of lipids, that alternate with layers of water. Bimolecular leaflets of lipids, together with protein, are also part of the structure of cell membranes and have been studied extensively in nerve tissue. Their arrangement as intracellular inclusion bodies makes the alveolar Type II cell unique.

The beginning of a lamellar body is shown in the inset in figure 1. As described by Williams and Mason (70), synthesis of one lamellar body component, presumably protein, may precede initiation of phospholipid synthesis. The electron-dense, homogeneous appearance of the granular matrix suggests that the content is largely protein. The number of lamellae increases as the forming lamellar body enlarges, but the mechanisms by which phospholipid is added to the growing granule are not certain. Autoradiographic studies of adult lung suggest that small lamellar bodies may shuttle phospholipid from Golgi to nascent lamellar bodies. Other morphologic observations clearly demonstrate that, later in development, multivesicular bodies participate in lamellar body formation, perhaps by fusion.

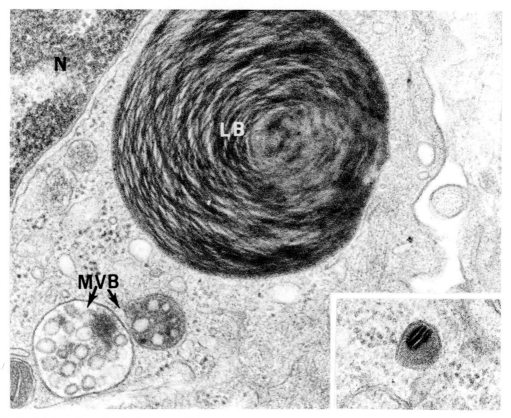

Fig. 1. Portion of an alveolar Type II cell from adult rat lung. N = nucleus. LB = large (mature?) lamellar body. MVBs = multivesicular bodies (Original magnification: × 29,000). Courtesy of Dr. Mary C. Williams. (*Inset*) Small dense granule in alveolar Type II cell of 21-day fetal rat lung. It contains acid phosphatase and a few lamellae. Such a granule is the earliest recognizable lamellar body in fetal lung; it precedes by several days the appearance of lamellae. (Original magnification: × 75,000.) Courtesy of Dr. Mary C. Williams.

What regulates the number and size of lamellar bodies is not known, although adrenal cortical hormones certainly play a role in maturing alveolar Type II cells to the stage of producing lamellar bodies. Some have evidence, not yet completely convincing, that the vagus nerves play a regulatory role.

What prompts mature lamellar bodies to seek the surface of the cell and slip through the cell wall into the air spaces (figure 2) is not known. Once there, the strands or membranes of a lamella unwind and become transformed into tubular myelin, a constant element of the extracellular lining layer of mammalian alveoli and a second form of surfactant; lamellar body membranes become continuous with those of the forming tubular myelin. If ever proof was needed that intracellular lamellar bodies become intra-alveolar lamellar bodies and these then become tubular myelin, it is provided by the continuities, shown in figure 3, between the unwind-

ing lamellae and the threads of the tubular myelin lattice-work (71). The centers of many secreted lamellar bodies are then seen to contain acid phosphatase-reactive material.

We've come a long way in 25 years from uncertainty about the very existence of a continuous cellular lining of alveoli (were the pulmonary capillaries naked?) to proof of a cell lining covered with a noncellular lining of super extraordinary juice.

Predicting Immature Lungs

There are many wondrous things about life. One of the most remarkable is how a single cell, the fertilized ovum, differentiates to form all of the highly specialized fluids, cells, tissues, and organs that make up a fetus, how the fetus develops into a newborn baby, how the baby grows into a pubescent child and the child matures into an adult—with each single event occurring on schedule, neither too early nor too late.

In the lungs, for example, the cuboidal cells that line what later on will be air-filled alveoli must become exquisitely thin, on schedule, to facilitate the postnatal transfer of gases between air and blood. And pulmonary capillaries, although little blood flows through them in fetal life, must, again right on schedule, multiply in close relationship to the future air sacs and be ready to accept the entire output of the heart each minute. Further, the alveolar surfaces must become prepared so that they permit inflation during inspiration and resist collapse during expiration. An essential item is surfactant, to prevent alveolar collapse after contraction of strong inspiratory muscles has brought the first breath of air deep into the baby's lungs and the time has come for the first expiration. The most remarkable part about this process of differentiation and development is not that once in a while something is off schedule, but that it almost always goes right *on* schedule.

What is the time schedule in the human fetus

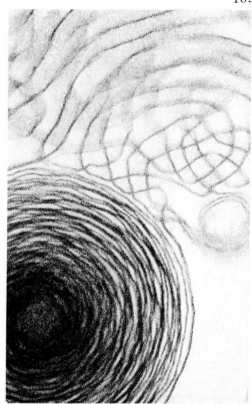

Fig. 3. Portion of a lamellar body that was extruded into a fluid-filled alveolar lumen of 21-day fetal rat lung. Note the continuities between the membranes of the lamellar body and tubular myelin (the lattice-like material on the right); these continuities suggest that a second material is formed within the alveolar lumen. Both the original and the new material are believed to be surfactants. (Original magnification: × 88,000) (From Williams [71]; reprinted by permission of publisher.)

for ensuring functioning surfactant? I say *functioning,* because as we have noted earlier, it can function only when it has spread as an extremely thin layer on the air side of the cells that line the alveoli. So there are really several schedules for surfactant: its synthesis; its packaging into lamellar bodies within alveolar Type II cells, its migration to the cell wall, its passage through the wall, and finally its transformation into an exceedingly thin surface layer. Total surfactant (intra- and extracellular) can be measured by mincing or homogenizing whole lung; intracellular surfactant can be estimated by counting the number of lamellar bodies (72); surface surfactant can be measured in lung washings or lung fluid, obtained without letting the insides of cells spill out.

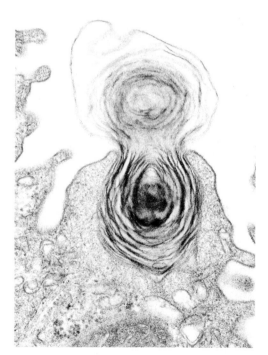

Fig. 2. Lamellar body being extruded from alveolar Type II cell into the lumen of an alveolus. 21-day fetal rat lung (Original magnification: × 35,000.) Courtesy of Dr. Mary C. Williams.

Intracellular surfactant in the human fetal lung appears long before there is a known need for it, at about the eighteenth to twentieth week, before a fetus is viable even if a physician could ventilate the lungs. However, it cannot usually be recovered from alveolar surfaces until about the thirtieth week and now the fetus *is* viable; at about the thirty-third week, the amount on surfaces begins to increase with a rush and by the end of a normal term, it is in abundance just where it ought to be.

Knowing the time when surfactant should normally arrive at its place of business could be very useful clinically if the physician had answers to two questions: (*1*) Does a particular fetus, apt to become a baby prematurely (either naturally or because of medical need for early delivery), have adequate surfactant ready to go to work? (*2*) If it does not, can anything be done about it?

First, *prenatal* tests. Fortunately, in the 1930s obstetricians learned from a radiologist (73) and from a biochemist (74) that, particularly in the last trimester of pregnancy, it was safe to insert a needle through the pregnant mother's abdomen directly into the amniotic sac and draw off a small sample of amniotic fluid for analysis. Until the 1960s, this could not be of any diagnostic use in a fetus with immature lungs because everyone "knew" since 1885 (75) that fetal lungs were filled with fluid and that this was mostly amniotic fluid (and whatever else was in it) that somehow or other had worked its way down the trachea into the lungs along with a little mucus secreted by glands lining the airways. But some had the idea that the flow of fluid between amniotic fluid and alveoli was mainly *out* of the lungs and *into* amniotic fluid and not the other way round, and they proved their point.

Jost and Policard in 1948 (76) showed, with some experimental overkill, that the lungs of the fetal rabbit became abnormally filled with fluid even after they had decapitated the fetus and securely tied off the neck, including the trachea; they proposed that the lungs contributed fluid to the amniotic fluid rather than the other way round. Setnikar, Agostoni, and Taglietti in 1959 (77), with a more sophisticated experimental technic, delivered the head of fetal goats from the mother's uterus, tied a tube in the trachea of the fetus, replaced the fetus in the uterus, and sewed up the incision in the uterus, leaving the other end of the tube on the outside. They were still able to collect tracheal fluid, thus confirming the studies of Jost and Policard; the

fluid could not possibly have come from amniotic fluid and must have originated in the lung.

In the 1960s, Forrest Adams and his associates (78) did a series of biochemical studies on lung fluid in fetal lambs that proved (*1*) that its chemical composition differed significantly from that of plasma or of amniotic fluid, (*2*) that fetal lung fluid contained surface-active materials not present in blood or pure amniotic fluid (79) (80), and (*3*) that the lung fluids flowed into amniotic fluid. This flow could occur either because the pressure developed by lung fluid as it formed was greater than that of amniotic fluid (81, 82) or because the fetus made breathing efforts *in utero* that brought some amniotic fluid into the lungs during inspiration and then expelled a mixture of lung fluid and amniotic fluid into the amniotic sac (83). Others showed that fetal alveolar liquid is not an ultrafiltrate of plasma but a special material formed by the fetal lung (84), and that the lung was the source of phospholipids present in tracheal fluid and probably of much of the phospholipids in amniotic fluid (81).

However, the first separation of lung fluids from amniotic fluid, without using tracheal tubes, came about in 1963, and with it came further proof that lung fluids flowed upward and outward and contained pulmonary surfactant. I have a brief report of it in my files in the form of an application, dated September 21, 1964, from a Senior Lecturer in Obstetrics at the National Women's Hospital in Auckland, New Zealand. The applicant's name was Dr. Graham Liggins (we come back to him later); he wanted to spend his sabbatical year working with Dr. Louis Holm, a physiologist at the University of California in Davis, and he needed $6,000 to help him survive our high cost of living for a year; this he received from the Lalor Foundation. Liggins's "plan of work" outlined in his application to the Lalor Foundation stated (in part):

> Using the facilities of the Animal Research Station, Ruakura, Hamilton [New Zealand], during the past three years, these techniques have been developed in the sheep.
>
> As the first step towards fetal transplantation in late pregnancy, the fetus is transferred from the uterus into a plastic bag within the maternal [sheep] abdomen, the cotyledons remaining undisturbed within the uterus. The allantoic and amniotic membranes are sealed over and *by suitable arrangements with plastic bags it is possible to collect the urinary and oropharyngeal contribu-*

tions separately [italics added]. At the same time, the amniotic and allantoic fluids (without fetal contribution) are available for sampling. Pregnancy continues normally in these circumstances.

Bilateral fetal adrenal ablation and hypophyseal ablation have been consistently achieved in sheep without interruption of the pregnancy. The adrenals are surgically exposed and then injected with a sclerosing fluid. The hypophysis is similarly ablated by blind introduction of a specially designed cannula.

It is intended that these techniques should be exploited in the following ways:

The geographical separation of the components of the liquor amnii provides an ideal basis for the study of feto-maternal and materno-fetal transfer of water, electrolytes and other solutes, employing isotope labelled materials.

The bag enclosing the fetal head has been found to contain a high concentration of surface-active material [italics added]. Collaboration with other workers in the field of lung surfactants is proposed . . .

The effect of fetal adrenal and hypophyseal ablation on parturition will be studied. The opportunity to extend work on the part which the fetal adrenal plays in estrogen metabolism will also be available.

The scope of this plan of work may seem too wide. However, it should be emphasised that it represents a period of intensive work on techniques which have been carefully prepared during the past 3 years so that delays from unexpected technical difficulties should be minimal.

None of the above techniques has been reported previously. It is known that unsuccessful attempts at fetal adrenalectomy and hypophysectomy (by decapitation) in larger animals have been made at centers in the United States. There is suggestive evidence from the known association of postmaturity with human anencephaly [congenital absence of the brain] and from the work of Holm (1961) in fetal calves with adrenal and hypophyseal hypoplasia that the onset of labor is closely related to fetal adrenal function, but direct experimental support for this hypothesis is lacking.

The field of fetal physiology has been a somewhat neglected one when compared with the work done on the neighbouring periods of life—embryonic and neonatal. This has been largely due to lack of suitable techniques by which to come to grips with the fetus in its protected environment. Until recently, experiments have been usually of an acute nature and often under most unphysiological conditions. Techniques such as those described above allow a direct approach while at the same time preserving a physiological state as far as possible.

Although none of those who studied the flow of lung fluids went so far as to propose a prenatal diagnostic test (possibly because there was none then known that would detect lung surfactant diluted by a large pool of amniotic fluid), they cleared the way to analyze human amniotic fluid and see if pulmonary surfactant was present. The first clinical prenatal test to identify immature lungs was devised by Gluck and his associates. Over a five-year period (1967 to 1972), they had done a careful analysis of the biochemical development of the mammalian fetal lung and published a series of papers in Pediatric Research. They noted that immature lungs were strikingly deficient in a major component of surfactant (lecithin) and that amniotic fluid analysis could be used not only to chart normal maturation of the lungs in utero but also to identify those fetuses who were almost certain to suffer from respiratory distress syndrome at birth. They used the ratio of lecithin (L) to sphingomyelin (S) in amniotic fluid. In babies with maturing lungs, the L concentration rises sharply at 35 weeks of gestation, usually to two times that of S, and continues to increase while S levels off or decreases. Gluck extracted phospholipids from about 5 ml of amniotic fluid and measured the L/S ratio by thin-layer chromatography; the analytic procedure required about 1½ to 2 hours (85). From this ratio he could now tell, before birth of the baby, whether the baby would (low ratio) or would not (high ratio) have respiratory distress syndrome. Knowing this greatly increased the baby's chances of survival if its mother was transported (by helicopter if need be) to a regional center staffed and equipped for, and dedicated to, intensive care of the newly born with respiratory distress syndrome (RDS), and the baby was born there.

It wasn't long before the need became apparent for a test that was as reliable as Gluck's, but faster, simpler, cheaper, and suitable for use in an office or even by a bedside. Clements and his group came up with one within the next year (86); it was based on Pattle's observation that where there was surfactant, there was stable foam. However, because other substances in amniotic fluid (proteins, bile salts, and salts of free fatty acids) can also form stable foam, Clements had to exclude these from the surface films; this he accomplished by adding a competitive (but nonfoaming) surfactant, ethyl alcohol. When he put equal volumes of 95 per cent alcohol and amniotic fluid in a tube and shook it, he found that when saturated lecithin (the kind that predominates in pulmonary surfactant) was present, foam formed and persisted for as long as several hours. Once one has obtained amniotic fluid, nothing could be simpler. The test does not require a highly trained biochemical technician; it needs only clean test tubes, pipettes, and 95 per cent alcohol. When amniotic fluid is not available, the test can be performed on fluid aspirated from the newborn's stomach, since this largely represents amniotic fluid, and maybe some tracheal fluid as well, that has been swallowed by the fetus.

Prevention of Respiratory Distress Syndrome

I said that basic data on the maturation of the lung might be clinically useful if (1) someone could develop a prenatal test that identified immature lungs (and two someones did), and (2) something could be done to make these lungs mature before or very shortly after delivery of the baby. Two "somethings" come to mind: (1) delay delivery, if possible and safe, for a day or two, and (2) hasten, by pharmacological means, maturation of the fetal lungs without harming other organs. The latter would be impossible if cells that normally form surfactant or systems that should release it from these cells are congenitally absent or defective. But it would be possible if all the parts of the machinery are there and ready to function but haven't yet got the signal from the programming system to get going.

We now come back to Graham Liggins, the obstetrician-researcher from New Zealand, who had started with the clinical observation that babies who were born without a brain (anencephalic) and therefore without a complete pituitary gland were often born postmature. Recall that in his 1964 application, he wanted to do a lot of things with his special sheep preparation (he allowed that "the scope of this plan of work may seem too wide") and one of these was to determine the effects on delivery of removal or destruction of the fetal pituitary gland and of the fetal adrenals (whose secretions depend on a functioning pituitary)—in short, did *fetal* hormones influence the time of delivery? When he got back to New Zealand in 1966, he continued to study the effect of ACTH and adrenal corticoids on the time of delivery; if removal of the fetal adrenals leads to postmature delivery, would injection of cortical hormones into the fetus lead to premature delivery? He injected dexamethasone into 10 lambs and in early 1969 reported these remarkable observations (88):

Gross examination of the lungs of ten lambs delivered spontaneously at 117–123 days after dexamethasone infusions showed that in six, none of which had been artificially ventilated, there was partial aeration. In most instances the aeration consisted of patchy expansion in the upper lobes, but in one lamb delivered at 123 days the lower lobes were also partly expanded. This lamb was found alive at least an hour after being born and survived for a further hour until killed. The body weight of 2349 g., the general appearance and the bone age determined by X-ray of the limbs corresponded with the duration of pregnancy calculated from the date of mating. During the period of observation the lamb bleated and showed some signs of respiratory distress. Histological examination of the lungs removed 4 hr. after death confirmed that alveolar expansion had been maintained. . . .

Cortisol is known to be capable of inducing precocious activity of a variety of enzymes in immature animals . . .

The observations on the foetal lungs of lambs at 117–123 days gestational age may represent another example of precocious induction of enzyme activity by corticosteroids. According to Howatt, Avery, Humphreys, Normand, Reid & Strang (1965), and Reynolds, Jacobson, Motoyama, Kikkawa, Craig, Orzalesi & Cook (1965), maintenance of alveolar expansion in the lamb is dependent on adequate surfactant activity. These authors and also Brumley, Chernick, Hodson, Normand, Fenner & Avery (1967), found that alveoli collapse and the lungs become airless at maturities of less than 125–127 days. Persistence of partial expansion of the lungs in the corticosteroid-treated lambs in the present series at 117–123 days strongly suggests accelerated appearance of surfactant, possibly as a result of premature activity of enzymes involved in a biosynthetic pathway. [Later studies (89) showed that fetal lambs have no or very little surfactant in their tracheal fluid at 124–133 days of age.]

Liggins now had a long list of studies that had to be done but decided to pass his observations on lung maturation on to others who had laboratories better equipped than his to do the necessary biochemical, biophysical, and electron microscopic studies. One of these was Avery, who visited New Zealand in March of 1968. On her return home she and her associates, first at Johns Hopkins and then at McGill (DeLemos, Kotas, Wang, Thurlbeck, and others), mounted a thorough attack on the problems (90–94), which confirmed and extended Liggins's observations and provided a morphological and biochemical framework for them.

Liggins decided instead to see if adrenal cortical hormones behaved in the human fetus as they did in the lamb—would they hasten the maturation of babies whose mothers were in spontaneous, premature labor? In 1972, he reported (95):

A controlled trial of betamethasone therapy was carried out in 282 mothers in whom premature delivery threatened or was planned before 37 weeks' gestation, in the hope of reducing the incidence of neonatal respiratory distress syndrome by accelerating functional maturation of the fetal lung.

Two hundred and thirteen mothers were in spontaneous premature labor. When necessary, ethanol or salbutamol infusions were used to delay delivery while steroid or placebo therapy was given. Delay for at least 24 hours was achieved in 77% of the mothers. In these unplanned deliveries, early neonatal mortality was 3.2% in the treated group and 15.0% in the controls (p 0.01). There were no deaths with hyaline membrane disease or intraventricular cerebral hemorrhage in infants of mothers who had received betamethasone for at least 24 hours before delivery. The respiratory distress syndrome occurred less often in treated babies (9.0%) than in controls (25.8%, p 0.003), but the difference was confined to babies of under 32 weeks' gestation who had been treated for at least 24 hours before delivery (11.8% of the treated babies compared with 69.6% of the control babies, p 0.02).

There may be an increased risk of fetal death in pregnancies complicated by severe hypertension-edema-proteinuria syndromes and treated with betamethasone, but no other hazard of steroid therapy was noted.

We conclude that this preliminary evidence justifies further trials, but that further work is needed before any new routine procedure is established.

Has further work established a role for pharmacological acceleration of lung maturation to prevent RDS? Apparently not if administered to a baby already born (because, postnatally, most infants with RDS have a marked increase in cortisol concentrations in plasma by 6 to 12 hours of age, presumably owing to the stress of the disease), but there *is* a role for adrenal cortical hormones given to mothers before delivery. There is agreement that the benefits clearly outweigh possible risks and that treatment with corticosteroids is indicated when prenatal tests of amniotic fluid are positive for RDS (negative for surfactant) and when delivery can be delayed safely for 24 hours (96).

Again, it is only fair to mention that someone else was the first. In 1950 (97), Provenzano treated a newborn baby with hypofunction of its adrenal cortex, using Upjohn's adrenocortical extract. Because Provenzano didn't begin this treatment until the 13th postnatal day, it is unlikely that the baby had RDS or immature lungs, but the baby's respiration improved, and its lungs (formerly collapsed) expanded. This encouraged Provenzano to use adrenal cortical extract in a controlled study with 118 untreated newborn babies and 118 treated with adrenal cortical extract (98); 16 untreated babies had prolonged and difficult grunting and retracting respirations and only 8 treated babies had these symptoms. He concluded by hoping "that other investigators will evaluate the use of this substance for newborn infants showing ill effects from anoxia...in order that the true value of adrenal cortex extract be established." I don't believe others did; Provenzano is not mentioned by Liggins, Avery, and others currently working on lung maturation by adrenal cortical hormones. If others had repeated his *postnatal* use of adrenal cortical extracts, they probably would have had disappointing results, for reasons just mentioned; it seems that the therapeutic value of corticoids had to be established by experimental obstetricians who studied the immature fetus *in utero*.

Buckingham and associates in an 18-line abstract published in 1968 (99) called attention to the work of Moog, who showed that maturation of fetal epithelial cells in the small intestine was enhanced by corticosteroids, and they wondered whether lung cells (which are derived embryologically from the same tissue as gut) might behave similarly. Buckingham died soon thereafter and there is no complete report. Liggins, who had already been working for several years with adrenal cortical hormones and fetal maturity, knew that cortisol could induce precocious activation of enzymes in immature animals and in his 1969 paper cited five references to this observation between 1955 and 1966. If he had not, Buckingham's few lines might have been the ones that triggered research in lung maturation.

Treatment of Respiratory Distress Syndrome

If all neonatal respiratory distress were due only to immaturity of fetal lungs at the moment of delivery, *if* neonatal diagnostic tests invariably spotted this, and *if* preventive measures (delaying delivery and speeding up lung maturation) always worked, there would be no need for *therapy*. But there are too many *ifs* involved and it is likely that intensive care will remain the backbone of treatment for another decade or two.

Intensive care involves many things: besides providing adequate pulmonary ventilation, it also means maintenance of nutrition, fluid balance, blood volume, and blood pressure, prevention or management of infections, maintenance of body temperature, and correction of congenital defects. Crucial to survival, of course, is providing adequate pulmonary ventilation. But even though all types of assisted, controlled, or mechanical ventilation useful in adults were tried in newly born babies with RDS, the mortality rate remained high. It is hard to compare mortality rates in different nurseries because each team has somewhat different criteria for the severity of RDS and for beginning a particular form of therapy, and of course each baby has its own complicating factors. And mortality rates are always higher in babies born early in gestation and lower in those born at or close to term, and physicians who compare the value of one procedure with another must always take gestational age into account. (It is usually estimated, though far from precisely, by the weight of the newly born baby.) Thus, in 1969, data collected by Swyer (100) from 6 hospitals on 289 babies with RDS who required artificial ventilation showed that of 2 babies who weighed less than 1,000 grams at birth, neither lived; of 64 babies who weighed between 1,001 and 1,500 grams, only 12.5 per cent lived; of 82 who weighed between 1,501 and 2,000 grams, 29 per cent lived, and of 141 who weighed more than 2,000 grams, 57 per cent lived.

In that same year, Gregory, Kitterman, Phibbs, Tooley, and Hamilton began to use continuous positive airway pressure (abbreviated CPAP and sometimes pronounced C-PAP), instead of intermittent positive pressure, in managing ventilation in babies with RDS; the method supplied a pressure of 6 to 12 mm Hg *throughout* the respiratory cycle while the infants breathed spontaneously, usually through an endotracheal tube. Their results, published as an abstract in 1970 (101) and as a full report in 1971 (102), were dramatic. Of 36 babies with RDS, all of whom had a Po$_2$ of arterial blood of 50 mm Hg or less despite the use of O$_2$ and positive pressure ventilation with a bag and mask, 32 (89 per cent) lived. Of their 12 RDS babies weighing between 1,000 and 1,500 grams, 83 per cent lived; of 11 babies weighing between 1,501 and 2,000 grams, 91 per cent lived; of 12 who weighed more than 2,000 grams, all lived. One who

weighed 930 grams died. Nothing had changed in their intensive neonatal care unit between 1965–1966, when only 11 per cent of their 1,000-1,500 gram babies had survived, and 1969–1971 when 83 per cent lived,† except for the use of CPAP. Soon nursery after nursery repeated and practically all confirmed the amazing results. *Medical World News* quoted Mary Ellen Avery in a January 1972 interview (103):

> Dr. Avery, who was one of the *NEJM* referees for Dr. Gregory's first report, has seen the results of CPAP at Montreal Children's Hospital.
> "You can't challenge this one when you see these babies," she says. "Everything Dr. Gregory says is absolutely true. Everyone around the country who has tried to use it comes up with eyes bugging and says, 'My goodness, it works!' What's so dramatic about it is that it happens within minutes. You can see it! I have no problem giving it unqualified endorsement. CPAP saves babies."

Now the main reason for using a retrospectroscope is to try to determine *why* certain advances in science occurred when they did—whether rapidly or slowly. Before 1959, there was no solid experimental basis for using CPAP in treating babies with RDS, but in 1959 there was. If you read or reread page 521 of Avery and Mead's 1959 report (104), you will find the statement:

> Thereafter [after the first inspiration], during expiration, the alveolar surface of the *normal* lung would have diminished tension, thus reducing the tendency of the air spaces to collapse. On the other hand, in a lung lacking this lining material, surface tension would tend to remain high during expiration; the air spaces would be unstable, and some would collapse.

And if you read page 720 of Brown, Johnson, and Clements's (105) report in the same year, under *Discussion* you will find:

> The uniformity of the results obtained in these several methods and preparations argues strongly for the presence of a peculiar material on the alveolar surface. Its minimum coefficient of compressibility is between 0.01 and 0.02 cm/d. This value places it in the category of 'liquid' films. The film can apparently be reversibly compressed to 50% of its initial area. After further compression, the film apparently ruptures on re-expansion. This suggests a solidification or gelation, or folding on marked compression which is irreversible.

These two paragraphs almost spell out the proper physical and physiological approach to ven-

---

† In 1975–76, 93 per cent in this weight group lived.

tilating the lungs of babies with RDS: Keep the alveoli open or they'll collapse on each expiration. If they do, the surface film will rupture irreversibly and not reform on the next inspiration. Alveolar collapse therefore places a severe strain on both the baby's inspiratory muscles and on its limited ability to synthesize new surfactant (to replace that destroyed during alveolar collapse).

With these observations pointing to the use of greater than atmospheric air pressure during expiration to counter the likelihood that the combined forces of elastic tissue recoil and surface tension would collapse alveoli, why were there no published reports of its successful use until 1970–71?**

One reason, in my opinion, was the old and continuing problem of the *name* of this disorder. Almost everyone called it hyaline membrane disease or respiratory distress syndrome (though one group called it the pulmonary hypoperfusion or pulmonary ischemia syndrome); few called it by its old name, atelectasis of the newborn. Perhaps if there had been no compulsion to change the name, more emphasis would have been placed on treatment designed to counteract alveolar collapse during expiration.

Another was that there were no modern intensive care units for the newly born until Mildred Stahlman's in 1963–64 and until then no one had systematically developed apparatus and tests for monitoring and measuring the physiological and biochemical state of these tiny and fragile creatures. Others soon followed Stahlman and permitted the scientific study and care of the newborn to spread.

A third reason was that some were intent on the wholly worthy effort of correcting the cause of the disease rather than treating it nonspecifically. When the chemical nature of surfactant became known (though in retrospect not fully) and pure dipalmitoyl lecithin became available, it seemed logical to try to replace natural surfactant by aerosols of DPL (107, 108). And when pulmonary ischemia was found to cause atelectasis associated with a deficiency of surfactant (109), it seemed desirable to improve pulmonary arterial blood flow.

But a fourth and probably more important reason was that World War II research pointed out several risks involved in the use of pressure breathing. Pressure breathing was tried between 1942 and 1945 as a means of permitting pilots of fighter planes to get to higher altitudes. After the war, it came into clinical use as controlled positive pressure ventilation of patients in operating rooms and as part of the management of several cardiopulmonary disorders in adults. Physiologists and anesthesiologists tested a variety of devices that produced a wide range of ventilatory patterns: short inspiration–long expiration, long inspiration–short expiration, rapidly versus slowly rising pressures during inspiration, rapidly versus slowly falling pressures during expiration, and positive pressure during inspiration coupled with negative (subatmospheric) pressure during expiration.

These studies showed that whatever increase in intra-alveolar pressure was transmitted through the lungs to the pleural cavity raised intrathoracic pressure, opposed the flow of blood into the intrathoracic venae cavae, and decreased venous return to the heart. This might be useful in treating patients with pulmonary vascular congestion but not in patients with low systemic arterial blood pressure. Figure 4, from a study by Cournand, Motley, Werkö, and Richards in 1948 (110), shows the effect of 3 different patterns of ventilation on mean pressure throughout the respiratory cycle; Werkö in his review article (111) summarized the situation succinctly by writing, "If no influence of pressure breathing on the circulation is desired, the mask pressure during the expiration should be kept as near atmospheric as possible." Beecher and associates were even stronger in their statement (112): "In animals [dogs] with poor circulation, increased pressure in the airway was deleterious and could cause death." Because premature babies with RDS are apt to have a low blood volume and suffer from circulatory shock, pediatricians were wary of positive pressure breathing and particularly of any variety of it that increased *mean* intra-alveolar pressure throughout the respiratory cycle, which of course is exactly what CPAP does.

But, in retrospect, these studies on adults or dogs didn't really apply to the lungs of babies

---

** I don't know how many pediatricians, obstetricians, or anesthesiologists tried CPAP (or some modification) without success and without reporting on their attempts. I know that Avery tried in at least one baby, Hamilton in two, Tooley in one, but none had enough success to continue at that time. And in 1972, Auld, Krauss, and Klain wrote a letter to the Editor of *Pediatrics* (106), telling of their unpublished 1968 attempt to treat four babies with RDS with continuous distending pressure with success for a few hours, followed by failure in three of the four.

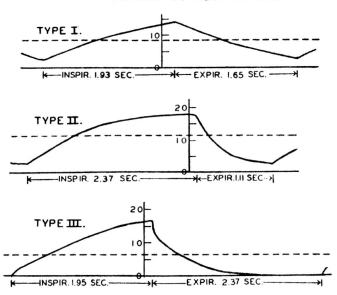

TYPES OF MASK PRESSURE CURVES
PRODUCED BY RESPIRATORS.

TYPE I.

|←——INSPIR. 1.93 SEC.——→|←—EXPIR. 1.65 SEC.——→|

TYPE II.

|←———INSPIR. 2.37 SEC.———→|←—EXPIR.1.11 SEC.—→|

TYPE III.

|←——INSPIR.1.95 SEC.——→|←——EXPIR. 2.37 SEC.———→|

Fig. 4. Three types of mask pressure curves observed during studies of *intermittent* positive pressure breathing. The dotted line is the *mean* mask pressure for the entire respiratory cycle. Note that rapidly rising and prolonged inspiration (type II) produces the highest mean pressure. (From Cournand and associates [110] ; reprinted by permission of publisher.)

with RDS in which pulmonary compliance was greatly increased and pretty uniformly so. Otis, Rahn, and Fenn (113) had pointed out in 1946 that the fraction of intra-alveolar pressure transmitted to the intrathoracic cavity was not a fixed and therefore predictable one but depended on the distensibility of the lungs. Further, Price and associates (114) made the clinical observation in 1951 that positive intrapulmonary pressure, as high as 22 to 25 cm H_2O, failed to decrease arterial blood pressure in patients profoundly anesthetized with cyclopropane, in part because the increased intra-alveolar pressure raised venous pressure only 9 to 11 cm H_2O in their patients as compared to 11 to 15 cm H_2O in conscious subjects.

Gregory and colleagues tested this point in their newborn babies with RDS and found that only 20 per cent of the air pressure applied to the airways was actually transmitted to the intrathoracic, extrapulmonary structures. Later, Herman and Reynolds (115) found almost no transmission of increased airway pressure to a balloon placed in the baby's esophagus and concluded that there is little risk of producing adverse circulatory effects by using high airway pressures during acute stages of severe RDS in babies; like Gregory and associates, they warned that air-

way pressures should be decreased when pulmonary compliance begins to return to normal values. Again, it is worth noting that the development of intensive care units for babies made possible such monitoring and measurements.

Who was Gregory and how did he become involved in this story? In 1961–62, William Hamilton, then Chairman of the Anesthesia Department at the University of Iowa, spent a sabbatical year at the University of California in San Francisco working with Clements and Tooley on atelectasis that occurs during temporary experimental occlusion of a right or left pulmonary artery in dogs, presumably because during the period of pulmonary ischemia, there is no substrate brought to alveolar cells that form pulmonary surfactant (116). As an anesthesiologist, he had been interested in ventilation of the lungs of patients with an open thorax and also in the causes and management of postoperative atelectasis and had occasionally used continuous positive airway pressure to relieve certain types of airway obstruction. From Clements and Tooley, he learned about pulmonary surfactant and a new type of atelectasis or alveolar collapse, and about problems arising from mismatched flow of air and blood to alveoli.

On his return to Iowa, he decided that when

the opportunity arose, he would use his "tight bag" technic to distend alveoli of babies with RDS. In 1963–64, several newborn babies were dying, despite the use of a respirator, and Hamilton worked throughout the night, maintaining a positive pressure in their airways. Babies about to die made a remarkable temporary recovery but became worse the next day; however, the *immediate* improvement made a lasting impression on Hamilton.

That same year Tooley, Clements, Klaus, and several colleagues decided to spend 6 months working in the delivery rooms and nurseries of the Kandang Kerbau Hospital in Singapore (where 40,000 babies were delivered each year, and more than 300 of these had RDS) to see whether they could replace the missing natural surfactant on the alveolar surfaces by aerosolized dipalmitoyl lecithin. Hamilton wanted to join the research team in Singapore to test the usefulness of his "tight bag" technic to distend lungs throughout the respiratory cycle, but the group concluded that it would be difficult enough to test one hypothesis (replacement therapy) in a 6-month period without trying to test two. The decision was of course correct in principle, although, in retrospect, it can be questioned (117).

Why this long parenthetical piece about Hamilton when I started to answer the question, "Who was Gregory?" Gregory had been a medical student at the University of California in San Francisco (M.D., 1963). He became interested then in RDS as a result of a lecture in obstetrics. After an internship at UCLA, he served 3 years as a resident at UCSF, one in surgery and two in anesthesia (1965 to 1967). During his anesthesia residency, he spent a lot of time in the delivery room and nursery with Tooley, Kitterman, and Phibbs, helping them in their attempts to improve the treatment of asphyxia. This was in the early days of intensive care units; Day in Kansas had organized the first coronary care unit in 1962–63 and Mildred Stahlman at Vanderbilt had developed the first genuine neonatal intensive care unit about 1963 or 1964. Tooley started his about 1965–66. Anesthesiologists were ideally trained to play an important role in these and were becoming interested and involved; Gregory was one of these.

Now at last we can connect Hamilton and Gregory. Stuart Cullen, Chief of Anesthesia at USCF, couldn't resist the "call" to be Dean in 1966, and in 1967, Hamilton, still deeply interested in RDS, came to San Francisco to take Cullen's old job as Chairman of Anesthesiology. Gregory was committed to a year's research fellowship in 1967–68, but at the end of that year, Hamilton assigned Gregory to a full-time position in the intensive care unit for the newborn with no responsibilities for giving anesthesia. For those not familiar with the economics of hospital care, I must add that it requires real conviction on the part of a professor of Anesthesia to assign one of his staff to work full time in the nursery instead of to regular duty in surgical operating and recovery rooms, but Hamilton was, at least vicariously, back in the RDS business.

One night there was no one in the nursery but Gregory, nurses, technicians, and a baby with RDS in its last minutes of life despite the use of O_2-intermittent positive pressure breathing. This was not the time to worry about transmission of pressure from airways to the intrathoracic space. (And there was really no need to because Phibbs and Kitterman at UCSF had long concentrated their efforts on correcting hypovolemia, low blood pressure, and decreased cardiac output in the newly born from the very moment of birth.) Gregory decided to use CPAP and the baby lived. An added dividend was that, because CPAP opened alveoli perfused with mixed venous blood and therefore oxygenated this blood, its use permitted treating the baby with lower (and safe) concentrations of inspired O_2 and thereby lessening or eliminating the toxic effects of O_2 on the lungs. (Frequent analyses of O_2 tension of arterial blood eliminated the other bugaboo of O_2 inhalation in the newly born—blindness due to retrolental fibroplasia.)

By 1970, the results of treating seven babies (six of whom survived), were reported to the Society for Pediatric Research, and in June 1971 the results of treating 36 babies (see page 506) were published in full. Why didn't it come in 1959–61 instead of 1969–71? I've mentioned some of the important reasons: need for the neonatal intensive care unit, need to test other forms of treatment, fear of adverse effects of CPAP on the circulation.

Why Gregory rather than A, B, or C? One reason was Hamilton's continuing faith in CPAP despite earlier setbacks. Another, of course, was Gregory's close relation with a large group of RDS investigators. Gregory gives several other reasons that influenced him.

One was that Harrison and his associates (118) had shown that babies who grunted (breathed out against an expiratory resistance, self-imposed) improved, but when Harrison introduced an endotracheal tube into these same babies, and they could no longer grunt, they got worse. A somewhat similar situation had been encountered by Smith and associates (119), who noted improvement in oxygenation of arterial blood of babies with RDS when a mechanical ventilator kept the intra-alveolar pressure above atmospheric for more than half of the baby's respiratory cycle.

Another was that newborn babies usually breathe rapidly—60/min or more. When a newborn baby was ventilated with a positive pressure device cycling at a rapid rate and there was not enough time during expiration for the alveolar and airway pressure to fall to atmospheric, the baby got better; when the machine malfunctioned at the high frequency and had to be used at a low frequency, the baby got worse. Gregory decided that when babies with RDS *did* breathe voluntarily, he would let them continue to do so (with a continuously imposed distending pressure) and not permit use of a slower rate of mechanical ventilation.

I suspect that in any case, CPAP was a treatment whose time had come. RDS was the most important life-or-death problem in pediatrics, more and more highly trained pediatricians were working in intensive care units for the newborn, and it was inevitable that someone in the proper environment would try CPAP, with the proper pressures. Llewellyn and Swyer came close in 1970 when they, like Gregory, reported their results to the Society for Pediatric Research (120); they added positive expiratory pressure (2.5 to 6 cm H_2O) to mechanical ventilation of 11 infants with RDS (mean birth weight 2,160 grams) and 7 (64 per cent) survived. Gregory used 8 to 16 cm H_2O pressure (6 to 12 mm Hg) continuously in babies breathing spontaneously without a ventilator.

Trials and Tribulations

Physicians engaged in clinical trials on the human fetus and newborn have special tribulations in addition to the usual ones. The special tribulations are that they are damned by some if they *don't* do research and damned by others if they *do*. The usual criticisms relate to the design of a therapeutic study and might be summed up by two questions: (*1*) Is the double blind, randomized clinical trial the only scientifically acceptable design? (*2*) Is this type of trial often scientifically unnecessary and ethically unacceptable?

Because there is currently a lively debate on these questions (121–125) and because the study of Gregory and his associates was not double blind and randomized, I should comment a bit on introducing new forms of treatment. I've done clinical investigation of therapeutic procedures as well as purely laboratory studies. One of my clinical studies with Dripps (the effect on healthy men of inhalation of O_2 for 24 hours versus inhalation of air for the same time) was as well controlled as a randomization enthusiast could want. But another was not. It was a non-randomized comparison of the efficacy of two methods of artificial ventilation. It couldn't possibly have been randomized because there wasn't any control group—each patient served as his own control. In 1946, when Dripps and I found that, in adult apneic patients, the Eve (tilting) method moved 500 ml air/breath and, in the same patient, the Schafer method moved only 75–117 ml (not enough even to clear the respiratory dead space), we realized that each-patient-as-his-own-control was the best way to determine which method was better. In our opinion, we would have served science poorly and morality even worse if we had randomly assigned each apneic patient to one of two groups and treated one with a method sure to fail (and now abandoned as worthless) and the other with a pretty good technic.

Statistician A. Bradford Hill (126) in 1951 pleaded for and obtained the controlled clinical trial; worshippers at his altar would do well to reread his original paper in which he stated:

> The first step in such a trial is to decide precisely what it is hoped to prove, and secondly whether these aims can be ethically fulfilled. It need hardly be said that the latter consideration is paramount and must never, on any scientific grounds whatever, be lost sight of. If a treatment cannot ethically be withheld then clearly no controlled trial can be instituted.
>
> ... Sometimes, not often, controls are indeed unnecessary. If in the past a disease has invariably and rapidly led to death there can be no possible need for controls to prove a change in the fatality rate. Thus the trial of streptomycin in tuberculous meningitis needed no control group. Given a precise and certain identification of the case, the success of treatment could be measured against the past 100% fatal conclusion. No controls, too, are essential to prove the value of a drug such as penicillin which quickly reveals dramatic effects in the treatment of a disease. Such dramatic effects occurring on a large scale and in many hands cannot be long overlooked.

It seems to me that there is a fairly sensible way of looking at clinical investigation that involves the medical or surgical management of patients: assuming that you agree with Bradford Hill that ethical considerations (the patient's right to life and happiness) supersede scientific ones, then do the very best study that *needs* to be done. Sometimes it will require no concurrent controls (e.g., when a drug or procedure leads to the almost invariable and complete cure of a disease previously almost invariably fatal); sometimes the best study requires treating all patients similarly, first with procedure A and then with procedure B, or vice versa (the sequential approach, or each-patient-as-his-own-control); sometimes the best study does indeed require a randomized, double blind, large scale and very expensive study to settle a question, such as whether gobbling huge doses of ascorbic acid daily prevents the common cold, and here the rigidly controlled trial ought to begin at least as early as the second patient is treated. But let's not live in constant fear of the great god Randomization; his (or her) appetite is huge, and, if fed continuously, could consume much of the nation's research dollars and personnel, and even the lives of some patients.

Clinical trials in the nursery differ somewhat from trials in children or adults. The blood pressure of an adult with hypertension is affected psychologically by his confidence in his physician; the life of a premature baby in the nursery is not. In the nursery, the color or taste of a placebo has no influence on the baby's will to live. In the nursery, the physician and nurse cannot be "blinded" to the therapy used, because they themselves must administer it; and they must know vital measurements minute by minute to carry out optimal therapy. In the nursery, immediate survival and preservation of organ function is all that counts.

Now let's look at the classic study of Gregory and his colleagues between 1969 and 1971. It *did* include two important controls: (*1*) It had the experience, over a period of years, of a highly expert group, schooled and skilled both in modern research technics and in intensive and continuous monitoring and care of the newborn so that it had unusually good records of the clinical, physiological, and biochemical state of both pre-CPAP treated and post-CPAP treated babies—in short, the group was unusually well equipped to identify and compare the results in RDS babies treated in 1966, 1967, 1968, 1969, etc. (see p. 506 and footnote). (*2*) At least initially, the group used each baby as its own control, first using modern intensive care and intermittent pulmonary ventilation and then the same modern intensive care with only one change, a switch to *continuous* positive airway pressure.

Let's ask how one would have obtained permission to do a randomized, controlled clinical study in the nursery in 1969 to 1971.

SCENARIO

Enter physician.

Physician to mother: Your baby has respiratory distress syndrome. We want to compare a new method of treatment, A, with the present management, B. Can we enter your baby in this study? It would be assigned randomly to treatment A or B.

Mother: In your opinion, does my baby have a better chance of living with treatment A or B?

Physician: We don't know. Maybe A, maybe B.

A space-age computer interrupts at this point: Not true. Physician incorrect. Answer unacceptable. He knows A is better because 5 babies in a row have lived with treatment A which is at least twice as good a record as treatment with B.

Physician (now speaking honestly): We're convinced that A is far better but we can't convince Drs. X, Y, and Z unless we have a randomized, controlled clinical study.

Mother: Thanks; I want a live baby more than anything else in the world—even more than convincing Drs. X, Y, and Z. *Please* be sure my baby gets the new treatment.

Exit Mother.

(Follow-up: The twins in figure 5 are happy that one of them was not assigned to a control group that was not treated with CPAP.)

Some believe that the time is now ripe for controlled studies, with randomization, designed to evaluate finer points of treatment, to achieve the lowest possible mortality and morbidity (127): what type of distending pressure is best? with what concentration of oxygen? when and for how long should it be applied?

WHERE ARE THEY NOW?

Neergaard, as mentioned earlier, died in 1947 before he had the satisfaction of seeing his work repeated, accepted, acclaimed, and canonized.

Gruenwald, after his 1946 research, made pressure-volume measurements of a very large series of lungs of infants who came to autopsy. In the early 1960s, while Associate Professor of Obstetrics, Pediatrics, and Pathology at Johns Hopkins, Gruenwald collaborated with Clem-

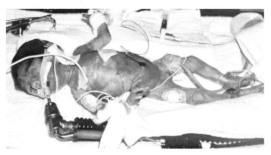 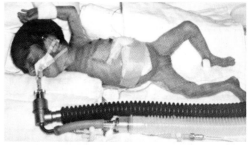

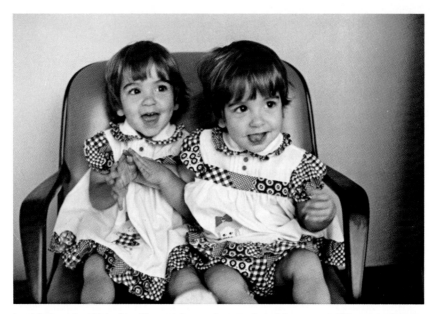

Fig. 5. Twin girls born in 1974 after 29 weeks' gestation. Birth weights were 1,100 and 1,160 grams. Both had assisted ventilation from birth. (*Upper left*) Twin A at 1 day of age, breathing against continuous positive pressure of 9 mm Hg. The tip of an umbilical artery catheter lies just above the bifurcation of the aorta; the catheter is used to obtain continuous measurements of arterial blood pressure and periodic samples of blood to measure its O_2 tension. (The size of each infant can be estimated from the diameter of the transparent corrugated tube [top right], which is 2.8 cm.) Twin A required ligation of a patent ductus arteriosus in her fourth day of life to relieve congestive heart failure. She received CPAP or positive end-expiratory pressure until the age of 24 days, when the endotracheal tube was removed. At 2 and 3 years of age, she performed within the normal range on standard infant intelligence tests. (*Upper right*) Twin B at 1 day of age breathing against a positive airway pressure of 10 mm Hg. She too required surgical ligation of a patent ductus arteriosus at 4 days of age. She was treated with CPAP or positive end-expiratory pressure until 21 days of age, when the endotracheal tube was removed. Intellectual performance at age 2 and 3 years was similar to that of Twin A. (*Lower*) Twins A and B at age of 2.

ents, then at Edgewood, Maryland, correlating the mechanical properties of infants' lungs with the surface activity of extracts made from them. He continued to publish papers on infant lungs throughout the 1960s. In 1968 he moved to Philadelphia, first to the Veterans Administration Hospital and the Department of Pathology at the University of Pennsylvania and, two years later, to Hahnemann. He has recently retired and is now Professor Emeritus of pathology at Hahnemann Medical College.

Macklin became Professor of Histology and Embryology at the University of Western Ontario

in 1921 (a position he held for the remainder of his academic career). He was elected to the Royal Society of Canada in 1924 and to numerous other societies in North America and Europe. His own university awarded him the honorary degree of D.Sc. in 1953 when he retired at age 70. Because the policy of his university denied its facilities to retired faculty members, he continued his studies at home "with old sections and an old microscope." He died suddenly from a coronary occlusion on November 23, 1959, at age 75.

Radford, after his first published paper, which dealt with alveolar surface area, made a number of additional lasting contributions to our knowledge of artificial respiration and the mechanical properties of the lungs. He then became interested in the air we breathe, in toxic substances in it (such as carbon monoxide and its effects on the heart) and in toxic chemicals in cigarette smoke (such as polonium-210 and its possible role in producing lung cancer). From time to time he returned to his first research interest (renal physiology, water metabolism, and the antidiuretic hormone). He has had positions at DuPont's Haskell Research Laboratories, again at Harvard, then at the University of Cincinnati, and now seems to be well settled at Johns Hopkins, where he has been Professor of Environmental Medicine since 1968, except for a year at Oxford (1975–76) as Visiting Professor to the Department of the Regius Professor of Medicine. As one would expect, he has served in many important roles as consultant on environmental medicine to state and national bodies and has always maintained his interest in teaching and training others.

Pattle has remained at the Chemical Defence Research Establishment where he has been Senior Principal Scientific Officer since 1963. He has continued research on inhaled toxic materials and on his first love—the action potential of nerve and muscle—but, since 1972, has published exclusively on lung surfactant: the effect of anesthetics and some chemical agents on it, electron microscopic studies, and comparative anatomy and physiology of surfactant.

In a recent letter to me (June 11, 1977), he wrote:

> Now one or two cautions. First, the words "surface active." In ordinary physical chemistry this means "tending to accumulate at a surface and lower surface tension." Unfortunately in specialist lung literature, it has come to mean "capable of forming a surface film which, when compressed, can assume a metastable state of high surface pressure and reduce the surface tension to a small fraction of its equilibrium value." I have floated the word "surpellic" to describe substances of the latter type and films formed from them. It is highly undesirable that we should use "surface active" in a sense different from the ordinary. It even seems to confuse writers on the lung. I hope that "surpellic" (from Latin "pellere," to push) will catch on (see J. Zool., *182*:125–136, 1977).

Secondly, some writers refer to a discovery based on observation of something which was not what was actually being investigated, as a "chance" or "accidental" discovery. This is *never* true. Observations are made because the observer is on the lookout for anything strange. The discovery of lung surfactant came about as the result of a peculiar concatenation of circumstances, but not as the product of chance or accident.

Von Neergaard deduced that the surfactant must exist, but he failed to find it for the following reason. He measured the surface tension by a method —i.e. measurement of the force necessary to pull a stirrup away from the surface—in which the surface was *stretched* at the moment of measurement. As the surfactant only shows its surpellic properties when the surface film is *compressed*, such a method could not detect it. In both the bubble and [Clements's] Wilhelmy trough methods the surface is *compressed*, so that the surfactant can be detected by these methods.

Clements left the Army Center for a year to be Visiting Professor in the Cardiovascular Research Institute, University of California, San Francisco, returned to Edgewood for a year, and then accepted a permanent faculty position in San Francisco where he still works as Professor of Pediatrics and Career Investigator of the American Heart Association. He was elected to the National Academy of Sciences in 1974 and has received many awards.

It may seem odd that Clements, who has always worked in the field of pulmonary and respiratory physiology, biochemistry, and biophysics, receives his lifetime professorial salary from the American Heart Association (AHA) rather than from the American Lung Association. The AHA started its Career Investigator program in 1951 and, over a period of years, its Research Committee has initiated about 14 lifetime awards. In 1962, the American Lung Association (ALA) (then the NTRDA) had not yet instituted a similar program (though the American Cancer Society had); a well-known pulmonary scientist sent a formal proposal to the American Thoracic Society (medical section of the ALA) asking that it and its parent body provide lifetime career professorships for innovative, creative scientists judged likely to be leaders throughout their scientific careers; the proposal also formally nominated Clements for such a position. The Society's committees considered the proposal sympathetically but turned it down in 1963 "because of the rather limited amount of money available." The American Heart Association awarded him a Career Investigatorship in 1964 despite the fact that Clements was and still is essentially a pulmonary biophysicist-physiologist.

It is of interest that both organizations derive their funds from contributions by the public and receive a somewhat similar amount each year. In 1963 the ALA received $31,093,111 (but had "limited funds"). In 1964 the AHA received $30,121,526 but went on to support its twelfth Career Investigator. The AHA interprets its mandate from the public one way; the ALA interprets its in another. The AHA's Committee on Research believed firmly that an important role for voluntary health agencies is the recognition and support of individuals with unusual talent for research, to free them for long periods from onerous responsibilities that interfere with their work. The ALA did not. It would be interesting some years from now to evaluate the results of these two different policies on the improvement of health.

Avery, after her research fellowship in Boston in 1957–59 with Mead, returned to Johns Hopkins where she became Associate Professor of Pediatrics in 1964. She left in 1969 to become Chairman of the Department of Pediatrics at McGill University, but since 1974 has been Chairman of Harvard's Pediatrics Department and Physician-in-Chief to Children's Hospital Medical Center in Boston. She has been a complete neonatologist and has done research on a wide variety of problems of the newborn; from 1970 on, however, she has been involved deeply and continuously in problems of lung maturation and ways of accelerating it and preventing RDS. In her spare time, she has written two widely used books, *The Lung and Its Disorders in the Newborn Infant,* now in its third edition, and (with A. J. Schaffer), *Diseases of the Newborn,* and chapters in 15 books.

Mead has never wandered from Harvard. He received his B.S. and M.D. there and, except for two years of Army service (1947–49), has been on the faculty of the Harvard School of Public Health continuously since 1950, Professor since 1965. Mead's first nine publications resulted from his Army experience and dealt with the relationship between temperature and peripheral blood flow. Once ensconced in Harvard, he turned to research on the physical properties of the lungs and has stayed with this problem continuously. He has been responsible for part or all of the research training of many now well-known scientists, and by his enthusiasm and dedication to research and his generosity with ideas, has catalyzed the research of many of his fellows and colleagues.

CONCLUDING REMARKS

Ritchie Calder divided scientists into two groups: those who make it *possible* and those who make it *happen* (128). In a period of 20-some years, respiratory distress of the newborn has advanced from a state of almost complete ignorance to one of the most completely characterized of all disorders—and both groups share the credit for this remarkable advance. Laplace, Young, Neergaard, Radford, Pattle, Clements, Liggins, and many others made it *possible,* and Avery, Gregory, Gluck, and many others made it *happen.* It's worth emphasizing that Laplace and Young lived 100 years before there was such a disorder as atelectasis of the newborn; that Neergaard did his classic study only to find out if the millions of tiny bubbles in the lungs (the air sacs) contributed a new and unsuspected type of recoil in expiration; that Radford wanted to measure the alveolar surface area just for the sake of acquiring new knowledge; that when Pattle was asked whether, by using antifoams, he could get rid of pulmonary edema foam (that blocked the airways of goats poisoned by phosgene), he was a physicist "who knew very little about the pulmonary or cardiovascular systems" and probably never heard of RDS; and that Clements was a physiologist-biophysicist who wanted primarily to learn whether Radford or Pattle was right. None of those "who made it possible" was at that time looking for something to help in the early diagnosis, prevention, or treatment of RDS.

Scarpelli, who in 1968 wrote the first scholarly monograph (129) on pulmonary surfactant (with more than 320 references to articles published at that time), summed up the story of discovery and application in one paragraph:

> In any science there are the discoverers and innovators whose contributions reside in their ability to look forward with true perspective. For the lung surfactant system these scientists are Drs. K. von Neergaard, R. E. Pattle, J. A. Clements, E. P. Radford, Jr., E. S. Brown, M. E. Avery, and J. Mead. There are those who extend and refine the science and continue to innovate. Their names are in the bibliography of this text. Then there is the reporter and author. His task is his responsibility and he can only hope that he has been objective, reasonable, and stimulating.

There's another lesson worth learning from the story of RDS. You've learned the lesson when you realize what all of the entries in the following list have in common:

measurement of molecular size and configuration
experimental ablation of pituitary gland

oxygen and carbon dioxide electrodes
measurement of intraesophageal pressure
high resolution electron microscope
chromatography and lipid chemistry
origin of amniotic fluid
nerve gas and respiratory paralysis
soap films and bubbles
laws of gravitation and planetary motion
electrophoresis; radioimmunology
conduction of electricity through stretched wire
phosgene poisoning and pulmonary edema
high altitude physiology
alveolar ventilation-blood flow ratios
pulmonary surface area
dipalmitoyl phosphatidyl choline
intensive coronary care units

Correct. Knowledge of each of the above, initially completely unrelated to RDS, was essential or helpful in saving the lives of babies born with premature lungs. So when someone asks you what's the good of all this research that's not specifically directed to immediately solving the problem of cancer or emphysema or congestive heart failure, tell him (or her) that essential clues, concepts, and methods often (usually) come from unrelated fields. And then show him the picture of twins A and B and ask if it isn't really all worthwhile. And if he (or she) isn't interested in human life but only in dollars, tell him that the March 1977 report of the Task Force on Respiratory Diseases of the NIH Division of Lung Diseases (130) includes an estimate that a primary prevention program for RDS (starting in 1977 at our present advanced position) would reduce the number of premature births in the United States each year from 500,000 to 350,000, would decrease the number of infants born with RDS from 50,000–70,000 to 35,000–47,000 and the number of deaths from 5,000–10,000 to 3,500–7,000, and reduce the costs of treatment by 75 to 150 million dollars.

One final remark. In the early 1900s, Boys had put his popular lectures, "Soap Bubbles" into book form ("meant for juveniles and for juveniles only") "in the hope that it may excite in a few young people some small fraction of the interest and enthusiasm . . . awakened in the author [by previous lectures of G. F. Rodwill]." In his introduction, Boys remarked, "I hope that none of you are yet tired of playing with bubbles, because, as I hope we shall see, there is more in a common bubble than those who have only played with them generally imagine." (131)

I wonder whether Neergaard was stimulated to do his experiments because of Boys's book. I also wonder how many more advances are still hidden inside an ordinary soap bubble.

NOTE: My sincere apologies to my many scientific associates and colleagues whose names should have but didn't appear in these three articles; I tried but found it impossible to write a scholarly review and interesting story in one and the same article.

Acknowledgment

I thank Drs. Avery, Clements, Gregory, Hamilton, Kitterman, Liggins, Pattle, Radford, and Tooley for telling me their recollections of people and events, Dr. Tooley for providing the before and after photographs of RDS twins treated with CPAP, and Dr. Mary C. Williams for providing previously unpublished electron micrographs showing the life and death of surfactant.

References

48. Macklin, C. C.: The pulmonary alveolar mucoid film and the pneumonocytes, Lancet, 1954, *1*, 1099-1104.

49. Pattle, R. E.: Properties, function and origin of the alveolar lining layer, Nature, 1955, *175*, 1125–1126.

50. Pattle, R. E.: Properties, functions and origin of the alveolar lining layer, Proc R Soc Lond [Biol], 1958, *148*, 217–240.

51. Clements, J. A.: Surface tension of lung extracts, Proc Soc Exp Biol Med, 1957, *95*, 170-172.

52. Pattle, R. E., and Thomas, L. C.: Lipoprotein composition of the film lining the lung, Nature, 1961, *189*, 844.

53. Buckingham, S.: Studies on the identification of an antiatelectasis factor in normal sheep lung, Am J Dis Child, 1961, *102*, 521-522.

54. Klaus, M. H., Clements, J. A., and Havel, R. J.: Composition of surface-active material isolated from beef lung, Proc Natl Acad Sci USA, 1961, *47*, 1858-1859.

55. Bondurant, S., and Miller, D. A.: A method for producing surface-active extracts of mammalian lungs, J Appl Physiol, 1962, *17*, 167-168.

56. Brown, E. S.: Isolation and assay of dipalmityl lecithin in lung extracts, Am J Physiol, 1964, *207*, 402–406.

57. Thannhauser, S. J., Benotti, J., and Boncoddo, N. F.: Isolation and properties of hydrolecithin (dipalmityl lecithin) from lung, its occurrence in the sphingomyelin fraction of animal tissues, J Biol Chem, 1946, *166*, 669–75.

58. Leathes, J. B.: Role of fats in vital phenomena, Lancet, 1925, *1*, 853–56.

59. King, R. J.: The surfactant system of the lung, Fed Proc, 1974, *33*, 2232–2237.

60. Clements, J. A., and King, R. J.: Composition of the surface active material, in *The Biochemical*

Basis of Pulmonary Function, R. G. Crystal, ed., Marcel Dekker, New York, 1976, pp. 363–387.

61. The Biochemical Basis of Pulmonary Function, R. G. Crystal, ed., Marcel Dekker, New York. 1976.

62. Pattle, R. E.: Surface lining of lung alveoli, Physiol Rev, 1965, *45*, 48–79.

63. Low, F. N.: The electron microscopy of sectioned lung tissue after varied duration of fixation in buffered osmium tetroxide, Anat Rec, 1954, *120*, 827–851.

64. Schlipköter, H.-W.: Elektronenoptische Untersuchungen ultradünner Lungenschnitte, Dtsch Med Wochenschr, 1954, *79*, 1658–1659.

65. Woodside, G. L., and Dalton, A. J.: The ultrastructure of lung tissue from newborn and embryo mice, J Ultrastruct Res, 1958, *2*, 28–54.

66. Buckingham, S., and Avery, M. E.: Time of appearance of lung surfactant in the foetal mouse, Nature, 1962, *193*, 688–689.

67. Klaus, M., Reiss, O. K., Tooley, W. H., Piel, C., and Clements, J. A.: Alveolar epithelial cell mitochondria as source of the surface-active lung lining, Science, 1962, *137*, 750–751.

68. Campiche, M.: Remarques sur l'ultrastructure des inclusions lamellaires de l'épithélium pulmonaire, Rev Méd Suisse Romande, 1965, *85*, 532–536.

69. Gil, J., and Reiss, O. K.: Isolation and characterization of lamellar bodies and tubular myelin from rat lung homogenates, J Cell Biol, 1973, *58*, 152–171.

70. Williams, M. C., and Mason, R. J.: Development of the type II cell in the fetal rat lung, Am Rev Respir Dis, 1977, *115* (Supplement, pp. 37–47).

71. Williams, M. C.: Conversion of lamellar body membranes into tubular myelin in alveoli of fetal rat lungs, J Cell Biol, 1977, *72*, 260–277.

72. Campiche, M. A., Gautier, A., Hernandez, E. I., and Reymond, A.: An electron microscope study of the fetal development of human lung, Pediatrics, 1963, *32*, 976–994.

73. Menees, T. O., Miller, J. D., and Holly, L. E.: Amniography: Preliminary report, Am J Roentgenol, 1930, *24*, 363–366.

74. Cantarow, A., Stuckert, H., and Davis, R. C.: The chemical composition of amniotic fluid, Surg Gynecol Obstet, 1933, *57*, 63–70.

75. Preyer, W.: Specielle Physiologie des Embryo, Grieben, Leipzig, 1885, p. 148.

76. Jost, A., and Policard, A.: Contribution expérimentale à l'étude du développement prénatal du poumon chez le lapin, Arch Anat Microsc, 1948, *37*, 323–332.

77. Setnikar, I., Agostoni, E., and Taglietti, A.: The fetal lung, a source of amniotic fluid, Proc Soc Exp Biol Med, 1959, *101*, 842–845.

78. Adams, F. H., Fujiwara, T., and Rowshan, G.: The nature and origin of the fluid in the fetal lamb lung, J Pediatr, 1963, *63*, 881–888.

79. Adams, F. H., and Fujiwara, T.: Surfactant in fetal lamb tracheal fluid, J Pediatr, 1963, *63*, 537–542.

80. Fujiwara, T., Adams, F. H., and Scudder, A.: Fetal lamb amniotic fluid: Relationship of lipid composition to surface tension, J Pediatr, 1964, *65*, 824–830.

81. Scarpelli, E. M.: The lung, tracheal fluid, and lipid metabolism of the fetus, Pediatrics, 1967, *40*, 951–961.

82. Adams, F. H., Desilets, D. T., and Towers, B.: Control of flow of fetal lung fluid at the laryngeal outlet, Respir Physiol, 1967, *2*, 302–309.

83. Howatt, W. F., Humphreys, P. W., Normand, I. C. S., and Strang, L. B.: Ventilation of liquid by the fetal lamb during asphyxia, J Appl Physiol, 1965, *20*, 496–502.

84. Adamson, T. M., Boyd, R. D. H., Platt, H. S., and Strang, L. B.: Composition of alveolar liquid in the foetal lamb, J Physiol, 1969, *204*, 159–168.

85. Gluck, L., Kulovich, M. V., and Borer, R. C., Jr.: Diagnosis of the respiratory distress syndrome by amniocentesis, Am J Obstet Gynecol, 1971, *109*, 440–445.

86. Clements, J. A., Platzker, A. C. G., Tierney, D. F., Hobel, C. J., Creasy, R. K., Margolis, A. J., Thibeault D. W., Tooley, W. H., and Oh, W.: Assessment of the risk of the respiratory-distress syndrome by a rapid test for surfactant in amniotic fluid, N Engl J Med, 1972, *286*, 1077–1081.

87. Evans, J. J.: Prediction of respiratory-distress syndrome by shake test on newborn gastric aspirate, N Engl J Med, 1975, *292*, 1113–1115.

88. Liggins, G. C.: Premature delivery of foetal lambs infused with glucocorticoids, J Endocrinol, 1969, *45*, 515–523.

89. Mescher, E. J., Platzker, A. C. G., Ballard, P. L., Kitterman, J. A., Clements, J. A. and Tooley, W. H.: Ontogeny of tracheal fluid, pulmonary surfactant, and plasma corticoids in the fetal lamb, J Appl Physiol, 1975, *39*, 1017–1021.

90. Avery, M. E.: Pharmacological approaches to the acceleration of fetal lung maturation, Br Med Bull, 1975, *31*, 13–17.

91. Farrell, P. M., and Avery, M. E.: Hyaline membrane disease, Am Rev Respir Dis, 1975, *111*, 657–688.

92. de Lemos, R. A., Shermeta, D. W., Knelson, J. H., Kotas, R., and Avery, M. E.: Acceleration of appearance of pulmonary surfactant in the fetal lamb by administration of corticosteroids, Am Rev Respir Dis, 1970, *102*, 459–461.

93. Wang, N. S., Kotas, R. V., Avery, M. E., and Thurlbeck, W. M.: Accelerated appearance of

osmiophilic bodies in fetal lungs following steroid injection, J Appl Physiol, 1971, *30*, 362–365.

94. Kotas, R. V., and Avery, M. E.: Accelerated appearance of pulmonary surfactant in the fetal rabbit, J Appl Physiol, 1971, *30*, 358–361.

95. Liggins, G. C., and Howie, R. N.: A controlled trial of antepartum glucocorticoid treatment for prevention of the respiratory distress syndrome in premature infants, Pediatrics, 1972, *50*, 515–525.

96. Lung Maturation and the Prevention of Hyaline Membrane Disease, Proceedings of the Seventieth Ross Conference on Pediatric Research, December 7–10, 1975, Columbus, Ohio, Ross Laboratories, 1976.

97. Provenzano, R. W.: Adrenocortical hypoplasia in the newborn infant: Report of a case with replacement therapy, N Engl J Med, 1950, *242*, 87–89.

98. Provenzano, R. W., McGovern, P., Schultz, R., and Hester, J.: Adrenal cortex extract in pediatrics, Am J Dis Child, 1951, *81*, 323–328.

99. Buckingham, S., McNary, W. F., Sommers, S. C., and Rothschild, J.: Is lung an analog of Moog's developing intestine? I. Phosphatases and pulmonary alveolar differentiation in fetal rabbits, Fed Proc, 1968, *27*, 328.

100. Swyer, P. R.: An assessment of artificial respiration in the newborn, in *Problems of Neonatal Intensive Care Units, Report of the Fifty-Ninth Ross Conference on Pediatric Research*, Columbus, Ohio, Ross Laboratories, 1969, pp. 25–35.

101. Gregory, G. A., Kitterman, J. A., Phibbs, R. H., Tooley, W. H., and Hamilton, W. K.: Continuous positive airway pressure with spontaneous respiration: A new method of increasing arterial oxygenation in the respiratory distress syndrome, Pediatr Res, 1970, *4*, 469–470.

102. Gregory, G. A., Kitterman, J. A., Phibbs, R. H., Tooley, W. H., and Hamilton, W. K.: Treatment of the idiopathic respiratory-distress syndrome with continuous positive airway pressure, N Engl J Med, 1971, *284*, 1332–1340.

103. Putting pressure on hyaline, Med World News, Jan 14, 1972, 27–32.

104. Avery, M. E., and Mead, J.: Surface properties in relation to atelectasis and hyaline membrane disease, Am J Dis Child, 1959, *97*, 517–523.

105. Brown, E. S., Johnson, R. P., and Clements, J. A.: Pulmonary surface tension, J Appl Physiol, 1959, *14*, 717–720.

106. Auld, P. A. M., Krauss, A. N., and Klain, D. B.: Continuous positive airway pressure (letter to the editor), Pediatrics, 1972, *49*, 468–469.

107. Robillard, E., Alarie, Y., Dagenais-Perusse, P., Baril, E., and Guilbeault, A.: Microaerosol administration of synthetic β-γ-dipalmitoyl-L-α-lecithin in the respiratory distress syndrome: A preliminary report, Can Med Assoc J, 1964, *90*, 55–57.

108. Chu, J., Clements, J. A., Cotton, E. K., Klaus, M. H., Sweet, A. Y., and Tooley, W. H.: Neonatal pulmonary ischemia. Part I: Clinical and physiological studies, Pediatrics, 1967, *40*, 709–782.

109. Finley, T. N., Tooley, W. H., Swenson, E. W., Gardner, R. E., and Clements, J. A.: Pulmonary surface tension in experimental atelectasis, Am Rev Respir Dis, 1964, *89*, 372–378.

110. Cournand, A., Motley, H. L., Werkö, L., and Richards, D. W., Jr.: Physiological studies of the effects of intermittent positive pressure breathing on cardiac output in man, Am J Physiol, 1948, *152*, 162–174.

111. Werkö, L.: The influence of positive pressure breathing on the circulation in man, Acta Med Scand *128*, Suppl. 193, 125 pp.

112. Beecher, H. K., Bennett, H. S., and Bassett, D. L.: Circulatory effects of increased pressure in the airway, Anesthesiology, 1943, *4*, 612–618.

113. Otis, A. B., Rahn, H., and Fenn, W. O.: Venous pressure changes associated with positive intrapulmonary pressures; their relationship to the distensibility of the lung, Am J Physiol, 1946, *146*, 307–317.

114. Price, H. L., King, B. D., Elder, J. D., Libien, B. H., and Dripps, R. D.: Circulatory effects of raised airway pressure during cyclopropane anesthesia in man, J Clin Invest, 1951, *30*, 1243–1249.

115. Herman, S., and Reynolds, E. O. R.: Methods for improving oxygenation in infants mechanically ventilated for severe hyaline membrane disease, Arch Dis Child, 1973, *48*, 612–617.

116. Tooley, W. H., Gardner, R. E., Hamilton, W. K., Maddison, F. E., Markel, G. G., Wright, R. R., and Bradley, B. L.: Unpublished observations, 1962.

117. Tooley, W. H.: Hyaline membrane disease—Telling it like it was, Am Rev Respir Dis, 1977, *115* (Supplement, pp. 19–28).

118. Harrison, V. C., Heese, H. de V., and Klein, M.: The significance of grunting in hyaline membrane disease, Pediatrics, 1968, *41*, 549–559.

119. Smith, P. C., Daily, W. J. R., Fletcher, G., Meyer, H. B. P., and Taylor, G.: Mechanical ventilation of newborn infants. I. The effect of rate and pressure on arterial oxygenation of infants with respiratory distress syndrome, Pediatr Res, 1969, *3*, 244–254.

120. Llewellyn, M. A., and Swyer, P. R.: Positive expiratory pressure during mechanical ventilation in the newborn, in *Program of the Society for Pediatric Research*, Atlantic City, New Jersey, 1970, p. 224.

121. Weinstein, M. C.: Allocation of subjects in

medical experiments, N Engl J Med, 1974, *291*, 1278–1285.

122. Gehan, E. A., and Freireich, E. J.: Non-randomized controls in cancer clinical trials, N Engl J Med, 1974, *290*, 198–203.

123. Chalmers, T. C.: Randomization of the first patient, Med Clin North Am, 1975, *59*, 1035–1038.

124. Silverman, W. A.: The lesson of retrolental fibroplasia, Sci Am, 1977, *236* (6), 100–107.

125. Byar, D. P., Simon, R. M., Friedewald, W. T., Schlesselman, J. J., DeMets, D. L., Ellenberg, J. H., Gail, M. H., and Ware, J. H.: Randomized clinical trials, perspectives on some recent ideas, N Engl J Med, 1976, *295*, 74–80.

126. Hill, A. B.: The clinical trial, Br Med Bull, 1951, *7*, 278–282.

127. Reynolds, E. O. R.: Management of hyaline membrane disease, Br Med Bull, 1975, *31*, 18–24.

128. Calder, R.: Profile of Science, George Allen & Unwin, London, 1951.

129. Scarpelli, E. M.: The Surfactant System of the Lung, Lea & Febiger, Philadelphia, 1968.

130. Respiratory Diseases, Task Force Report on Prevention, Control, Education, Division of Lung Diseases, National Heart, Lung and Blood Institute, Washington, D.C., DHEW Publication No. (NIH) 77–1248, March 1977.

131. Boys, C. V.: Soap-Bubbles, Their Colours and the Forces which Mould Them, Society for Promoting Christian Knowledge, London, 1890; ed. 2, 1911, reprinted by Dover Publications, New York, 1959.

Index